# Handbook of Psychiatric Diagnostic Procedures

# Handbook of Psychiatric Diagnostic Procedures

# Vol. I



**RICHARD C. W. HALL, M.D.**
Medical Director, Psychiatric Programs
Florida Hospital, Orlando
Director of Research, Monarch Health Corp.
Clinical Professor of Psychiatry
University of Florida, Gainesville

**THOMAS P. BERESFORD, M.D.**
Chief, Psychiatric Service
Veterans Administration Medical Center
Associate Professor of Psychiatry
University of Tennessee Center for the Health Sciences
Memphis, Tennessee

MTP PRESS LIMITED
*International Medical Publishers*

Published in the UK and Europe by
MTP Press Limited
Falcon House
Lancaster, England

Published in the US by
SPECTRUM PUBLICATIONS, INC.
175-20 Wexford Terrace
Jamaica, NY 11432



ISBN: 0-85200-656-X

Printed in the United States of America

THIS BOOK IS DEDICATED TO:

Anne and Ryan

and

Carol, Eddie, Hal, and Charlie

# Contributors

**Thomas P. Beresford, M.D.** Chief, Psychiatry Service, Veterans Administration Medical Center; Associate Professor of Psychiatry, University of Tennessee Center for the Health Sciences, Memphis, Tennessee

**Bernard J. Carroll, M.D., Ph.D.** Professor and Chairman, Department of Psychiatry, Duke University Medical Center, Durham, North Carolina

**John M. Davis, M.D.** Director of Research, Illinois State Psychiatric Institute; and Gilman Research Professor in Psychiatry, University of Illinois College of Medicine, Chicago, Illinois

**Neil Edwards, M.D.** Associate Professor, University of Tennessee Center for the Health Sciences; Director, Clinical Services, Department of Psychiatry, University of Tennessee, Memphis, Tennessee

**Jan Fawcett, M.D.** Professor and Chairman, Department of Psychiatry, Rush-Presbyterian St. Luke's Medical Center, Chicago, Illinois

**Donald L. Feinsilver, M.D.** Assistant Professor of Psychiatry and Emergency Medicine, Medical College of Wisconsin, Milwaukee, Wisconsin

**Arthur M. Freeman III, M.D.** Professor and Vice-Chairman, Department of Psychiatry, University of Alabama in Birmingham, Birmingham, Alabama

**Mark S. Gold, M.D.** Director of Research, Fair Oaks Hospital, Summit, New Jersey

**Richard C. W. Hall, M.D.** Medical Director, Psychiatric Programs, Florida Hospital, Orlando; Clinical Professor of Psychiatry, University of Florida, Gainesville; Director of Research, Monarch Health Corp.

**Javaid I. Javaid, Ph.D.** Assistant Director of Biological Services, Research Department, Illinois Psychiatric Institute, Chicago, Illinois

**James W. Jefferson, M.D.** Co-Director, Lithium Information Center, and Professor of Psychiatry, University of Wisconsin Center for the Health Sciences, Madison, Wisconsin

**Howard M. Kravits, D.O.** Assistant Professor, Department of Psychiatry, Psychology, and Social Sciences, Rush-Presbyterian St. Luke's Medical Center, Chicago, Illinois

**Michael H. Kronig, M.D.** Staff Physician, Department of Psychiatry, Research Facilities, Fair Oaks Hospital, Summit, New Jersey

**William Matuzas, M.D.** Assistant Professor of Psychiatry, University of Chicago, Chicago, Illinois

**Robert J. Perchalski, M.D.** Research Chemist, Veterans Administration Medical Center; Assistant Professor, Department of Medicinal Chemistry, College of Pharmacy, University of Florida, Gainesville, Florida

**Hector C. Sabelli, M.D., Ph.D.** Assistant Professor, Department of Psychiatry, and Director, Psychobiology Laboratory, Rush-Presbyterian St. Luke's Medical Center, Chicago, Illinois

**Carl B. Shory, M.D.** Department of Psychiatry, University Hospital, Birmingham, Alabama

**B. J. Wilder, M.D.** Chief, Neurology Service, Veterans Administration Medical Center; Professor of Neurology and Neuroscience, University of Florida College of Medicine, Gainesville, Florida

# Contents

# Introduction

## The Science of Psychiatry

We live in exciting times. Psychiatrists practicing their specialty are beset as never before with news of developments in the field. The conduits of news to the practicing clinician are usually either stories written in the popular medical press such as news circulars and advertisements from commercial concerns, or from detailed scientific articles written for the scientific community. In both forms, the news has been coming thick and fast.

The problem encountered most often by practicing psychiatrists and clinicians responsible for hospital facilities is integrating this material into a coherent whole, with sufficient technical detail to permit the appropriate development or use of the new tests and procedures in the clinical setting.

The two volumes comprising the *Handbook of Psychiatric Diagnostic Procedures* represent an attempt to provide a clinically useful review of the current accepted applicability of these tests and procedures, to enable the clinician to properly implement and evaluate the procedures as well as the results obtained.

A few chapters, such as that by Dr. Salzburg, deal with highly technical mathematical constructs as they relate to signal analysis. Such material is not immediately applicable to clinical practice. Other chapters, however, such as Weinberger's chapter on the CT scan, Hall's chapter on laboratory diagnosis in psychiatry, Carroll's on dexamethasone suppression tests, Gold's on comprehensive thyroid evaluation, and Fawcett's on CNS amine metabolites, have a broader clinical application to general psychiatric practice. Included also is a section dealing with laboratory evaluation for special groups of patients, such as alcoholics, the elderly, and substance abusers.

Psychiatry no longer views itself as the domain of the single practitioner sitting quietly in the consultation room with no need of diagnostic instruments and rarely of a prescription blank. Research into the biological cuases and correlations of mental illness, foreseen by Adolph Meyer and Sigmund Freud long ago, is coming of age and moving from the laboratory and academic center to the general hospital. To name but a few areas of import, current research is examining the usefulness of MHPG as a clinical indicator in depression, the use of 5-HIAA as a predictor of suicidal behavior, adrenal and thyroid function in depression, brain receptor physiology in the major psychotic illnesses, sleep measurement and its relation to depression and other mental illnesses, the clinical usefulness of serum and intracellular levels of psychoactive drugs, and the physiology of the brain itself seen through new technologies such as the PETT scan, nuclear magnetic resonance, and sophisticated new methods of signal analysis.

The office practitioner is bombarded by glossy literature from commercial concerns who already offer tests designed to provide the clinician with data useful in his office practice. The number of tests offered by the more sophisticated commercial laboratories catering to the office psychiatrist approximates a hundred. Similarly, few medical news publications cross the practitioner's desk without some mention of a new investigation in neuropsychiatry. The busy psychiatrist will generally react in one of two ways to the latest medical sales pitch or news story.

The first is enthusiasm. Truly, the new diagnostic and treatment methods being brought to fruition are causes of wonder. Perhaps the most striking example is the cinematic display provided by the PETT scan. This graphic display of altered brain physiology in mental illness is both dramatic in its technicolor presentation and convincing in its evident concreteness. Only the technical difficulty and sophisticated equipment required for performing the PETT scan save it from becoming an extension of the mass media.

The practitioner's second reaction may be one of apathy disguised as studied skepticism. The PETT scan may be colorful, but what does it mean? The PETT scan may demonstrate altered brain physiology in schizophrenia but how does that help in treating the schizophrenic patient and his family? Technology is all very well, but psychiatry will require several more years, if not decades, to properly integrate it.

Our hope in providing these volumes is that a compromise between these two positions is possible. The office clinician must be aware of his own enthusiasm and the harm it could do his patients were he to listen to it uncritically. At the same time the practicing psychiatrist is the very person who must do the hard work of integrating the new knowledge science brings us into the careful treatment of patients. We have assembled a series of discussions of new diagnostic approaches and their technologies by physicians and scientists well versed in their respective subjects. We have specifically requested each of them to address their comments in the language of the office practitioner or scientist rather than the language of either the lay news media or the technical journalist. Each has, in our view, responded to the greatest extent in their specific fields.

Our hope is that this volume will provide an accessible reference to the office practitioner of psychiatry and that it will take advantage both of enthusiasm and of critical intelligence. Our aim is an informed discussion of the new techniques and the new views of familiar techniques that can be effectively brought to bear upon the diagnosis and treatment of psychiatric patients.

We believe the following chapters provide a common source which is current, state-of-the-art, and widely applicable. They can be used by the clinician to expand his or her horizons concerning the technical aspects of psychiatric diagnosis and treatment, to provide new areas of inquiry and thereby facilitate differential diagnosis, to assist in the biological sub-grouping of patients, to provide a means for following improvement and prognosticating treatment endpoints, and to predict which patients are likely to relapse. We believe these chapters are valuable in synthesizing the current state of knowledge in each respective area and providing the clinician with sufficient clinically important material to order these tests appropriately and to correctly interpret their results. The timeliness of the volume is also its major limitation. Since this field is changing so rapidly, it is anticipated that many of the chapters will be upgraded in future editions.

We have dound the chapters that follow most exciting. The excitement results from the enlightenment that each of them provides in understanding mental illness. We offer them in that same sense of skeptical enthusiasm.

## ACKNOWLEDGMENTS

We would like to express special appreciation to Glenda Price for her assistance in the preparation of this book.

**RICHARD C. W. HALL, M.D.**
**THOMAS P. BERESFORD, M.D.**

# Neuroendocrine Diagnostic Tests

CHAPTER 1

# Dexamethasone Suppression Test

BERNARD J. CARROLL

## INTRODUCTION

The overnight dexamethasone suppression test (DST) was first proposed as a diagnostic aid for endogenous depression or melancholia in 1976 [1,2] and was further standardized in 1981 [3]. It has attracted wide interest in the past few years as its use passed out of investigational units into clinical practice. As with other examples of technology transfer from research to clinical settings, second-generation reports that either strongly confirm or seriously question the utility of the DST can be found in recent literature. In many ways, this situation reminds us of the era soon after the tricyclic antidepressant drugs were introduced: About one third of the reported studies failed to demonstrate the antidepressant efficacy of imipramine [4]. Many of the same reasons for confusion at that time (diagnostic heterogeneity and reliability issues) are responsible for the uncertainty today about the DST. There are also technical issues related to the test itself that have not always been properly understood.

This review summarizes the current status and potential of the DST for clinical practice, with special attention to methodologic aspects that must be clearly understood by clinicians who use the test. As with any diagnostic index (be it a laboratory test, a psychological test, a discriminant index based on clinical features, or a nonstatistical algorithm such as DSM III criteria) an understanding of applied con-

*Handbook of Psychiatric Diagnostic Procedures,* vol. 1, edited by R. C. W. Hall and T. P. Beresford. 

ditional probability theory is essential. These aspects of Bayesian theory for clinicians have been reviewed extensively elsewhere [5-7] and will not be reiterated here.

## HISTORICAL BACKGROUND

Endocrine disturbances in depressed and manic patients had been proposed for many years before the DST was developed. In particular, activation of the adrenal cortex in depressed patients was repeatedly described by the endocrine assessment methods available in the 1940s and 1950s [8.9]. These observations were generally interpreted within the prevailing stress paradigms of that period, even until the early 1970s in some centers [10], and their specificity for particular diagnostic categories was never documented. As new developments emerged in basic and clinical endocrinology during the 1960s, psychiatrists exploited the evolving concepts and techniques to articulate the neuroendocrine strategy for research in depression and other disorders. The important conceptual innovation was the use of dynamic function tests to assess the integrity of neuroendocrine systems. This approach rapidly replaced the earlier, relatively unrewarding practice of simply measuring the amounts of hormones and their metabolites present in blood and urine.

The logic of this new strategy can be summarized succinctly. Neuroendocrine function is regulated by the limbic system and hypothalamus, which are thought to be the site(s) of primary pathology in the affective disorders. Direct, invasive studies of the limbic system in human patients are not feasible, but the study of neuroendocrine function can be used to obtain indirect knowledge about the integrity of the limbic system. In principle, this strategy could reveal specific disturbances of limbic-neuroendocrine function in patients with melancholia. It could also be used to test theories about the neurotransmitter basis of melancholia and, by extension, to study the mode of action of thymoleptic drugs. Over the past fifteen years this approach has yielded much valuable information, reviewed in detail elsewhere [8, 11].

The DST was introduced in 1960 for the study of Cushing's disease [12]. Several variants of the test followed, one of which, the overnight DST with a single morning blood sample [13-15], became a popular screening test among clinical endocrinologists because a normal response rules out the presence of Cushing's disease with high confidence. Patients with abnormal results are then evaluated by more extensive procedures.

The overnight DST was applied to depressed patients independently by Stokes [16,17] and by the author in Melbourne [18-20]. Both groups found evidence of abnormal results. At about the same time, two other groups, also working independently, used another variant of the DST and found abnormal results in depressed patients [21,22]. Several other groups later studied the overnight DST, with generally consistent findings [8,23]. Overall, about 40% of depressed patients had abnormal DST results. Further development of the test did not occur, however, until three critical points were established.

First, the idea was refuted that abnormal DST results are simply psychological stress responses. This theory prevailed in the early 1970s, mainly due to the work of Mason [24] and Sachar et al. [10], who at that time had not actually used the DST. We found that abnormal DST results did not occur in schizophrenic patients even though they had severe "breakdown of ego defenses," as rated by Sachar's method [20,25]. Later, Sachar and associates [26] obtained evidence from their own studies which led them to change their earlier view and to agree that disinhibited HPA activity in melancholic patients reflects a limbic system disturbance.

Second, the overnight DST procedure was improved [1]. From the results of 48-hour venous catheter studies, it was apparent that melancholic patients have a more subtle HPA disturbance than patients with Cushing's disease. Many melancholic patients have normally suppressed plasma cortisol concentrations in the early morning but escape from suppression later in the day. Normal subjects remain suppressed for at least 24 hours after an overnight dose of dexamethasone. In melancholic patients an abnormally early escape from suppression was found in the afternoon or evening. These results led us to propose a new procedure for the DST in psychiatric units [1,2]. Instead of obtaining only one postdexamethasone blood sample, at 8 AM, we added samples at 4 PM and 11 PM. An elevated plasma cortisol concentration in any of the three samples indicated abnormal disinhibition of HPA activity.

Third, the specificity of abnormal DST results in melancholic patients was described, and it was explicitly suggested that the DST might be a useful diagnostic laboratory test for melancholia [2]. The specificity of the test was apparent in our original report [18] and also in the later study [20]. The full significance of this finding was not realized, however, until a much larger number of nonmelancholic patients was tested in 1976. At this time we showed that patients with nonendogenous depression had normal DST results [2].

## DST PROCEDURE AND LABORATORY ASSAY

In the recommended procedure [3] for the DST in psychiatric practice a 1-mg tablet of dexamethasone is taken at 2300 hours. The next day, blood samples for determination of plasma cortisol are drawn at 1600 and 2300 hours. For convenience, only the 1600-hours sample is obtained from outpatients. An increased plasma concentration of cortisol in *either* blood sample signifies an abnormal or positive test result. The cutoff for normal plasma concentrations of cortisol is 5 μg/dL with the competitive protein binding (CPB) assay used in my laboratory. Strictly speaking, this assay measures total plasma corticoids [27] rather than "plasma cortisol" alone.

When other CPB or radioimmunoassay (RIA) methods of measuring plasma cortisol are used, special care is needed to ensure that the assay has good precision and accuracy in the low range of plasma cortisol concentrations. Recently, concern has arisen about the wide variation among routine (nonspecialized) laboratories in the accuracy of plasma cortisol assays, especially at low concentrations around 5 μg/dL [28]. The need to correct this potential source of error cannot be stressed too strongly.

The antibodies in commercial RIA reagent kits are not uniformly specific for cortisol, so different cutoff values will result. With highly specific antibodies in research laboratories the cutoff value may be as low as 3.5, 4 or 4.5 μg/dL [29-31]. With other RIAs the cutoff value may be as high as 10 μg/dL [32]. Each laboratory should, therefore, standardize its own assay procedure and should define its own cutoff value based on a local study of normal subjects and nondepressed psychiatric patients. It is *not* appropriate to simply adopt the cutoff value of 5 μg/dL for assays that differ from the CPB assay used in our standardization study [3]. We have completed a study of 16 commercial RIA kits for cortisol and found that thirteen of them yielded cutoff values *higher* than 5 μg/dL [33].

Clinical chemists should keep in mind that the typical assay for cortisol in hospital laboratories is *not* designed to provide maximum precision and accuracy in the low range of cortisol values. This goal can readily be achieved, however, by modifying the assay system. In my laboratory, for example, we have modified the clinical CPB procedure to yield a sensitivity intermediate between the microscale and ultramicroscale assay procedures originally described by Murphy [27]. This is accomplished by decreasing the concentration of the pooled human plasma reagent (the source of corticosteroid binding globulin) from 5% to 2%. This adjustment shifts the sensitivity of the assay to the left, so that most values in the range of 5 μg/dL fall on the steepest portion of the binding curve. For the first assay of every sample we use duplicate aliquots of the ethanolic extracts of patient's plasma. The standards (run in triplicate) are 0, 0.5, 1, 2, 4, 10, 15, and 20 ng of cortisol per tube. We also use magnesium silicate (Florisil) rather than Fuller's earth as the adsorbent and we use tritiated corticosterone rather than tritiated hydrocortisone as the radioactive tracer [33]. Quality control plasma pool samples at low, intermediate, and high concentrations are always included.

When the first reported value is $< 3$ or $> 7$ μg/dL, that value is reported. When the first value is between these limits, the sample is reassayed with three different-sized aliquots of the ethanolic extract of plasma, to provide at least two separate and duplicate estimates on the steep portion of the binding curve. The mean of these four values is reported. Although this double-checking is usually redundant, it improves the precision of assay of borderline-abnormal samples.

With the above procedure, the sensitivity (true positive rate) of the DST for melancholia is about 65% and the specificity (true negative rate) is about 95% [3]. With the outpatient protocol (only one blood sample), the sensitivity will be about

50%. On the basis of these results, an abnormal DST result will carry a high diagnostic confidence (predictive value) for melancholia; *a negative test result, however, will not rule out the diagnosis of melancholia.* This point must be clearly understood by clinicians who use the test. Just as a normal EEG reading will not rule out epilepsy when the clinical features are otherwise consistent, so also a normal DST will not rule out endogenous depression or melancholia when the clinical features are consistent with the diagnosis.

## EXCLUSION CRITERIA

All the current approaches to laboratory diagnosis of depression, such as the DST, TRH test, and sleep EEG, are *functional* assessments of aspects of central nervous system activity. Like other functional tests, therefore, such as the glucose tolerance test, they may be affected by drugs or metabolic factors unrelated to depression. Aside from drug considerations, the basic principle to remember is that *patients should be medically healthy and physiologically stable when the test is performed.* The prevalence of these interfering conditions is higher than many clinicians appreciate. In our own report, for example, we excluded 20% of available inpatients and 9% of outpatients, mostly on account of interfering drugs [3]. The conditions presently known to cause spuriously positive or negative DST results are listed in Table 1.

The drugs that cause false positive results accelerate the hepatic metabolism of dexamethasone by liver enzyme induction, and their influence on the test may take up to three weeks to subside after intake of the drugs is stopped. It follows that valid DST results cannot be obtained, then, in patients with epilepsy who are not withdrawn from their anticonvulsant drugs. Clinicians should also check carefully for unreported use of barbiturates, which patients sometimes obtain from a different physician. Compound barbiturate preparations such as Donnatal and Fiorinal also should not be overlooked. In some countries compound preparations containing barbiturates are freely available without a prescription and are even sold over the counter within hospitals. This factor was identified as the cause of unexpected positive tests in at least one European study (J. P. deVigne, M.D., personal communication). High levels of estrogen, as in pregnancy or in the treatment of prostatic cancer with stilbestrol, elevate plasma transcortin concentrations and thus interfere with the test. Low doses of estrogen in oral contraceptive preparations or in menopausal estrogen replacement therapy do not seem to have been associated with unexpected results in our experience.

Diabetic patients who experience hypoglycemic episodes [37] or develop ketoacidosis will have invalid test results. Recently, patients with controlled insulin dependent diabetes mellitus also were found to have a high frequency of abnormal results [38].

**Table 1. Factors That Interfere with the DST**

| | |
|---|---|
| *False positive result* | |
| Drugs | Phenytoin, barbiturates, meprobamate, carbamazepine, glutethimide, methaqualone, methyprylon, heavy alcohol use, ? reserpine |
| Endocrine | Cushing's disease or syndrome; pregnancy or high dose estrogen treatment; diabetes mellitus (especially with hypoglycemia or ketoacidosis) |
| Medical | Major medical disorders such as: infections; uncontrolled cardiac failure or hypertension; advanced renal or hepatic disease; cancer |
| Metabolic | Acute withdrawal from alcohol; fever, dehydration, severe nausea, vomiting; low body weight (anorexia nervosa, malnutrition); ongoing weight loss (rigid dieting); circadian phase advance (suspected, e.g., shift workers, airline travellers) |
| Other | Electroconvulsive therapy (on post-dexamethasone day?), grand mal seizures (on post-dexamethasone day?) temporal lobe disease? brain tumor? Alzheimer disease and multiinfarct dementia. Other endocrine disease (? hypercalcemia, hypothyroidism) |
| *False negative result* | |
| Drugs | Synthetic corticosteroid therapy<br>Indomethacin [34]<br>High dose cyproheptadine<br>? High dose benzodiazepines [35]<br>? Tricyclic antidepressants [36]<br>? 1-tryptophan [36] |
| Endocrine | Hypopituitarism<br>Addison's disease<br>Abnormal slow metabolism of dexamethasone |

Dehydration is an important factor to consider in catatonic or recently admitted psychotic patients. Their physiologic status must first be stabilized and, in general, it is unwise to conduct the DST within the first 48 hours after a psychotic patient enters the hosptial.

Severe weight loss in the clinical contexts of malnutrition [39] or anorexia nervosa [40] is a well established cause of abnormal DSTs, though the mechanism is not known. More recently, 30-40 percent of subjects on rigid weight reduction diets were found to have abnormal DSTs even though their absolute body weights were within normal limits [41,42]. Since weight loss is an important feature of depression itself, questions have arisen whether this feature alone is responsible for abnormal DSTs in depressed patients [43,44]. Neither multivariate cross-sectional analyses that covary weight loss with age and severity of depression [45] nor longitudinal testing of individual patients in relation to weight loss and clinical change [46] suggest that this is the case in depressed patients. Until further studies are done to clarify this issue a more or less conservative interpretation should be placed on abnormal test results in patients with ongoing weight loss, depending on the clinical context in which the test was requested.

In Table 1 several other factors that can potentially interfere with the test are indicated. Circadian phase advances greater than 3 hours in rotating shift workers or airline travellers could lead to spurious positive test results, based on studies by Krieger et al. [47], in which low doses of dexamethasone were given at various times in the 24 hour cycle. A phase advance of 3 hours, however, apparently does not affect the test [18,48].

Conditions affecting the central nervous system have not been studied extensively in relation to the DST. We have no data on the effect of electroconvulsive treatments given on the post-dexamethasone day, nor do we know what effect spontaneous epilepsy with grand mal seizures has on the test. Temporal lobe disease or degenerative disease involving the limbic system (Alzheimer's disease and multi-infarct dementia) could obviously affect the neural circuits involved in normal maintenance of suppression after dexamethasone.

The causes of false negative results are fewer in number and they are mostly obvious (hypopituitarism, chronic steroid therapy, Addison's disease). High dose cyproheptadine is listed because this drug has been used to reverse the clinical and endocrine features of diencephalic Cushing's disease [49]. No definite evidence has yet been presented to support suggestions that benzodiazepines l-tryptophan or tricyclic antidepressants cause false-negative DSTs. The commonly used psychotropic drugs such as lithium, tricyclic antidepressants, monoamine oxidase inhibitors, neuroleptic drugs, and chloral hydrate do *not* cause false-positive DST results. Whether, and how often, they can cause false-negative results is still being evaluated.

To avoid the effects of cumulative steroid administration, the DST should not be given more often than every five to seven days. From a clinical perspective, testing at less than weekly intervals would seldom be appropriate.

## FUNCTIONAL MEANING OF ABNORMAL DST RESULTS

Provided the technical issues discussed above are controlled, what does an abnormal DST result tell the clinician? In endocrine terms it signifies disinhibited function of the limbic system-hypothalamo-pituitary-adrenal (LHPA) axis. This functional disturbance is thought to originate in the limbic areas of the brain that regulate neuroendocrine function. The same regions of the brain also regulate emotions and affective states [50].

The plasma cortisol suppression response to dexamethasone is, of course, one step removed from the anterior pituitary which, in turn, is one step removed from the brain. The presumption is that the limbic system dysfunction causes excessive release of corticotropin releasing factor (CRF, corticoliberin). In turn, CRF is presumed to override the action of dexamethasone in the anterior pituitary causing the release of adrenocorticotrophic hormone (ACTH), and ACTH in turn stimulates the release of cortisol from the adrenal gland [1]. To date, attempts to confirm this sequence by measures of plasma ACTH are fragmentary and inconclusive [51-53], and there is considerable doubt about the sensitivity of the ACTH assays used by some investigators.

The most conservative position at present is that the abnormal DST gives the clinician *indirect* evidence of disturbed function of the limbic system in depressed patients. The neuroendocrine disturbance may be regarded as a "limbic system noise" phenomenon. The lack of absolute sensitivity of the DST may then be more readily understood. So may the fact that in some patients the test is intermittently positive.

Some comparisons from clinical neurology may be helpful at this point. The sensitivity of the routine electroencephalogram (EEG) for adult-onset epilepsy is about 70%. Like the DST in depression, the EEG in epilepsy is only an indirect index of the underlying pathologic process. Indeed, the best way to regard the DST in depression may be to view it as *the neuroendocrine equivalent of an EEG of the limbic system.* Clinicians experienced in the care of patients with complex partial seizures (temporal lobe epilepsy) also know that depth electrode recordings in this condition may be intermittently abnormal.

Although it is an indirect marker of dysfunction in the limbic system the DST can give the clinician useful information. Its diagnostic utility for psychiatrists comes from its temporal association with episodes of melancholic depression and from its specificity in relation to other depressions. This face validity is supported by several other lines of converging evidence for its predictive validity and construct validity [50,54].

## RELATION TO DIAGNOSTIC SUBTYPES OF DEPRESSION

Clinicians are familiar with several current schemes for the diagnosis and classification of depression by clinical features [55-57]. These are all only provisional conventions. They enable different centers to describe their depressed patients with some reliability, but their validity has not been established [58]. The broad category termed "major depressive disorder" in the recent Third Edition of the Diagnostic and Statistical Manual (DSM III) of the American Psychiatric Association [57] is extremely heterogeneous. The "melancholia" subtype of DSM III also has been criticized by several groups [58,59]. Any proposed clinical classification will need to be validated by studies of family history, natural history, treatment response, and biological markers. The DST might serve as one such marker, along with others [5]. Eventually, these markers may help us to improve or choose among the various clinical classifications. In time, new definitions of depressive subtypes may emerge that give the laboratory markers diagnostic weight along with traditional clinical features. Historically, the same process has occurred in many other areas of medicine.

Results of the DST are often abnormal in melancholic patients, as this term is used in my investigative unit [3,59,60]. By contrast, patients with equally severe but nonendogenous depression have normal DST results [3,59]. The concept of melancholia we use is essentially Kraepelinian. In making the diagnosis we consider not only the current profile of symptoms but also features that are ignored by DSM III. These include family history, phasic course of the illness, response and quality of response to previous treatments, and any history of manic or hypomanic episodes. We include patients with unipolar, bipolar and mixed manic-depressive states in the category melancholia. Like many European groups [e.g., 61] we regard depressed patients with a bipolar history as melancholic unless there are exceptional reasons for thinking otherwise. In keeping with this Kraepelinian approach we also recognize that melancholic depressions may present in mild or attenuated forms that do not necessarily manifest the fixed loss of reactivity, the completely pervasive anhedonia or the full symptom profile required by DSM III.

The final diagnostic judgement, then, relies on information from many sources and is based on much more than the cross-sectional profile of symptoms. As we have emphasized before [59], the cognitive process of clinical diagnosis is a complex pattern recognition task and it is not necessarily reducible to a simple algorithm. Using the statistical procedure of discriminant function analysis we have provided a diagnostic index based on clinical features that classifies the majority of unipolar melancholic and nonendogenous depressed patients with high probability and that also predicts the DST result as well as our clinical diagnoses do [60]. Whether other groups will be able to use this discriminant index with equal success will depend in large measure on how rigorous are their phenomenologic judgments of clinical features.

Some groups report abnormal DST results in primary depression but not in secondary depression [62,63]. There is disagreement on this point. Our own results suggest that the rate of abnormal DSTs for patients with secondary depression depends on the proportion of melancholic patients in this group [50]. Current studies with DSM III [57] or the Research Diagnostic Criteria (RDC) [56] suggest that, by these conventions, the DST does not distinguish between melancholia and nonendogenous depression [63-65]. It remains to be seen whether this represents a problem for the DST or for the DSM III and RDC (or for the elastic way these criteria are often used in practice [66]). The entire field has reached an interesting dialectic phase right now as we go through the iterative process of testing the DST first as a dependent variable, and then as an independent variable, in relation to the clinical diagnostic categories of depression.

## VARIANCE IN THE INDEPENDENT VARIABLE

The key issue to keep in mind as this debate continues is that significant and sometimes alarming variance is known to exist in the clinical diagnoses now used as the independent variables. For example, even in careful research studies the coefficient of diagnostic concordance (Cohen's kappa [67]) is seldom greater than about 0.55 to 0.65 for diagnoses of endogenous depression [68,69]. In more routine clinical settings the diagnostic reliability is likely to be even less secure, and kappa values of about 0.4 would be expected. The effect of this variance in the independent variable (diagnostic unreliability) on the apparent performance of a laboratory test can easily be computed (Table 2). Even when the diagnostic reliability is acceptable by current clinical standards (kappa 0.50) the apparent performance of a quite good test will be weaker than its true performance. The apparent loss of specificity is particularly serious. If the clinical diagnoses are even less secure then the apparent test performance will be even more affected. If the inter-diagnostician agreement is only 65% (kappa 0.30) then the apparent sensitivity will be only 49% and the apparent specificity will drop to 69%.

These considerations raise sobering problems of epistemology and methodology for the development and validation of diagnostic tests. So long as the clinical diagnoses (independent variables) with a given center are themselves insecure, and so long as there is known variability among clinical centers in the accurate use of diagnostic criteria, then apparently discrepant reports from different programs must

**Table 2. Effect of Diagnostic Error on the Apparent Performance of a Laboratory Test**

| | Actual | Apparent[a] |
|---|---|---|
| Sensitivity (%) | 70 | 55 |
| Specificity (%) | 90 | 75 |
| Predictive value (%) (abnormal result) | 88 | 69 |

[a]The apparent sensitivity, specificity and positive predictive value of a laboratory test are seriously impaired, even when the clinical diagnostic assessment are only moderately unreliable. The calculations are based on a test with a true sensitivity of 70% and a true specificity of 90%, used in a group of patients for whom the diagnostic reliability (Cohen's kappa) is 0.50 in relation to the true diagnosis. This requires 75% overall diagnostic accuracy. The calculations assume a standardized 50% prevalence rate for the index diagnosis.

be interpreted with caution. For example, the apparently poor specificity of the DST in the NIMH Collaborative Study of the Psychobiology of Depression [65] could readily be attributed to diagnostic reliability problems in the study, which involved multiple psychiatrists at six different centers.

## CLINICAL APPLICATIONS

The DST is *not* recommended as a screening test for all psychiatric patients, but should be used in a clinical context where it may help to resolve a specific question [5,50,70]. As with all laboratory tests, if the DST is used in a population where the prevalence of the index disorder (melancholia) is low, then the predictive value of an abnormal test result will be greatly reduced [71,72]. Further, among melancholic patients abnormal DST results occur in close relationship to episodes of depression, but usually not in the euthymic intervals. Thus the DST is not useful as a trait marker of subjects predisposed to develop melancholia.

The clinical applications discussed below are supported by positive reports, usually from more than one center. However, larger-scale and well-designed studies are still needed to document the clinical utility of the test in these areas. Certainly, use of the DST by general clinicians must be regarded as *optional,* as is true of many other laboratory tests in medicine.

## CONFIRMATION OR SUPPORT OF A CLINICAL DIAGNOSIS

The DST can be useful in confirming a diagnosis of melancholia, even if the clinician is confident of the diagnosis. Such confirmatory use of laboratory tests by other medical specialties is routine, because the laboratory measures can provide a degree of objectivity that is impossible to achieve with clinical methods alone. Taken by itself, the diagnostic significance of an abnormal DST is superior to that of any of the "vegetative" clinical features clinicians now use for the positive diagnosis of melancholia (J. Davidson, M.D., and K. R. Krishnan, M.D., personal communication, 1983).

In patients with less certain or disputed diagnoses, the finding of an abnormal DST result may contribute strongly to the final assessment, especially when there is clinical disagreement about the importance of apparent psychogenic precipitants. Despite the new diagnostic criteria that deemphasize precipitants, many clinicians still have difficulty making the diagnosis of melancholia when clear precipitants are thought to be present.

An example is provided by the case of a young woman in her late 20s who was admitted to our unit 2 weeks after being assaulted and raped. Clinically, she exhibited symptoms of severe depression. The staff was divided as to her diagnosis.

One group believed that the depressive symptoms were reactions to an important precipitating event and that the depression should be treated by psychotherapy to help the patient deal with her feelings of anger, shame, and demoralization. Others believed that, despite the obvious traumatic precipitant, the patient now had an autonomous, nonreactive melancholic depression that would require somatic treatment. The patient underwent 6 weeks of intensive psychotherapy, during which time she was enrolled in a blinded DST study. When it became evident that she was not responding to psychotherapy, we added desipramine to her treatment regimen. Within 3 weeks she made a good recovery and was discharged. Subsequently, it was found that she had had six consecutive abnormal DST results during her treatment with psychotherapy alone, and a rapid return to normal on the DST when the tricyclic antidepressant drug treatment was started. Thus, the DST can help to resolve diagnostic disagreements when a clinical assessment is ambiguous.

Some patients are more willing to accept the diagnosis, to form a treatment alliance, and to comply with antidepressant drug treatment when their DST results are abnormal. For other patients, the knowledge of abnormal laboratory findings helps them resist the pressure of guilty and self-deprecatory ideas about their illness. Still others will interpret the test results in a negative, pessimistic way. All patients, therefore, need careful explanation, education, and support by the physician when the results of the test are reviewed with them. The *psychological meaning* of the test result to the patient needs to be addressed and can be used to advantage by the physician in the treatment relationship.

## SELECTION OF TREATMENT

Depressed patients with abnormal DST results will require somatic antidepressant treatment in addition to whatever psychotherapeutic and supportive measures are thought necessary. In my experience these patients will not respond to psychotherapy alone. The patient just described illustrates this recurrent clinical experience. More systematic study of cognitive psychotherapy seems to confirm this clinical impression (A. John Rush, M.D., personal communication, 1983). So far, there is not good evidence that abnormal DST results predict response to any particular antidepressant of the tricyclic or the monoamine oxidase inhibitor classes. When indicated on clinical grounds, electroconvulsive therapy should be given.

## MONITORING RESPONSE TO TREATMENT

As patients improve with treatment their DST responses gradually approach normal values [73,74]. When the test results convert to normal before significant clinical change is evident, this is usually a good prognostic sign that the patient will

Table 3. DST Normalization and Clinical Outcome

| | DST normalized | | DST not normalized | |
|---|---|---|---|---|
| | Poor outcome | Good outcome | Poor outcome | Good outcome |
| Carroll 1972 [20] | – | – | 7 | 0 |
| Greden, 1980 [70] | 2 | 8 | 4 | 0 |
| Papakostas, 1981 [77] | 0 | 5 | 3 | 1 |
| Holsboer, 1982 [76] | 0 | 16 | 4 | 0 |
| Targum, 1982 [78] | 3 | 16 | 3 | 3 |
| Yerevanian, 1983 [79] | 0 | 4 | 10 | 0 |
| Nemeroff, 1983 [80] | 2 | 11 | 5 | 2 |
| TOTALS[a] | 7 | 60 | 36 | 6 |

[a]Chi squared $p < 0.0001$.

eventually respond [73.74]. This information may be helpful in maintaining patients on a given course of treatment so that changing treatments prematurely is avoided. Some patients improve clinically but the test results remain abnormal; such patients frequently have early relapse [20,75-80]. On the other hand, it has *not* been established that normalization of the DST result is in itself a sufficient indication to stop active somatic antidepressant treatment.

Seven studies of DST conversion in relation to clinical response are summarized in Table 3. All the cases included in these studies had abnormal DSTs on admission. At the time of discharge the test was repeated. In the six more recent studies 35 of 102 patients (34%) still had abnormal DSTs on discharge. Of these, 83% had a poor outcome even though treatment was continued in most cases. In two studies suicides were recorded among these patients with persistently abnormal DSTs [75, 79]. In contrast, 90% of the patients whose DSTs normalized had a good short-term response to treatment and were free of relapse for up to 6 months. In several of these studies the non-normalizers were recognized to be incompletely recovered even though discharge from inpatient treatment was felt to be a reasonable clinical decision. The reports of Targum [78] and of Holsboer et al. [76] are the most convincing, since the rated severity of depression at discharge was equivalent in the normalizing and non-normalizing groups. Taken together, these results indicate that a persistently abnormal DST result, despite apparent clinical improvement, identifies a group of patients at high risk of continued impairment of functioning, suicide, and relapse. This application of the test in monitoring the response to treatment is another reason for obtaining a DST during the initial evaluation of depressed patients.

## PREDICTION OF NEW EPISODES

In rapidly cycling bipolar patients the DST results become abnormal one to three days before the onset of the depressive phase [81]. In our only study to date of a patient with the more usual episodic course, the test results became abnormal three weeks before the recurrence of a depressive episode. If this pattern is confirmed by further studies, then the DST might be used to anticipate new episodes of depression in selected patients.

Intermittently abnormal test results have recently been reported for patients maintained on long-term preventive treatment with lithium carbonate [82]. The abnormal test results did not necessarily precede relapses in these patients. If confirmed, this observation tells us several important things about the DST in depressives and about the action of lithium. For example, it suggests that these patients developed recurrent disturbance of limbic system function that, without lithium treatment, would have led to relapse. This is consistent with the clinical course of patients who are withdrawn from preventive treatment with lithium: They revert to the same frequency of episodes as before the lithium was given. Second, Coppen's observation suggests that lithium acts to suppress the clinical manifestation of the recurrent pathology in the limbic system at a site "below" the primary lesion. For these reasons, abnormal DST results in longitudinal monitoring of patients taking preventive lithium carbonate may *not* necessarily indicate an imminent relapse.

## SUICIDE ALERT

At least two groups [83,84] report that nearly all melancholic patients who committed suicide had abnormal DST results. The test might thus alert clinicians to the risk of suicide in melancholic patients. The test would *not* be useful for other patients at high risk of suicide, such as alcoholics and schizophrenics because these patients have normal DST results.

Among melancholic patients, abnormal DST results will usually be observed in association with other established clinical risk factors for suicide (active suicidal ideas, previous suicide attempts, delusional depression, hopelessness, and so forth). When these risk factors are present, then the clinical staff should be even further alerted by the finding of an abnormal test result. In no way, however, should their alertness be diminished by a normal test result if the patient appears clinically at risk to attempt suicide. This caveat parallels the warning stated earlier against using the DST result alone to rule out the diagnosis of melancholia.

## SPECIAL DIAGNOSTIC PROBLEMS

As noted earlier, the best established diagnostic use of the DST is in the differentiation between melancholic and nonendogenous depression, especially when the importance of psychogenic precipitants is unclear or disputed. Several other difficult diagnostic problems frequently arise in clinical practice, however, for which objective laboratory markers like the DST might be very useful.

### Catatonic Patients

Preliminary reports suggest that abnormal DST results occur in mute and catatonic depressive but not in catatonic schizophrenic patients [85,86]. Such patients must be adequately hydrated when tested. Indeed, as I emphasized long ago [1], an important principle for all psychotic patients is that the test should not be given within the first two days after admission to the hospital. Such patients often have been living in chaotic circumstances before admission, and they are frequently ketotic and dehydrated when first seen. They should receive adequate nutritional supplements and rehydration before one attempts to obtain a valid DST result.

### Geriatric Depressive Pseudodementia

If the correct diagnostic distinction is not made between true dementia and depressive pseudodementia in elderly patients, many treatable cases will be missed. Some preliminary reports suggest that the DST can help with this differential diagnosis [87,88], but further systematic studies of demented patients are needed before this application of the DST is accepted. Two recent studies of patients with senile dementia of the Alzheimer type found abnormal DST results in almost 50% [89,90]. The clinical significance and mechanism of this neuroendocrine disturbance in demented patients is being pursued for the possibility that it may help us understand the mechanism in depressed patients.

Pseudodementia presents diagnostic problems mainly when there is apparent dementia *of recent onset.* The two studies of Alzheimer-type dementia cited above involved patients with longstanding disease. A standard diagnostic principle of geriatric medicine is to carefully exclude a treatable cause of recent-onset dementia. Depression is one of the most common such causes. I recommend, therefore, that we look very carefully for a treatable depression whenever a patient with apparent dementia of recent onset has an abnormal DST result. The case reports mentioned above [87,88] confirm the value of this approach for some patients. A more recent study of outpatients with senile dementia of the Alzheimer type found no abnormal DST results [112]. In contrast to the earlier reports on severely affected, nonverbal demented patients [89,90] these outpatients could be rated more reliably for a possible mood disturbance.

### Depression in Adolescents

Many clinicians fail to recognize and diagnose episodes of melancholia in adolescent patients. Although the diagnosis can usually be made if the right questions are asked, the diagnostic "set" of the clinician is often the limiting factor. Some depressed adolescents, however, present with unusual clinical features that obscure the affective disorder. They may be diagnosed initially as having a schizophreniform disorder, but are later reclassified as affective disorder on follow-up. Their DST results are consistent with affective disorder from the beginning [91]. Other adolescent patients with more typical melancholia have abnormal DST results with the same frequency as adult melancholic patients [3,92].

### Depression in Childhood

The existence of syndromal depressions in prepubertal children is gradually being recognized. As with adolescents, however, most clinicians still do not consider the diagnosis in dysphoric children. In one recent report a 0.5-mg-dose DST was studied in children aged 6-12 years. The sensitivity and specificity of this procedure for prepubertal melancholia were similar to the values reported for the 1-mg-dose DST in adults [93].

### Masked Depression

Some depressed patients present a prominent somatic focus of complaint and do not discuss their mood disturbance. When the clinician also fails to ask about the patient's mood and related features, a case of "masked depression" is created. A recent study of patients referred to a chronic pain clinic revealed a significant group with clinical depression, abnormal DST results, abnormal sleep EEG features consistent with depression, and good response to amitriptyline [94].

### Complicated Depression

When patients with another chronic psychiatric disorder (such as borderline personality disorder) develop a superimposed episode of melancholia, the clinician often fails to recognize the new condition and to treat it effectively. Such patients, with two distinct but interacting disorders, are among the most difficult melancholic patients to manage. The character disorder will often cause serious unreliability in the assessment of specific melancholic features.

Two studies in patients with borderline personality disorder and depressed mood have confirmed that many such patients do have abnormal DST results [95,96]. In principle, concurrent treatment with antidepressant drugs (tricyclics or monoamine oxidase inhibitors) should supplement the psychotherapeutic management of these patients. Controlled trials of this matter are needed.

## SPECIFICITY QUESTIONS

A number of recent reports have questioned the specificity of the DST for melancholic or endogenous depression. Readers attempting to evaluate these reports are advised to keep some key principles in mind. First, some studies have failed to observe the *technical exclusion factors* discussed above, such as drug use or recent withdrawal from alcohol [97,98]. Second, other investigators have based their arguments on a surprisingly rigid (and quite unjustified) assumption about the *validity of DSM III criteria* for melancholia [e.g., 64,65]. The author's use of the term melancholia is more consistent with the Kraepelinian tradition than is the DSM III version, which is overly restrictive. These reports of a high frequency of abnormal DSTs in non-melancholic depression could equally be signalling a problem with the DSM III criteria as indicating nonspecificity of the DST. Indeed, the Kraepelinian concept of melancholia is quite broad and it includes attenuated forms of the classical disorder (dysthymic and cyclothymic states) as well as atypical presenting forms such as delusional or paranoid depression, catatonic depression, and depressive pseudodementia.

Third, the *reliability of diagnostic practice* in these reports is rarely stated. As pointed out earlier (Table 2) a quite specific diagnostic test will appear nonspecific when the clinical diagnoses are not very secure. This problem exists even in first rate academic centers. A good illustration is found in a recent report on diagnostic reliability from Copenhagen [99]. A group of psychiatrists interviewed 35 depressed patients (average 6 to 7 psychiatrists present at each interview). In 31 cases no more than one rater disagreed that the diagnosis was major depression by DSM III and in 34 cases at least half of the raters agreed that this was the diagnosis. The corresponding figures for DSM III melancholia diagnoses, however, were 9 and 18! In other words, the "certainty index" for major depression was 91% (31 of 34) but for melancholia it was only 50% (9 of 18). The formal kappa values for diagnostic concordance were 0.64 and 0.57, equivalent to state-of-the-art reliability in other units, as reviewed earlier.

Fourth, some authors have found a high incidence of abnormal DSTs in *mania* and have questioned the test's specificity for this reason [65,100]. In the author's unit patients with cycling bipolar disorder usually have abnormal test results when depressed, but normal results when manic or hypomanic [81]. Euphoric manic patients usually have normal DSTs (85%). The few abnormal DSTs in mania, in our experience, have occurred in patients with dysphoric-irritable mania or in subjects who soon switched to a depressive phase. In other reports to date it is not always clear which type of mania was associated with abnormal DSTs, nor even whether mixed manic-depressive cases were included. The author has always classified such cases as melancholic: They certainly have a high frequency of abnormal DST results [101,102]. In any event, simple mania does not pose significant diagnostic problems for clinicians and *the DST would not be requested in this context.* In other words, regardless of the theoretical importance of what happens to the DST in mania, the issue is of no practical consequence for the differential diagnosis of depression from mania. More recent data from the McLean Hospital group [103] suggest that, if indeed there is a high frequency of abnormal DSTs in mania, then the test may be useful for the frequently difficult differential diagnosis of mania from schizophrenia.

Fifth, there is an old legal axiom that difficult or unusual cases make for bad laws. Similarly, insecure diagnostic entities make for unreliable estimates of specificity. Reports of abnormal DSTs in *schizoaffective disorder* or *atypical psychosis* [103,104] need to be considered in this light. These conditions are the subject of persistent nosologic debate and their diagnostic criteria in DSM III are either lacking (schizoaffective) or incomplete (atypical psychosis). They may be related to affective disorder as the author has discussed for schizoaffective illness [50], or the diagnosis may change to affective disorder on follow-up in the case of atypical psychosis [86,105]. The same finding was reported for patients with *schizophreniform disorder* and abnormal DSTs [91]. Once again, if one adopts a rigid view of the validity of DSM III categories then the DST could appear nonspecific. Another reasonable interpretation of the data, however, would be that the DST is signalling heterogeneity within these DSM III categories that contain a significant proportion of cases with atypically presenting affective disorders.

Sixth, some reviewers seem to be confused about the distinction between Axis I and Axis II of DSM III when discussing the abnormal DSTs reported in dysphoric patients with *borderline personality disorders.* The author's full discussion of this matter [54,95] should be consulted and readers should understand that the reliability of Axis I diagnoses in borderline patients may be even worse than it is in uncomplicated melancholia. The most recent study of borderline patients found abnormal DSTs in 58% of those with concomitant depressive features (7 of 12 cases) but in only 8% of those without depression (1 of 12 cases) (K. R. Krishnan, M.D., personal communication, 1983).

Seventh, some investigators place undue confidence in the primary-secondary classification of depressed patients. For example, a report of *obsessive-compulsive disorder* [106] described abnormal DSTs mainly in cases with secondary depression. Although the authors of this report were very cautious in their conclusions, others have been less critical in their interpretation of this study. There is, in fact, no longer any reason to believe that the primary-secondary distinction is meaningful. From a practical point of view it has no importance in selection of treatment. From a theoretical point of view it is agnostic, atheoretical, and implies nothing about etiology [66]. From an empirical point of view it has no relationship to the DST [30,50], though the Iowa City group do not agree [63].

Eighth, reports of new associations of the DST with other disorders raise the issue of how a diagnostic entity is identified and validated. In *bulimia,* for example, a large proportion of patients apparently have abnormal DST results [107,108]. Proposals have been made that, therefore, bulimia is an atypical form of affective disorder. While this may be a worthwhile research question, others should be careful not to beg the question by assuming that bulimia is nosologically related to depression. Undue enthusiasm on this issue is just as inappropriate as is undue negativism in the case of schizoaffective disorder or atypical psychosis. In each case, converging evidence from several directions is required to begin to answer the question. The classical validating dimensions for nosology, of course, aside from clinical features, are natural history, family history, response to specific treatments, and laboratory markers.

Ninth, many recent reports have uncritically adopted the 5 μg/dL cortisol cutoff value without validating their local cortisol assay, despite repeated cautions [6,20,50,54,70,72] against assuming that all cortisol assays are equivalent in the critical range for DST results. As pointed out earlier in this review, most clinical cortisol assays actually have higher cutoff values than 5 μg/dL. Meltzer and Fang [28] pointed out that errors of this type will produce spuriously low estimates of specificity. In a recent study from England, for example, the authors adopted a cutoff level of 5 μg/dL even though their data pointed to the need to raise this criterion value, since only 89% of their control subjects suppressed below the cutoff level [82]. The correct statistical principle is to set the cutoff level so that 95% of normal subjects fall below this value with the local assay. Consequently, the specificity results in other diagnoses of this report will need to be revised upwards, but it is impossible to judge by how much since the report does not present the data needed for these calculations.

Tenth, it is clear that when we lowered the recommended dose of dexamethasone from 2-mg to 1-mg [3] we approached the limit of low dosage to discriminate melancholia from other disorders or from normal subjects. In an attempt to reduce the dose even lower Rush and associates tested both 1-mg and 0.75-mg doses in normal subjects [109]. The specificity was 95% with 1-mg but only 76% with 0.75-mg, so clearly the dose cannot be lower than 1-mg for routine use. These considerations raise the questions of *bioavailability* of different dexamethasone formulations and standardization of this aspect of the test. Obviously, preparations with reduced bioavailability could be responsible for impaired apparent specificity of the DST. Additional research with measures of plasma dexamethasone concentrations will be needed to answer these questions.

## SUMMARY

The DST is a practical laboratory test that can be used in outpatient or inpatient settings. The required laboratory technology is available at most hospitals. No subjective, behavioral, or metabolic side effects occur with the single-dose administration of dexamethasone, and the test is well tolerated by patients. The test is not affected by most of the usual psychotropic drugs and no special dietary precautions are needed. The recommended procedure for inpatients yields good sensitivity (67%) and high specificity (96%).

Like many laboratory tests, the DST will be most useful if there is a moderate probability that the disorder being considered (melancholia) is actually present [5, 71]. If the prevalence of melancholia in the population tested is at least 35%, then the predictive value (diagnostic confidence) of an abnormal test result will be at least 90%. If the prevalence is very low, however, then the predictive value also will be much lower. Thus, the DST is not suitable for screening unselected patients but should be used when the clinician thinks it might help to answer a specific diagnostic question.

While some questions remain, there is now reason to recommend use of the DST in diagnosis and patient management. An important goal for the future will be to develop other laboratory markers for use in combination with the DST, so that the proportion of melancholic patients who can be positively identified is raised to an even higher level. Eventually, we may expect the emergence of a new definition of melancholia that includes appropriate weighting of the laboratory findings in addition to the usual clinical features.

Gillespie wrote, in 1929, that "it is clear that no one sign . . . is going to serve as a touchstone for diagnosis, or prognosis, or as a therapeutic indication" [110]. The same is true of laboratory tests in the 1980s. They do not replace the thought and care the clinician must invest in evaluating a patient, but they can give useful information that must be ordered, interpreted, and assessed in the clinical context with good judgement and common sense. There will be times when an unexpected laboratory result will force the clinician to go back and take a fresh look at the patient and perhaps see a diagnostic pattern that was not apparent before.

The author has repeatedly warned against simplistic or concrete interpretation of the test results and has stressed the need to integrate the laboratory data with clinical findings. All physicians are taught the principle that they treat patients rather than laboratory test results: It would be ironic if psychiatrists overlook this basic axiom as laboratory diagnostic aids become available to supplement their clinical assessments of patients. Just as physicians gradually had to learn how to use the glucose tolerance test wisely for the diagnosis of diabetes mellitus [111], so psychiatrists will need time to gain experience and perspective on the use of the DST. As in the area of diabetes, "much heat, and little light, has been generated in the last five years over . . . diagnostic criteria" [111]. Perhaps the most important value of the DST will be to stimulate additional research on the mechanisms of neuroendocrine disturbance in depressed and other groups of patients, so that a more refined understanding emerges of the etiology of limbic system pathology.

We are in an interesting dialectic stage in which we are moving from DSM III to DSM IV by an iterative process. We are going from standard clinical descriptive notions to examining patterns of abnormal laboratory markers and back again to refine our clinical notions. Eventually, with increasing experience, the real place of the sleep EEG, TRH test, and DST will become clear, and DSM IV will incorporate biologic markers with clinical description. When that day comes, we will be in a stronger position to identify homogeneous groups of patients for selective antidepressant therapy and for research studies.

## REFERENCES

1. Carroll BJ, Curtis GC, Mendels J: Neuroendocrine regulation in depression. I. Limbic system-adrenocortical dysfunction. Arch Gen Psych 33:1039-1044, 1976
2. Carroll BJ, Curtis GC, Mendels J: Neuroendocrine regulation in depression. II. Discrimination of depressed from non-depressed patients. Arch Gen Psych 33:1051-1057, 1976
3. Carroll BJ, Feinberg M, Greden JF et al: A specific laboratory test for the diagnosis of melancholia. Standardization, validation and clinical utility. Arch Gen Psych 38:15-22, 1981
4. Morris JB, Beck AT: The efficacy of antidepressant drugs. Arch Gen Psych 30:667-74, 1974
5. Carroll BJ: Implications of biological research for the diagnosis of depression. In J Mendlewicz (ed): New Advances in the Diagnosis and Treatment of Depressive Illness. Excerpta Medica, Amsterdam, 1980
6. Carroll BJ: Clinical application of neuroendocrine research in depression. In H VanPraag (ed.): Handbook of Biological Psychiatry: Part III, Brain Mechanisms and Abnormal Behavior. M Dekker, New York, 1980.
7. Galen RS, Gambino SR: Beyond Normality: The Predictive Value and Efficiency of Medical Diagnoses. Wiley, New York, 1975
8. Carroll BJ, Mendels J: Neuroendocrine regulation in affective disorders. In EJ Sachar (ed): Hormones, Behavior and Psychopathology. New York, Raven Press, 1976
9. Carroll BJ: Neuroendocrine function in mania. In B Shopsin (ed): Manic Illness: A Profile in Psychobiological Research. New York, Raven Press, 1979
10. Sachar EJ, Hellman L, Fukushima DK, et al: Cortisol production in depressive illness. A clinical and biochemical clarification. Arch Gen Psych 23:289-298, 1970
11. Carroll BJ: Neuroendocrine function in psychiatric disorders. In MA Lipton, A DiMascio, KF Killam (eds): Psychopharmacology: A Generation of Progress. New York, Raven Press, 1978
12. Liddle GE: Tests of pituitary-adrenal suppressibility in the diagnosis of Cushing's Syndrome. J Clin Endocrinol Metab 20:1539-1560, 1960

13. Pavlatos FC, Smilo RP, Forsham PH: A rapid screening test for Cushing's Syndrome. JAMA 193:720-723, 1965
14. Nugent, CA, Nichols T, Tyler FH: Diagnosis of Cushing's Syndrome. Single dose dexamethasone suppression tests. Arch Intern Med 116:172-176, 1965
15. McHardy-Young S, Harris PWR, Lessoff MH, et al: Single-dose dexamethasone suppression test for Cushing's Syndrome. Br Med J 1:740-744, 1967
16. Stokes PE: Pituitary suppression in psychiatric patients. The Endocrine Society (USA), 48th Meeting Abstracts, 1966
17. Stokes, PE: Studies on the control of adrenocortical function in depression. In TA Williams, MM Katz, JA Shields (eds): Recent Advances in the Psychobiology of the Depressive Illnesses. Washington, DC, US Government Printing Office, 1972
18. Carroll BJ, Martin FIR, Davies BM: Resistance to suppression by dexamethasone of plasma 11-OHCS levels in severe depressive illness. Br Med J 3:285-288, 1968
19. Carroll BJ, Davies BM: Clinical associations of 11-hydroxycorticosteroid suppression and non-suppression in severe depressive illness. Br Med J 1:789-791, 1970
20. Carroll BJ: The hypothalamic-pituitary-adrenal axis in depression. In B Davies, BJ Carroll, RM Mowbray (eds): Depressive Illness: Some Research Studies. Springfield, Charles C Thomas, 1972
21. Butler PWP, Besser GM: Pituitary-adrenal function in severe depressive illness. Lancet 2:1234-1236, 1968
22. Fawcett JA, Bunney WE: Pituitary adrenal function and depression: An outline for research. Arch Gen Psych 16:517-535, 1967
23. Carroll BJ: The hypothalamus-pituitary-adrenal axis in depression. In G Burrows (ed): Handbook on Depression. Amsterdam, Excerpta Medica, 1977
24. Mason JW: A review of psychoendocrine research on the pituitary-adrenal cortical system. Psychosom Med 30:576-607, 1968
25. Carroll BJ: Limbic system-pituitary-adrenal cortex regulation in depression and schizophrenia. Psychosom Med 38:106-121, 1976
26. Sachar EJ, Hellman L, Roffwarg H, et al: Disrupted 24 hour patterns of cortisol secretion in psychotic depression. Arch Gen Psych 28:19-24, 1973
27. Murphy BEP: Some studies of the protein-binding of steroids and their application to the routine micro and ultramicro measurement of various steroids in body fluids by competitive protein-binding radioassay. J Clin Endocrinol Metab 27:973–990, 1967
28. Meltzer HY, Fang VS: Cortisol determination and the dexamethasone supresion test. Arch Gen Psych 40:501–505, 1983
29. Rubin RT, Poland RE, Blodgett ALN, et al: Cortisol dynamics and dexamethasone pharmacokinetics in primary endogenous depression: preliminary findings. In F Brambilla, G Racagni, D DeWied (eds): Progress in Psychoneuroendocrinology. Amsterdam, Elsevier, 1980
30. Rush AJ, Giles D, Parker CR, et al: Sleep EEG and dexamethasone suppression findings in depression. Biol Psychiatry 17:327–342, 1982
31. Wilens TE, Arana GW, Baldessarini RJ et al: Comparison of solid-phase radioimmunoassay and competitive protein binding method for post-dexamethasone cortisol levels in psychiatric patients. Psych Res 8:199–206, 1983
32. Aggernaes H, Kirkegaard C, Krog-Meyer I, et al: Dexamethasone suppression test andTRH test in endogenous depression. Acta Psychiatr Scand 67:258–264, 1983

33. Ritchie JC, Olton P, Presty S, et al: Plasma cortisol determination for the dexamethasone suppression test. Comparison of competitive protein binding and commercial radioimmunoassay methods. In press, 1984
34. Mathe AA: False normal dexamethasone suppression test and indomethacin. Lancet ii:714, 1983
35. Langer G, Schonbeck G, Koinig G, et al: Hyperactivity of hypothalamic–pituitary–adrenal axis in endogenous depression. Lancet, ii:524, 1979
36. Nuller JL, Ostroumova MN: Resistance to inhibiting effect of dexamethasone in patients with endogenous depression. Acta Psychiatr Scand 61:169–177, 1980
37. Hofeldt FC, Levin SR, VonWerder K, et al: Altered hypothalamic-pituitary-adrenal responsiveness to dexamethasone–insulin tolerance test in active acromegaly. J Clin Endocrinol Metab 41:399–401, 1975
38. Cameron OG, Kronfol Z, Greden J, et al: The dexamethasone suppression test (DST) in diabetes. Society of Biological Psychiatry, 38th Annual Meeting, New York, 1983
39. Smith SR, Bledsoe T, Chhetri MK: Cortisol metabolism and the pituitary–adrenal axis in adults with protein calorie malnutrition. J Clin Endocrinol Metab 40:43–52, 1975
40. Bethge H, Nagel AM, Solbach HG, et al: Zentrale Regulationsstorung der Nebennierenrindenfunktion bei der Anorexia Nervosa. Mat Med Nordmark 22:204–214, 1970
41. Edelstein CK, Roy-Byrne P, Fawzy IF, et al: Effects of weight loss on the dexamethasone suppression test. Am J Psychiatry 140:338–341, 1983
42. Berger M, Doerr P, Lund R, et al: Neuroendocrinological and neurophysiological studies in major depressive disorders: are there biological markers for the endogenous subtype? Biol Psych 17:1217–1242, 1982
43. Berger M, Pirke KM, Doerr P, et al: Influence of weight loss on the dexamethasone suppression test. Arch Gen Psych 40:585–586, 1983
44. Fichter MM, Pirke KM, Doerr P, et al: Effect of behavior therapy and weight gain on behavior, attitudes and endocrine parameters in anorexia nervosa. In C Perris, G Struwe, B Jansson (eds): Biological Psychiatry 1981. Holland, Elsevier, 1981
45. Feinberg M, Carroll BJ: Biological markers for melancholia: effect of age, severity of illness, weight loss, and polarity. In press, 1984
46. Holsboer F, Steiger A, Maier W: Four cases of reversion to abnormal dexamethasone suppression test response as indicator of clinical relapse: a preliminary report. Biol Psychiatry 18:911–916, 1983
47. Krieger DT, Allen W, Rizzo F, et al: Characterization of the normal temporal pattern of plasma corticosteroid concentrations. J Clin Endocrinol Metab 32: 266, 1971
48. Pepper GM, Davis KL, Davis BM, et al: DST in depression is unaffected by altering the clock time of its administration. Psych Res 8:105–109, 1983
49. Krieger DT: Serotonin regulation of ACTH secretion. In DT Krieger, WF Ganong (eds.): ACTH and Related Peptides: Structure, Regulation and Action. New York, New York Academy of Science, 1977
50. Carroll BJ: The dexamethasone suppression test for melancholia. Br J Psychiatry 140:292–304, 1982
51. Fang VS, Tricou BJ, Robertson A, et al: Plasma ACTH and cortisol levels in depressed patients: relation to dexamethasone suppression test. Life Sciences 29:931–938, 1981

52. Reus VI, Joseph MS, Dallman MF: ACTH levels after the dexamethasone suppression test in depression. The New England Journal of Med 306:23, 1982
53. Yerevanian BI, Woolf PD: Plasma ACTH levels in primary depression: relationship to the 24-hour dexamethasone suppression test. Psych Res 9:45–51, 1983
54. Carroll BJ: Neuroendocrine diagnosis of depression: the dexamethasone suppression test. In PJ Clayton, JE Barrett (eds): Treatment of Depression: Old Controversies and New Approaches. New York, Raven Press, 1983
55. Feighner JP, Robins E, Guze SB, et al: Diagnostic criteria for use in psychiatric research. Arch Gen Psych 26:57–63, 1972
56. Spitzer RL, Endicott J, Robins E: Research Diagnsotic Criteria for a Selected Group of Functional Disorders, 3rd ed, New York State Psychiatric Institute, New York, 1977
57. Diagnostic and Statistical Manual of Mental Disorders, 3rd ed., American Psychiatric Association, Washington, DC, 1980
58. Nelson JC, Charney DS: The symptoms of major depressive illness. Am J Psychiatry 138:1–13, 1981
59. Carroll BJ, Feinberg M, Greden JF, et al: Diagnosis of endogenous depression: comparison of clinical, research and neuroendocrine criteria. J Affective Disorders 2:177–194, 1980
60. Feinberg M, Carroll BJ: Separation of subtypes of depression using discriminant analysis. Br J Psychiatry 140:384–391, 1982
61. Matussek P, Feil WB: Personality attributes of depressive patients. Arch Gen Psych 40:783–790, 1983
62. Schlesser MA, Winokur G, Sherman BM: Hypothalamic–pituitary–adrenal axis activity in depressive illness. Arch Gen Psych 37:737–743, 1980
63. Coryell W, Gaffney G, Burkhardt MS: DSM III and the primary–secondary distinction: a comparison of concurrent validity by means of the dexamethasone suppression test. Am J Psych 139:120–120, 1982
64. Meltzer HY, Fang VA, Tricou BJ, et al: Effect of dexamethasone on plasma prolactin and cortisol levels in psychiatric patients. Am J Psych 139:763–768, 1982
65. Stokes P, Stoll P, Maas J, et al: Dexamethasone suppression test: clinical utility. History, physiology, clinical utility: An overview. American Psychiatric Association Syllabus and Scientific Proceeding, Abstract 35A, p 100, 1983
66. Carroll BJ: Neurobiologic dimensions of depression and mania. In Angst J (ed): The Origins of Depression: Current Concepts and Approaches. Berlin, Springer–Verlag, 1983
67. Fleiss JL: Statistical Methods for Rates and Proportions, 2nd ed., Wiley, New York, 1981
68. Helzer JE, Clayton PJ, Pambakian R, et al: Reliability of psychiatric diagnosis. II. The test–retest reliability of diagnostic classification. Arch Gen Psych 34:136–141, 1977
69. Spitzer RL, Endicott J, Robins E: Research diagnostic criteria. Rationale and reliability. Arch Gen Psych 35:773–782, 1978
70. Carroll BJ: Clinical applications of the dexamethasone suppression test for endogenous depression. Pharmacopsychiatria 15:19–25, 1982
71. Galen RS, Gambino SR: Beyond Normality: The Predictive Value and Efficiency of Medical Diagnoses, Wiley, New York, 1975

72. Carroll BJ: Use of the dexamethasone suppression test in depression. J Clin Psych 43:44–48, 1982
73. Albala AA, Greden JF, Tarika J, et al: Changes in serial dexamethasone suppression tests among unipolar depressives receiving electroconvulsive treatment. Biol Psychiatry 16:551–560, 1981
74. Greden JF, Gardner R, King D, et al: Dexamethasone suppression tests in antidepressant treatment of melancholia. Arch Gen Psych 40:493–500, 1983
75. Greden JF, Albala AA, Haskett RF, et al: Normalization of dexamethasone suppression tests: A probable index of recovery among endogenous depressives. Biol Psych 15:449–458, 1980
76. Holsboer F, Liebl R, Hofschuster E: Repeated dexamethasone suppression tests during depressive illness: normalization of test result compared with clinical improvement. J Affective Disorders 4:93–101, 1982
77. Papakostas Y, Fink M, Lee J, et al: Neuroendorcine measures in psychiatric patients: course and outcome with ECT. Psychiatr Res 4:56–64, 1981
78. Targum SD: Persistent neuroendocrine dysregulation in major depressive disorder: A marker for early relapse. Biol Psychiatry 19:305–318, 1984
79. Yerevanian BI, Olafsdottir H, Milanese E, et al: Normalization of the dexamethasone suppression test at discharge from hospital. J Affective Disorders 5:191–197, 1983
80. Nemeroff CB, Evans DL: Correlation between the DST in depressed patients and clinical response. Am J Psych 141:247–249, 1984
81. Greden JF, DeVigne JP, Albala AA, et al: Serial dexamethasone suppression tests among rapid cycling bipolar patients. Biol Psychiatry 17:455–462, 1982
82. Coppen A, Abou-Saleh M, Milln P, et al: Dexamethasone suppression test in depression and other psychiatric illness. Brit J Psychiat 142:498–504, 1983
83. Carroll BJ, Greden JF, Feinberg M: Suicide, neuroendocrine dysfunction and CSF 5-HIAA concentrations in depression. In B Angrist (ed): Recent Advances in Neuropsychopharmacology. Oxford, Pergamon, 1981
84. Coryell W, Schlesser MA: Suicide and the dexamethasone suppression test in unipolar depression. Am J Psych 138:1120–1121, 1981
85. Greden JF, Carroll BJ: The dexamethasone suppression test as a diagnostic aid in catatonia. Am J Psych 136:1199–1200, 1979
86. Carman JS, Wyatt ES, Crews EL, et al: Dexamethasone non-suppression: predictor of thymoleptic response in catatonic and schizo-affective patients. In C Perris, G Struwe, B Janssen (eds): Biological Psychiatry 1981. Amsterdam, Elsevier, 1981
87. Rudorfer MV, Clayton PJ: Depression, dementia and dexamethasone suppression. Am J Psych 138:701, 1981
88. McAllister TW, Ferrell RB, Price TRP, et al: The dexamethasone suppression test in two patients with severe depressive pseudodementia. Am J Psych 139: 479–481, 1982
89. Spar JE, Gerner R: Does the dexamethasone suppression test distinguish dementia from depression? Am J Psych 139:238–240, 1982
90. Raskind M, Pesking E, Rivard F, et al: Dexamethasone suppression test and cortisol circadian rhythm in primary degenerative dementia. Am J Psych 139: 1468–1471, 1982
91. Targum SD: Neuroendocrine dysfunction in schizophreniform disorder: correlation with six-month clinical outcome. Am J Psych 140:309–313, 1983

92. Crumley FE, Clerenger J, Steinfink D, et al: Preliminary report on the dexamethasone suppression test for psychiatrically disturbed adolescents. Am J Psych 139:1062–1064, 1982
93. Poznanski EO, Carroll BJ, Banegas MC, et al: The dexamethasone suppression test in prepubertal depressed children. Am J Psych 139:321–324, 1982
94. Blumer D, Zorick F, Heilbronn M, et al: Biological markers for depression in chronic pain. J Nerv Ment Dis 170:425–428, 1982
95. Carroll BJ, Greden JF, Feinberg M, et al: Neuroendocrine evaluation of depression in borderline patients. Psychiatr Clin North America 4:89–99, 1981
96. Extein I, Pottash Al, Gold M: Neuroendocrine tests in depressed borderlines. American Psychiatric Association, 134th Annual Meeting, 1981
97. Haier RJ, Keitner GI: Sensitivity and specificity of 1 and 2 mg dexamethasone suppression tests. Psych Res 7:271–276, 1982
98. Swartz CM, Dunner FJ: Dexamethasone suppression testing of alcoholics. Arch Gen Psych 39:1309–1312, 1982
99. Bech P, Gjerris A, Andersen J, et al: The melancholia scale and the Newcastle scales: item-combinations and inter-observer reliability. Brit J Psych 143: 58–63, 1983
100. Graham PM, Booth J, Boranga G, et al: The dexamethasone suppression test in mania. J Affective Disorders 4:201–211, 1982
101. Krishnan RR, Maltbie AA, Davidson JRT: Abnormal cortisol suppression in bipolar patients with simultaneous manic and depressive symptoms. Am J Psych 140:203–205, 1983
102. Evans DL, Nemeroff CB: The dexamethasone suppression test in mixed bipolar disorder. Am J Psych 140:615–617, 1983
103. Arana GW, Barreira PJ, Wilens T, et al: Clinical studies of the dexamethasone suppression test in psychotic illnesses. American College of Neuropsychopharmacology, Abstracts 21, 79, 1982
104. Greden JF, Kronfol Z, Gardner R, et al: Neuroendocrine evaluation of schizoaffectives with the dexamethasone suppression test. In C Perris, G Struwe, B Jansson (eds): Biological Psychiatry 1981. Amsterdam, Elsevier, 1981.
105. Pope HG: Distinguishing bipolar disorder from schizophrenia in clinical practice: Guidelines and case reports. Hosp and Comm Psych 34:322–328, 1983
106. Insel TR, Kalin NH, Guttmacher LB, et al: The dexamethasone suppression test in patients with primary obsessive-compulsive disorder. Psych Res 6: 153–160, 1982
107. Gwirtsman HE, Roy-Byrne P, Yager J, et al: Neuroendocrine abnormalities in bulimia. Am J Psych 140:5 559–563, 1983
108. Hudson JI, Pope HG, Jonas JM, et al: Hypothalamic–pituitary–adrenal–axis hyperactivity in bulimia. Psych Res 8:111–117, 1983
109. Rush AJ, Schlesser MA, Giles DE, et al: The effect of dosage on the dexamethasone suppression test in normal controls. Psych Res 7:277–285, 1982
110. Gillespie RD: The clinical differentiation of types of depression. Guy's Hospital Reports, 79:306–344, 1929
111. Alberti KGMM, Hockaday TDR: Diabetes mellitus. In DH Weatherall, JGG Ledingham, DA Warrell (eds): Oxford Textbook of Medicine. Oxford, Oxford University Press, 1983
112. Carnes M, Smith JC, Kalin NH, et al: The dexamethasone suppression test in demented outpatients with and without depression. Psych Res 9:337–344, 1983

CHAPTER 2

# Comprehensive Thyroid Evaluation in Psychiatric Patients

MARK S. GOLD and
MICHAEL H. KRONIG

## THE HYPOTHALAMIC-PITUITARY-THYROID AXIS

The thyroid gland is one link in the neuroendocrine system known as the Hypothalamic-Pituitary-Thyroid (HPT) axis [1-3]. Within this axis, circulating thyroid hormones are tightly regulated by both central nervous system input and peripheral feedback control. The hypothalamus secretes Thyrotropin Releasing Hormone (TRH) into the portal system of the adenohypophysis. TRH stimulates the pituitary thyrotrope cells to release Thyroid Stimulating Hormone (TSH), which in turn increases the rates of iodide uptake, hormone synthesis, and release of thyroxine ($T_4$) and triiodothyronine ($T_3$).

Hypothalamic input is essential for normal thyroid function [2,3]. Experimental lesions which destroy or disconnect the hypothalamus from the pituitary result in hypothyroidism [4]. It appears, then, that the major hypothalamic input is stimulatory. Hypophyseal portal blood was found to stimulate the pituitary to release TSH [5]. The active substance, TRH, was determined to be a tripeptide

*Handbook of Psychiatric Diagnostic Procedures*, vol. 1, edited by R. C. W. Hall and T. P. Beresford. 

hormone [6]. By a variety of techniques such as microlesions, biopsies, electrical stimulation and, finally, immunoassay, TRH was found in the highest concentrations in the paraventricular nuclei of the hypothalamus [2,7,8]. It is also present in other sections of the hypothalamus and, of great theoretical interest, TRH is widely distributed throughout the brain and spinal cord [7,8]. In fact, it is estimated that as much as 80% of TRH is extrahypothalamic.

In rats, lesions of the hypothalamus which result in a marked reduction of hypothalamic TRH do not affect the extrahypothalamic TRH pool [9]. Thus, it appears that extrahypothalamic TRH is synthesized in situ and may be a peptide neurotransmitter [6,9]. Using single-cell recording techniques, TRH has been shown to have both inhibitory [10,11] and excitatory [11] influences on different neurons. There are animal studies that show behavioral stimulation upon TRH injection [12,13], but others show no effect or behavioral quieting [14]. TRH injected into rats causes an increased norepinephrine turnover as measured by fluorescence histochemistry [15], and there are reports of antidepressant actions in humans [16]. However, TRH infused daily for 7-10 days in a group of depressed patients failed to produce a clinical antidepressant response [17].

The release of TRH is controlled at least in part by monoamine neurotransmitters [2,3,6,18]. In vitro studies in the mouse indicate that dopamine and norepinephrine increase TRH release, whereas serotonin inhibits TRH release. The acetylcholine analogue carbachol has no effect [18]. There is little human data available at this time, except for one study which tends to support the fact that serotonin inhibits TRH release [19]. It is not known whether a "short-loop" negative feedback system exists whereby pituitary TSH inhibits TRH, nor have hypothalamic TRH autoreceptors been described. It is known that thyroid hormone increases catecholamine receptor sensitivity [20]; if anything, this would tend to increase TRH release and thus be a positive feedback at the hypothalamic level. There is one animal study supporting a positive feedback of $T_4$ on TRH; the presence of TSH was necessary for this effect [21].

TSH is found in specific basophilic (thyrotrope) cells of the anterior pituitary which are discrete from those cells which secrete gonadotropins and ACTH [1-3]. It is a glycoprotein (molecular weight 28,000) with two subunits. Once released into the blood, it circulates unbound and has a half-life of 50-60 minutes [22]. TSH levels in man have a circadian rhythm with the highest levels from 4 AM to 8 AM [23].

TRH interacts with high-affinity receptors at the pituitary [24] to stimulate the release of TSH, probably via a cyclic AMP "second messenger" system [25]. The TRH induced TSH response can be inhibited by somatostatin [26], another hypothalamic hormone; the mechanism is unclear, but may involve a discrete somatostatin receptor. Other hormones modify the TSH response to TRH. Estrogen enhances, whereas growth hormone and glucocorticoids inhibit, TSH release [2,26, 27].

In addition to control from hypothalamic centers, the release of TSH is under negative feedback from circulating thyroid hormones. Circulating $T_3$ and $T_3$ made locally (within the thyrotrope) from the monodeiodination of $T_4$ interact with a receptor on the cell nucleus. Presumably, a protein is synthesized which competitively interferes with the thyrotrope's responsiveness to TRH [28]. TSH release is suppressed, and stimulation of the thyroid gland decreases.

The thyroid gland secretes primarily $T_4$, but also $T_3$ [29,30]. $T_4$ is deiodinated by the liver, kidneys, and other peripheral tissues to $T_3$ [31]. Most of the thyroid hormone bioactivity is provided by $T_3$ [24,30]. Only a small percentage of $T_3$ and $T_4$ circulate free, with the major part bound to proteins such as Thyroid Binding Globulin (TBG) and Thyroid Binding Prealbumin (TBPA). The presence of dietary iodide ($I^-$) is crucial for the production of thyroid hormones. Insufficient iodide leading to hypothyroidism and goiter was previously common in certain sections of the U.S., but is now rare because of the addition of iodide to salt and packaged foods [32].

## LABORATORY EVALUATION OF THYROID FUNCTION

In the past, the only laboratory methods available were the measurement of circulating thyroid hormones. This situation has changed, and the clinician should be familiar with the newer thyroid tests.

### $T_3$, $T_4$, and $T_3$ Resin Uptake

Circulating thyroid hormones used to be measured by protein-bound iodine (PBI) or $T_4$ by column chromatography. These methods lack sensitivity and specificity, and are of historical interest only. The most widely used assays for $T_4$ are the competitive protein binding assay and the radioimmunoassay. Because both of these techniques measure total $T_4$, they are influenced by changes in the number of binding sites. Binding capacity is increased in conditions such as pregnancy, hepatitis, and with the use of certain medications (estrogens, perphenazine). It is decreased in major illness, nephrotic syndrome, and with other medications (salicylate, phenytoin) [30].

To help correct for these changes in binding capacity, the $T_3$ resin uptake ($T_3$ RU) determination is performed. This is a measurement of the number of thyroid hormone binding sites available. A standardized amount of the patient's serum is mixed with radioactively labeled $T_3$ ($T_3$*) and with a resin which absorbs thyroid hormones. The $T_3$* which is not absorbed by binding sites in the patient's serum is absorbed by the added resin, which is then measured. If the patient has an excess of thyroid hormone (hyperthyroidism), or a decrease in binding sites, most of the patient's binding sites are already filled and there is a surplus of $T_3$* absorbed by the resin. The opposite is true in hypothyroidism, or when binding sites are increased. Interpretation of the $T_3RU$, then, is as follows: ↑$T_3RU$ indicates ↓ in available binding sties, and ↓$T_3RU$ indicates ↑ in available binding sites.

Other measures are free $T_4$ by a dialysis technique, $T_3$ by radioimmunoassay, and free $T_3$ by dialysis. The free thyroxin index (FTI) is the product of total $T_4$ and $T_3RU$. It is a calculated value which correlates well with free $T_4$ as measured by dialysis.

## Reverse $T_3$

$T_4$ is deiodinated to $T_3$ by removing an iodide atom from the "outer" (phenol) ring. However, as much as 30%–40% of $T_4$ is deiodinated on the "inner" (tyrosine) ring to form Reverse $T_3$ ($RT_3$). This is an apparently inactive form of $T_3$ which can be measured by radioimmunoassay [33]. Its importance is just being investigated. One theory is that an abnormal increase in deiodination to $RT_3$, rather than $T_3$, would result in hypothyroid states.

## TSH

Circulating levels of TSH can now be measured routinely by radioimmunoassay. The TSH level yields a measure of compensatory pituitary function and responsiveness to feedback [29,30]. If circulating free $T_4$ and $T_3$ decrease for any reason, the pituitary thyrotrope loses its $T_3$-induced inhibition. It becomes more sensitive to TRH, and the release of TSH increases relative to the person's previous baseline or normal. The thyroid gland is then stimulated in an attempt to maintain output in the normal range. If the thyroid fails to produce sufficient hormone, this cycle continues and eventually the clinical picture of hypothyroidism emerges. At this point the laboratory data will reveal decreased $T_4$ and elevated TSH. Rarely is TSH elevated except when the thyroid is failing. There do exist TSH-secreting tumors which are autonomous of thyroid hormone inhibition. Here the clinical picture is of elevated TSH, increased $T_4$, and hyperthyroidism.

## TRH-Thyroid Test

The TRH stimulation test is a provocative test of the HPT axis at the pituitary level, which can also shed light on the state of the thyroid gland itself [30,34]. In this test, the responsiveness of the thyrotrope to a TRH challenge is measured. Our technique is as follows: The patient is fasted overnight. At about 8:30 AM the patient is asked to lie in a comfortable position and a butterfly needle is inserted in standard fashion. The vein is kept patent by a slow drip of normal saline. Blood is drawn for TSH, $T_4$, $T_3RIA$, and $T_3RU$ at 8:59. Then, a 500 mg bolus of synthetic TRH (protirelin) is injected over 30–60 seconds. Side effects noted are transient and include a feeling of warmth, desire to urinate or defecate, nausea, metallic taste, headache, dry mouth, chest tightness, and a pleasant genital sensation. Blood is drawn for TSH 15, 30, 60, and 90 minutes after the TRH is infused. The baseline TSH value is subtracted from the peak TSH to give the ΔTSH. In normals ΔTSH is from 7–15 μIU/ml. Hypothyroid patients have supersensitivity to the TRH, and therefore an elevated ΔTSH; hyperthyroid patients are subsensitive and have a decreased ΔTSH. The TRH test in psychiatric patients will be discussed more fully below.

### Thyroid Autoantibodies

The immune system, under certain circumstances, makes antibodies directed against thyroid substances [35]. Two commonly measured substances are anti-microsomal (anti-M) and anti-thyroglobulin (anti-T) antibodies. Investigators are determining whether the primary defect is in genetically transmitted antigen-specific suppression T lymphocytes which attack the thyroid [36]. High titers, which may be transient or permanent, are evidence of autoimmune disease. In one Australian study of a "random" population of 2838 subjects, the prevalence of anti-M antibodies was 9.8% in women and 2.8% in men. Women in the sixth decade had a prevalence of 15% [37]. The presence of anti-M antibodies was related to thyroid disease as measured by lymphocytic-infiltration of the thyroid and elevated TSH levels. A Finnish study yielded similar results [38].

## HYPOTHYROIDISM AND DEPRESSION

It has long been known that many signs and symptoms of overt thyroid disease, such as anergia, constipation, and appetite and weight changes, overlap with those of depression [29,39,40,41] (see Figure 1). Because both thyroid disease and depression carry a good prognosis when treated correctly, it is crucial to make an accurate diagnosis prior to treatment. Psychiatric diagnostic systems, such as the DSM III [42] and RDC [43] emphasize differential diagnosis among psychiatric syndromes and stress the importance of ruling out organic causes [44]. The DSM III category of Organic Affective Syndrome is described by the same clinical features as Major Depressive Episodes, except that in addition to mood disturbance only two "associated features" are needed instead of four. This highlights the need to pursue a thorough general medical, neurologic, metabolic, and endocrinologic evaluation for patients presenting with "depressive" syndromes.

Most psychiatrists routinely include hypothyroidism in the differential diagnosis of depressive states. Although this has not been studied systematically, the average workup probably comprises a $T_4$ and $T_3$RU. Occasionally, a baseline TSH is ordered. These tests will certainly pick up patients with overt thyroid

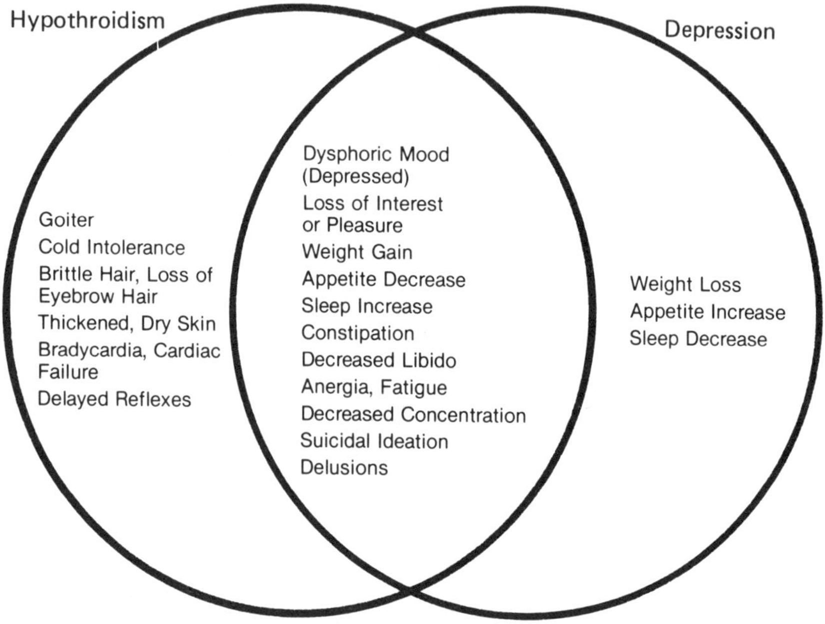


**Figure 1.** Signs and symptoms of hypothyroidism and depression.

failure and some with lesser degrees of thyroid dysfunction, but will not detect mild degrees of hypothyroidism. Recent evidence indicates that this latter group is highly represented in psychiatric patients presenting with depression. The grossly hypothyroid patients are readily identified and treated by other physicians and rarely present to psychiatrists.

Endocrinologists no longer describe hypothyroidism as an "all or nothing" phenomenon. Rather, thyroid dysfunction is seen as a spectrum illness, with various grades of disease [45–49]. TRH testing has been a major tool in this conceptual development and in the early diagnosis of hypothyroidism.

## Grade 1 Hypothyroidism

Grade 1 is overt hypothyroidism. These patients have the classical signs and symptoms of hypothyroidism which are found in any medical text: lethargy, weakness, slowed mentation, sluggish reflexes, constipation, weight gain, hair and skin changes. Laboratory values show $\downarrow T_4$, $\uparrow$TSH, and $\uparrow\Delta$TSH.

### Grade 2 Hypothyroidism

This is mild hypothyroidism. Grade 2 patients have a few clinical symptoms, such as lethargy and early skin or hair changes, or more numerous nonspecific complaints. $T_4$ is normal, but baseline TSH is marginally elevated. TRH testing reveals ↑ΔTSH.

### Grade 3 Hypothyroidism

Grade 3 is also known as "subclinical" hypothyroidism, which may be a misnomer. These patients have few clinical symptoms, and laboratory testing is normal except for ↑ΔTSH on TRH stimulation.

The TRH test has been used in psychiatric settings for about a decade. Prange and associates, intrigued with the finding that some depressed women had a better response to imipramine when also given $T_3$, tested 10 unipolar depressed women with the TRH test. Two of their initial 10 patients had a blunted TSH response (↓ΔTSH) to TRH [50]. This finding has been replicated by many investigators, with about 20-40% of patients with major depression having a blunted ΔTSH [51-56]. Further studies by Gold et al [57] and Extein et al [58], but not Linkowski et al [59], have shown that ↓ΔTSH is generally confined to unipolar depressed patients.

The finding of a blunted TSH response to TRH infusion contradicts the notion that depressed patients may be hypothyroid. If anything, mild hypothyroidism would render the pituitary supersensitive to TRH, with a resulting augmentation of TSH response (↑ΔTSH). The reason for this finding is unclear. One theory is that the ↓ΔTSH is secondary to alterations in monoaminergic systems.

Gold et al [19] found an inverse correlation between CSF 5-HIAA (the major serotonin metabolite) and ΔTSH, indicating that increased serotonergic activity inhibits the TSH response. Kirkegaard et al [60] injected patients with the serotonin precursor 5-hydroxytryptophan prior to TRH testing; ΔTSH was unaffected by this manipulation. Another postulate is that the blunted ΔTSH in unipolar depressive is secondary to elevated glucocorticoid levels; this has not been found in two separate studies [51,57].

Gold and colleagues [61] evaluated a large series of 250 patients with the TRH test. All patients were referred for depression and/or anergia. None were referred specifically for thyroid evaluation or replacement, nor had any been treated with thyroid hormones for at least 12 months. Patients were medication-free for one week. Of these patients, 20 (8%) had some degree of hypothyroidism as evidenced by TRH testing. As defined above, Grade 1 (overt) hypothyroidism was present in 2 patients (<1%); Grade 2 (mild) hypothyroidism in 8 patients (3.2%), and Grade 3 (subclinical) hypothyroidism in 10 patients (4.0%). This is a much higher percentage of thyroid disease than has been previously reported. What is also impressive is that, in open trials, some refractory patients had an excellent response to thyroid replacement. Sternbach and colleagues [62] followed the inpatient study with a series of 44 outpatients evaluated for complaints of depression and/or anergia. Of these patients, 6 (13.5%) had an augmented TSH response to TRH infusion consistent with thyroid dysfunction. Five of these 6 patients had other evidence of thyroid disease (↑ baseline TSH and/or positive anti-thyroid antibodies).

An important question is the etiology of the thyroid dysfunction. A well-recognized entity in the endocrinologic literature is called Symptomless Autoimmune Thyroiditis (SAT) [48,63]. This entity affects 5–15% of the general population and is especially prevalent in elderly women; it is defined by the presence of lymphoplasmocytic infiltration of the thyroid and the presence of antithyroid antibodies. A high proportion (65%) of patients with SAT have elevated ΔTSH on TRH testing. Gold et al [64] tested 100 consecutive patients complaining of depression and/or anergia; in this study, 15% had some degree of hypothyroidism. Of these 15 patients, 9 (60%) were positive for anti-M antibodies. Putting these studies together, the conclusion is that many psychiatric patients presenting with depression and/or anergia are hypothyroid, and that the most common etiology is SAT. In other words, thyroid failure that is "symptomless" to the endocrinologist may be "depression" to the psychiatrist.

Treatment alternatives for these patients have not yet been studied in double-blind fashion. Clearly, all patients with Grade 1 (overt) disease need thyroid replacement. Recent reports in the endocrinologic literature indicate that patients with Grade 2 (mild) hypothyroidism should be treated routinely with thyroid replacement. It is felt that hypothyroidism is progressive, and there are some reports that patients with mild hypothyroidism are at increased risk for cardiac disease and myocardial infarction [65]. There are proven beneficial cardiac responses to thyroid replacement in patients with Grade 2 hypothyroidism [66]. It is likely, although unproven in large trials, that thyroid replacement will improve mood in patients with mild hypothyroidism who present with depression and/or anergia. At this time, we recommend thyroid replacement in all such patients, with the addition of antidepressants if response to thyroid hormone alone is incomplete. Treatment for depressed patients with Grade 3 (subclinical) hypothyroidism is less clear. At this point, patients should be treated on an individualized basis; certainly those who do not respond to 21 consecutive days at therapeutic blood-levels of an antidepressant should be tried on thyroid hormone in addition to the antidepressant. We have generally used $T_3$ (liothyronine sodium, Cytomel) for replacement, beginning with a daily dosage of 25 $\mu$g, and closely monitor the patient's clinical condition. A good biochemical end-point for thyroid replacement is normalization of the TRH stimulation test.

Prange et al [67] and others [68–71] have reported that $T_3$ has antidepressant properties singly and in combination with tricyclics. It is interesting to speculate that this effect may be due to reversal of subclinical thyroid failure, but further data are needed.

## HYPERTHYROIDISM AND PSYCHIATRIC ILLNESS

The classic psychiatric presentation of hyperthyroidism is generalized anxiety [39,40]. When other clinical signs such as weight loss with increased appetite, tachycardia, fine tremor, and exophthalmos are present, the diagnosis is self-evident. What is not clear is the prevalence of hyperthyroidism among patients presenting with a chief complaint of anxiety.

Manic and schizophrenic syndromes have also been associated with thyroid hormone. In one series of 100 committed inpatients [72], three patients were hyperthyroid and met RDC for manic depressive illness and three were hyperthyroid and met RDC for schizophrenia. In another series of 191 inpatients [73], seven were hyperthyroid: five presented as affective psychosis, one as neurotic depression, and one as schizophrenia. There are recent cases reported in the literature of mania following the administration of exogenous thyroid. One case occurred during a treatment study of resistant depression with imipramine plus $T_3$ [70]. A 37-year-old woman on imipramine 50 mg po TID developed mania three hours after the addition of 25 mg of $T_3$. It was not stated whether or not she had a bipolar history, nor whether this relatively small amount of $T_3$ made her chemically hyperthyroid. Another case [74] involved a 34-year-old woman with a history of treated Grave's disease who became hypothyroid and was treated with $T_4$ 150 mg daily for 4 days, at which time she became clinically manic. She had a prior history of hypomania, but it is not clear whether that was related to her prior hyperthyroid state. In reviewing the literature, Josephson and MacKenzie [75] found 25 cases of "mania" following thyroid replacement for hypothyroidism. They analyzed 18 case reports and determined that 15 of these patients were psychotic prior to thyroid replacement; the significance of this is not clear. Hyperthyroidism can also present as depression. There is a case report of thyrotoxicosis presenting as a delusional depression which resolved only upon treatment of the endocrine disorder [76].

Bipolar, lithium-free manics have a blunted TSH response to TRH infusion [59,77,78]. Extein et al [78] have postulated that increased noradrenergic or dopaminergic transmission in mania causes increased TRH release at the hypothalamic level. Pituitary TRH receptors then "down regulate" in an attempt to maintain homeostasis. Therefore, the pituitary is less sensitive to the infused TRH, with resultant blunted TSH response. In this model amphetamine and cocaine states are model systems for mania [79]; cocaine, amphetamine, l-dopa and mania all blunt the TRH-induced TSH response. An alternate theory, which is by no means incompatible with Extein's, is that some manic patients are mildly hyperthyroid. Increased $T_3$ would make the pituitary thyrotrope cells less sensitive to infused TRH with the same result. Lithium's efficacy in hyperthyroidism also supports this notion [80].

As reviewed above, hypothyroidism is now being viewed along a continuum. There is no reason to assume that hyperthyroidism is not also a spectrum illness

As reviewed above, hypothyroidism is now being viewed along a continuum. There is no reason to assume that hyperthyroidism is not also a spectum illness ranging from subclinical to overt. This issue has not been studied in either the endocrinologic or psychiatric spheres. It is conceivable that subsets of anxious or manic patients have mild forms of hyperthyroidism which is either the primary etiology or a major exacerbating factor to the illness.

## THYROID-CATECHOLAMINE INTERRELATIONSHIPS

The amino acid tyrosine is the precursor for both thyroid hormones and the catecholamine neurotransmitters, norepinephrine (NE) and dopamine (DA). Whybrow and Prange [20] hypothesize that the functional outcome of this phenomenon may be the interaction between thyroid and catecholamine receptors. They note the studies of enhanced response to tricyclics when $T_3$ is administered. Among depressed patients, evidence of increased thyroid activity correlates with rapid recovery when patients are given drugs that increase catecholamine availability, but not when serotonin precursors are administered. Thyroid hormones increase B-adrenergic receptor sensitivity, which would increase NE transmission along these CNS pathways. A deficiency of thyroid hormone would decrease B-receptor sensitivity with a resultant decline in effective B-adrenergic activity. This decrease in thyroid hormone would be relative and not absolute, decreased thyroid for the person reflected in ΔTSH but not thyroid hormone levels until illness had progressed. By the classic catecholamine hypothesis of depression [81], this would result in or contribute to depression. Conversely, in mania it is hypothesized that there is an increase of noradrenergic and/or dopaminergic activity. Hyperthyroidism, by increasing receptor sensitivity, could theoretically be associated with increased transmission and therefore mania.

Lithium is a potent antimania agent both for acute episodes and for prophylaxis of recurrent illness [82]. It is also a potent antithyroid agent [83,84]. The thyroid concentrates lithium, which reduces the synthesis and release of $T_3$ and $T_4$. Circulating thyroid hormones are decreased within a few days of beginning lithium. It is postulated that lithium's antimanic actions are significantly related to this decrease in available thyroid hormone, which would secondarily decrease catecholaminergic transmission in the CNS.

## THYROID WORKUP OF THE PSYCHIATRIC PATIENT

Clearly, the practicing psychiatrist must screen all patients for physical illness. Many investigators have found in psychiatric populations a high percentage of patients with physical illnesses which either caused or exacerbated the "psychiatric"

**SIGNS and SYMPTOMS OF THYROID DYSFUNCTION**

| | Present | Absent |
| --- | --- | --- |
| Goiter | ________ | ________ |
| Thyroid Bruit | ________ | ________ |
| Fine Tremor | ________ | ________ |
| Weight Loss | ________ | ________ |
| Increased Appetite | ________ | ________ |
| Lid Lag | ________ | ________ |
| Depressed Mood | ________ | ________ |
| Sweating | ________ | ________ |
| Heat Intolerance | ________ | ________ |
| Positive Family History | ________ | ________ |
| Lethargy/Anergia | ________ | ________ |
| Weight Gain | ________ | ________ |
| Hoarseness | ________ | ________ |
| Dry Skin | ________ | ________ |
| Nervousness | ________ | ________ |
| Hair Loss | ________ | ________ |
| Cold Intolerance | ________ | ________ |
| Delayed Reflexes | ________ | ________ |
| Constipation | ________ | ________ |
| Exophthalmos | ________ | ________ |
| Recent M. I. | ________ | ________ |
| Coronary Artery Disease | ________ | ________ |
| Arrhythmias | ________ | ________ |
| Pulse>90/minute | ________ | ________ |
| Hypertension | ________ | ________ |
| **TOTAL** | ________ | ________ |

Patient with 5 or more signs/symptoms have high degree of suspicion of hypothalamic-pituitary-thyroid axis dysfunction.

**Figure 2.** Thyroid dysfunction checklist.

conditions (for review see Estroff and Gold in Gold, Carmen, Lydiard) [85]. As has been reviewed in this chapter, hypothyroidism is common in "depressed" patients and hyperthyroidism should also be considered in anxiety and manic disorders. In evaluating patients with suspected thyroid disease, the clinician needs to rely on history, physical examination, and laboratory testing. DSM III diagnosis does not differentiate primary from secondary depression especially in patients with thyroid disease [61,62].

The history elicited from a patient with thyroid disease will depend on both the severity of illness and the rigor with which thyroid referable complaints are elicited. It is important to remember that hypothyroid patients may present with only complaints of depression or anergia, and hyperthyroid patients perhaps just with anxiety. A helpful tool is a standardized checklist of symptoms and signs of thyroid disease, such as the one presented in Figure 2. Four or five positives on this list is highly suggestive of thyroid disease. A patient with a positive family history for thyroid disease should always be evaluated.

Physical examination is too often neglected by the psychiatrist. Even a brief examination can give invaluable clues as to the patient's thyroid status. Vital signs will screen for altered blood pressure, tachycardia or bradycardia, and dysrhythmias. Inspection of the patient may reveal tremor, exophthalmos, diaphoresis, or loss of hair. The patient's clothing may reveal weight changes or heat or cold intolerance. Skin and hair changes may be palpable, and the thyroid should be checked for size, tenderness, and presence or absence of bruits. A neurologic examination will pick up lid lag, tremor, and delayed or brisk ankle jerks.

Presence of positive items on history or physical strongly increases the possibility of thyroid disease, and a full laboratory workup is mandatory. We feel that all patients presenting with anergia or depression require at least $T_4$, $T_3$RIA, $T_3$RU, and TSH. This will pick up patients with Grade 1 hypothyroidism and will be suggestive in Grade 2 disease. Patients suspected of Grade 2 or Grade 3 hypothyroidism should have the TRH infusion test to confirm the diagnosis and help guide treatment. Patients with an abnormally high $\Delta$TSH $\geq 20$ should be screened for anti-M and anti-T antibodies.

Although the prevalence of hyperthyroidism in patients with generalized anxiety or mania is not fully known, it seems most prudent to screen such patients with $T_4$, $T_3$RIA, $T_3$RU, and TSH. The TRH infusion is clearly of value in differentiating mania from acute schizophrenia, and a normal $\Delta$TSH will help rule out hyperthyroidism. A blunted $\Delta$TSH will not, however, differentiate "primary" mania from mania in which hyperthyroidism is etiologically responsible. Likewise, a normal TRH infusion test in a patient presenting with anxiety will rule out hyperthyroidism, but there is no definitive interpretation of a blunted TRH infusion test in such a patient.

Lithium-treated bipolar or recurrent unipolar patients present a unique problem. These patients are by definition predisposed to depressive episodes. In addition, they are at risk for lithium-induced hypothyroidism which can cause or increase susceptibility to depression. How should the psychiatrist work up the bipolar depressed patient who is taking lithium? A TRH infusion test can be of considerable help. Following a $\Delta$TSH in the patient from before treatment to lithium maintenance is of considerable importance in the early identification of lithium-induced Grade 3 disease. An increasing $\Delta$TSH should raise the possibility of Grade 2 or 3 hypothyroidism, and thyroid replacement should be considered before starting antidepressants.

## SUMMARY

The interactions between thyroid hormones, catecholamines, and mental states are complex. Many questions remain unanswered concerning the interpretation of thyroid tests and subsequent treatment in borderline cases. There is a familiar adage in internal medicine, "If you don't take a temperature, you won't find a fever." An analogous situation holds true in psychiatry. The psychiatrist who ignores the thyroid will find no thyroid illness, whereas the psychiatrist who keeps a high index of suspicion will find the yield of complete thyroid evaluations to be significant. This will result in increased diagnostic accuracy, and most importantly, improved therapeutic results for his or her patients.

## REFERENCES

1. Demeester-Mirkline N, Dumont JE: The hypothalama-pituitary-thyroid axis. In DeVisscher M (ed): The Thyroid Gland. New York, Raven Press, 1980
2. Martin JB, Reichlin S, Brown GM: Clinical Neuroendocrinology. Philadelphia, FA Davis Company, 1977
3. Morley JE: Neuroendocrine control of thyrotropin secretion. Endocr Rev 2: 396–436, 1981
4. Martin JB, Boshans R, Reichlin S: Feedback regulation of TSH secretion in rats with hypothalamic lesions. Endocrinology 87:1032–1040, 1970
5. Wilber JF, Porter JC: Thyrotropin and growth hormone releasing activity in hypophysial portal blood. Endocrinology 87:807–811, 1970
6. Jackson IMD: Thyrotropin-releasing hormone. N Eng J Med 306:145–153, 1982
7. Hokfelt T, Fuxe K, Johansson O, et al: Distribution of thyrotropin-releasing hormone (TRH) in the central nervous system as revealed with immunochemistry. Eur J Pharmacol 34:389–392, 1975
8. Hokfelt T, Johansson O, Ljungdahl A, et al: Neurotransmitting and neuropeptides: distribution patterns and cellular localization as revealed by immunocytochemistry. In Nobel Symposium, 42d Stockholm, 1978. Central Regulation of the Endocrine System. New York, Plenum Press, 1979
9. Jackson IMD, Reichlin S: Brain thyrotropin-releasing hormone is independent of the hypothalamus. Nature 267:853–854, 1977
10. Renaud LP, Martin JB: Thyrotropin-releasing hormone (TRH): depressant action on central neuronal activity. Brain Res 86:150–154, 1975
11. Braitman DJ, Auker CR, Carpenter DO: Thyrotropin-releasing hormone has multiple actions in cortex. Brain Res 194:244–248, 1980
12. Porter CC, Lotti VJ, DeFelice MJ: The effect of TRH and a related tripeptide, L-N-(2-oxopiperidin-6-yl-carbonyl)-L-histidyl-L-thiazolidine-4-carboxamide (MK-771, OHT), on the depressant action of barbiturates and alcohol in mice and rats. Life Sci 21:811–820, 1977
13. Stanton TL, Beckman AL, Winokur A: Thyrotropin-releasing hormone effects in the central nervous system: Dependence on arousal state. Science 214:678–681, 1981

14. Costall B, Hui S-CG, Metcalf G, et al: A study of the changes in motor behavior caused by TRH on intracerebral injection. Euro J Pharmacol 53:143–150, 1979
15. Constantinidis J, Geissbuhler F, Gaillard JM: Enhancement of Cerebral noradrenaline turnover by thyrotropin-releasing hormone: evidence by fluorescence histochemistry. Experientia 30:1182–1183, 1974
16. Kastin AJ, Ehrensing RH, Schalch DS, et al: Improvement in mental depression with decreased thyroid response after administration of thyrotropin-releasing hormone. Lancet 2:740–742, 1972
17. Ehrensing RH, Kastin AJ, Schalch DS, et al: Affective states and thyrotropin and prolactin responses after repeated injections of thyrotropin-releasing hormone in depressed patients. Am J Psychiatry 131:714–718, 1974
18. Grimm Y, Reichlin S: Thyrotropin-releasing hormone (TRH): Neurotransmitter regulation of secretion by mouse hypothalamic tissue in vitro. Endocrinology 93:626–631, 1973
19. Gold PW, Goodwin FK, Wehr T, et al: Pituitary thyrotropin response to thyrotropin-releasing hormone in affective illness: Relationship to spinal fluid amine metabolites. Am J Psychiatry 134:1028–1031, 1977
20. Whybrow PC, Prange AJ: A hypothesis of thyroid-catecholamine-receptor interaction: Its relevance to affective illness. Arch Gen Psychiatry 38:106–113, 1981
21. Roti E, Christianson D, Harris AC, et al: "Short" loop feedback regulation of hypothalamic and brain thyrotropin-releasing hormone content in the rat and dwarf mouse. Endocrinology 103:1662–1667, 1978
22. Okuno A, Taguchi T, Nakayama K, et al: Kinetic analysis of plasma TSH dynamics after TRH stimulation. Horm Metab Res 11:293–295, 1979
23. Vanhaelst L, Van Cauter E, Degaute JP, et al: Circadian variations of serum thyrotropin levels in man. J Clin Endocrinol Metab 35:479–482, 1972
24. Grant G, Vale W, Guillemin R: Interaction of thyrotropin-releasing factor with membrane receptors of pituitary cells. Biochem Biophys Res Commun 46:28–34, 1972
25. Larsen PR: Thyroid-pituitary interaction: feedback regulation of thyrotropin secretion by thyroid hormones. N Eng J Med 306:23–32, 1982
26. Sowers JR, Carlson HE, Brautbar N, et al: Effect of dexamethasone on prolactin and TSH responses to TRH and metoclopramide in man. J Clin Endocrinol Metab 44:237–241, 1977
27. Re RN, Kourides IA, Ridgway EC, et al: The effect of glucocorticoid administration in human pituitary secretion of thyrotropin and prolactin. J Clin Endocrinol Metab 43:338–346, 1976
28. Siler TM, Yen SSC, Vale W, et al: Inhibition by somatostatin on the release of TSH induced in man by thyrotropin-releasing factor. J Clin Endocrinol Metab 38:742–745, 1974
29. Ingbar SH, Woeber KA: The thyroid gland. In Williams RH (ed): Textbook of Endocrinology. Philadelphia, WB Saunders Company, 1974
30. Blum M: Easier understanding of the new thyroid tests. Resident and Staff Physician 27:72–90, 1981
31. Warren DW, LoPresti JS, Nicoloff JT: A new method for measurement of the conversion ratio of thyroxine to triiodothyronine in euthryoid man. J Clin Endocrinol Metab 53:1218–1222, 1981
32. Taylor F: Iodine: going from hypo to hyper. FDA Consumer 15–18, 1981

33. Ingbar SH, Woeber KA: The thyroid gland In Williams RH (ed): Textbook of Endocrinology. Philadelphia, Saunder, 129–131, 1981
34. Ormston BJ, Garry R, Cryer RJ, et al: Thyrotropin-releasing hormone as a thyroid-function test. Lancet 2:10–14, 1971
35. Fink JN, Beall GN: Immunologic aspects of endocrine disease. JAMA 248: 2696–2700, 1982
36. Fournier C, Chen HP, Leger A, et al: T cell functions in autoimmune thyroid diseases. Hormone Res 16 (No 5) Sept-Oct.:348, 1982
37. Hawkins BR, Dawkins RL, Burger HG, et al: Diagnostic significance of thyroid microsomal antibodies in randomly selected population. Lancet 2:1057–1059, 1980
38. Gordon A, Maatela J, Miettinen A, et al: Serum thyrotropin and circulating thyroglobulin and thyroid microsomal antibodies in a Finnish population. Acta Endocrinologica 90:33–42, 1979
39. Whybrow PC, Prange AJ, Treadway CR: Mental changes accompanying thryoid gland dysfunction: A reappraisal using objective psychological measurement. Arch Gen Psychiatry 20:48-63, 1969
40. Haskett RF, Rose RM: Neuroendocrine disorders and psychopathology. Psychiatr Clin North Am 4:239–252, 1981
41. Gold MS, Pottash ALC, Extein I, et al: Diagnosis of depression in the 1980's. JAMA 245:1562–1564, 1981
42. Diagnostic and Statistical Manual of Mental Disorders (3rd edition). Washington, DC, American Psychiatric Association, 1980
43. Spitzer RL, Endicott J, Robins E: Research Diagnostic Criteria (RDC) for a Selected Group of Functional Disorders. New York, New York State Psychiatric Institute, 1980
44. Skodol AE, Spitzer RL: The development of reliable diagnostic criteria in psychiatry. Ann Rev Med 33:317–326, 1982
45. Billewicz WZ, Chapman RS, Crooks J, et al: Statistical methods applied to the diagnosis of hypothyroidism. Q J Med 150:255–266, 1969
46. Evered DC, Ormston BJ, Smith PA, et al: Grades of hypothyroidism. Br Med J 1:657–662, 1973
47. Harvey RF: Grades of hypothyroidism (let). Br Med J 2:488–489, 1973
48. Bastenie PA, Bonnyns M, Vanhaelst L: Grades of subclinical hypothyroidism in asymptomatic autoimmune thyroiditis revealed by the thyrotropin-releasing hormone test. J Clin Endocrinol Metab 51:163–166, 1980
49. Wenzel KW, Meinhold H, Raffenberg M, et al: Classification of hypothyroidism in evaluating patients after radioiodine therapy by serum cholesterol, $T_3$-uptake, total $T_4$, $FT_4$-index, total $T_3$, basal TSH and TRH-test. Eur J Clin Invest 4:141–148, 1974
50. Prange AJ, Lara PP, Wilson IC: Effects of thyrotropin-releasing hormone in depression. Lancet 2:999–1002, 1972
51. Targum SD, Sullivan AC, Byrnes SM: Compensatory pituitary-thyroid mechanisms in major depressive disorder. Psychiatry Res 6:85–96, 1982
52. Kirkegaard C, Bjorum N: TSH responses to TRH in endogenous depression (let). Lancet 1:152, 1980
53. Prange AJ, Loosen PT: Some endocrine aspects of affective disorders. J Clin Psychiatry 41:29–34, 1980
54. Gold MS, Pottash ALC, Extein I, et al: The TRH test in the diagnosis of major and minor depression. Psychoneuroendocrinology 6:159–169, 1981

55. Ettigi PG, Brown GM: Psychoneuroendocrinology of affective disorder: An overview. Am J Psychiatry 134:493–501, 1977
56. Sternbach H, Gerner RD, Gwirtsman HE: The thyrotropin-releasing hormone stimulation test: A review. J Clin Psychiatry 43:4–6, 1982
57. Gold MS, Pottash ALC, Ryan N, et al: TRH-induced TSH response in unipolar, bipolar and secondary depressions: Possible utility in clinical assessment and differential diagnosis. Psychoneuroendocrinology 5:147–155, 1980
58. Extein I, Pottash ALC, Gold MS et al: The thyroid-stimulating hormone response to thyrotropin-releasing hormone in mania and bipolar depression. Psychiatry Res 2:199–204, 1980
59. Linkowski P, Brauman H, Mendlewicz J: Thyrotropin response to thyrotropin-releasing hormone in unipolar and bipolar affective illness. J Affective Disord 3:9–16, 1981
60. Kirkegaard C, Bjorum N, Cohn D, et al: Studies on the influence of biogenic amines and psychoactive drugs on the prognostic value of theTRH stimulation test in endogenous depression. Psychoneuroendocrinology 2:131–136, 1977
61. Gold MS, Pottash ALC, Extein I: Hypothyroidism and depression: evidence from complete thyroid function evaluation. JAMA 245:1919–1922, 1981
62. Sternbach HA, Gold MS, Pottash ALC, et al: Thyroid failure and protirelin (thyrotropin-releasing hormone) test abnormalities in depressed outpatients. JAMA 245:1618–1620, 1983
63. Bonnyns M, Vanhaelst L, Bastenie PA: Asymptomatic atrophic thyroiditis. Horm Res 16:338–344, 1982
64. Gold MS, Pottash ALC, Extein I: "Symptomless" autoimmune thyroiditis in depression. Psychiatry Res 6:261–269, 1982
65. Bastenie PA, Vanhaelst L, Bonnyns M, et al: Preclinical hypothyroidism: A risk factor for coronary-heart disease. Lancet 1:203–204, 1971
66. Ridgway EC, Cooper DS, Walker H, et al: Peripheral responses to thyroid hormone before and after L-thyroxine therapy in patients with subclinical hypothyroidism. J Clin Endocrinol Metab 53:1238–1242, 1981
67. Prange AJ, Wilson IC, Rabon AM, et al: Enhancement of imipramine antidepressant activity by thyroid hormone. Am J Psychiatry 126:457–469, 1969
68. Wilson IC, Prange AJ, McClane TK, et al: Thyroid-hormone enhancement of imipramine in nonretarded depressions. N Eng J Med 282:1063–1067, 1970
69. Wheatley D: Potentiation of amitriptyline by thyroid hormone. Arch Gen Psychiatry 26:229–233, 1972
70. Earle BV: Thyroid hormone and tricyclic antidepressants in resistant depressions. Am J Psychiatry 126:143–145, 1970
71. Whybrow PC, Coppen A, Prange AJ, et al: Thyroid function and the response to liothyronine in depression. Arch Gen Psychiatry 26:242–245, 1972
72. Hall RCW, Gardner ER, Stickney SK, et al: Physical illness manifesting as psychiatric disease. II. Analysis of a state hospital inpatient population. Arch Gen Psychiatry 37:989–995, 1980
73. Carney MWP, Macleod S, Sheffield BF: Thyroid function screening in psychiatric inpatients. Br J Psychiatry 138:154–156, 1981
74. Josephson AM, MacKenzie TB: Appearance of manic psychosis following rapid normalization of thyroid status. Am J Psychiatry 136:846–847, 1979
75. Josephson AM, MacKenzie TB: Thyroid-induced mania in hypothyroid patients. Br J Psychiatry 137:222–228, 1980

76. Kronfol Z, Grenen JF, Condon M, et al: Application of biological markers in depression secondary to thyrotoxicosis. Am J Psychiatry 139:1319–1322, 1982
77. Extein I, Pottash ALC, Gold MS, et al: Differentiating mania from schizophrenia by the TRH test. Am J Psychiatry 137:981–982, 1980
78. Extein I, Pottash ALC, Gold MS, et al: Using the protirelin test to distinguish mania from schizophrenia. Arch Gen Psychiatry 39:77–81, 1982
79. Gold MS, Byck R: Endoprhins, lithium and naloxone: Their relationship to pathological and drug-induced manic-euphoric states. In Peterson RC (ed): The International Challenge of Drug Abuse, Monograph 19. Rockville, MD, National Institute on Drug Abuse, 1978
80. Temple R, Berman M, Robbins J, et al: The use of lithium in the treatment o of thyrotoxicosis. J Clin Invest 51:2746–2756, 1972
81. Schildkraut JJ: The catecholamine hypothesis of affective disorders: A review of supporting evidence. Am J Psychiatry 122:509–522, 1965
82. Davis JM: Overview: maintenance therapy in psychiatry: II. Affective disorders. Am J Psychiatry 133:1–13, 1976
83. Reisberg B, Gershon S: Side effects associated with lithium therapy. Arch Gen Psychiatry 36:879–887, 1979
84. Peselow E, Lautin A, Gershon S: Prophylactic and therapeutic profile of lithium. Bibl Psychiatr 161:1–31, 1981

# Tests Involving CNS Amine Metabolites

CHAPTER 3

# CNS Amine Metabolites


## JAN FAWCETT, HOWARD M. KRAVITZ, and HECTOR C. SABELLI


> Things are either what they appear to be; or they are not, nor do they appear to be; or they are, yet do not appear to be; or they are not, and yet appear to be
>
> . . . Epiticus c. 50–150

There is an extensive body of indirect evidence from animal studies which indicates that the "biogenic amines" act as central nervous system (CNS) neurotransmitters, particularly in critical integrative brain pathways. The catecholamines (CA) norepinephrine (NE) and dopamine (DA), the indoleamine (IA) serotonin (5-HT), and the quaternary alkyl-amine acetylcholine (ACh) are the brain amines on which most interest has been focused. In addition, the brain has also been found to contain and form other adrenergic amines, such as phenylethylamine (PEA) and octopamine, and indoleamines such as tryptamine, etc. One or more of these amines may act as co-transmitters, modulators, or regulators of synaptic transmission mediated by chemically related transmitters. Thus, tryptamine may be a modulator of serotonergic synapses [1] and PEA may be a modulator of CA synapses [1,2], as evidenced by studies on the ocular sympathetic system [3]. Octopamine appears to be co-transmitter in sympathetic nerves [4]. Based on the metabolic and functional unity of the neuron [5], Dale [6] proposed that a neuron releases the same trans-


*Handbook of Psychiatric Diagnostic Procedures*, vol. 1, edited by R. C. W. Hall and T. P. Beresford.

**Table 1. CNS Metabolite Studies. Sources of Variance Which Affect Specificity**

- Patient Variables
  - Naturalistic versus controlled studies
  - Heterogeneous patient groups (diagnostic classification) and "normal" controls
    - Age differences
    - Sex differences
    - Genetic differences
  - Clinical state variables versus state-independent clinical differences (traits)
    - Depression
    - Psychosis
    - Anxiety and/or stress, including subjective distress
    - Phase of illness
    - Biological rhythms and circadian periodicity/diurnal variation (especially with respect to sampling time of specimen obtained and amine measured)
    - Homeostatic balance (dynamic state versus regulatory and adaptive processes)
    - Compensatory changes (tonic and phasic changes)
  - Pathophysiology of illness
    - Correlation of physiological measures with measures of amine metabolism and turnover
      - Physical activity and psychomotor activity (agitation, retardation)
      - Anorexia (results in an indoleamine-deficit state)
  - Specimen related variables
  - Dietary alterations (low monoamine diet versus uncontrolled or precursor supplement
  - Source of specimen (blood, urine, CSF, brain tissue)
  - Sampling technique (including preservative used)
  - Assay differences
  - Probenecid dose
  - Probenecid CSF levels achieved
  - Extraneous drug effects, including steroid interactions and specific psychoactive drugs
- Amine-specific Variables
  - Affect of changes in one monoamine system on another (including neurotransmitter, co-transmitter, and neuromodulator/neuroregulator changes)
  - Nonselective effects of pharmacologic changes
  - Receptor changes

mitter at all its endings. Although Dale's law has been interpreted to mean that there is only one transmitter, this latter assumption does not appear to hold true. Sabelli and associates [7] have thus proposed to extend Dale's principle as follows: Each neuron releases at all its endings the same transmitter and metabolically related co-transmitters, and contains the same receptors throughout its surface membrane. In addition, there may be cells which contain the metabolic machinery for producing more than one family of transmitters; for instance, sympathetic neurons contain not only CA and metabolically related amines (octopamine, PEA) but also

ACh [7-12] and possibly histamine [7,12,13]. Thus, we may have to allow for complex interactions at the synapse. One biogenic amine may affect the metabolism or levels of another, and there may be complex interactions between monoaminergic systems and other neurotransmitters or neuromodulator systems.

Data from pharmacological studies have been extrapolated to form hypotheses that functional abnormalities in one or more of these amines may be involved in human psychiatric disorders. Further, the assumption has been made that the concentration of amine metabolites in body fluids and tissue reflects the functional status of central monoaminergic systems. There are also questions of specificity: Does a specific abnormality characterize or distinguish an illness? Many of the potential sources of variance in these studies are outlined in Table 1.

However, it would be misleading to reject a role for the biogenic amines in the pathogenesis of these disorders, despite the discrepancies, without taking into consideration the complexities of the tasks involved in generating preclinical-clinical correlations. (A thorough review of preclinical issues is beyond the scope of this chapter.) Problems arising from the interpretation of these indirect findings have led to techniques which may allow more direct investigation of central amine function by measuring levels of amine metabolites in various readily available tissues and body fluids. The most direct way to investigate these amines, and hypotheses generated by their presence, has been to study amine metabolites in cerebrospinal fluid (CSF), blood and urine, and in postmortem brain tissue.

We will present the current state of the art in the clinical use of CNS amine metabolites, as measured by ourselves and others, including their diagnostic and treatment relevance.

## AFFECTIVE DISORDERS

### Introduction

Theories suggesting that the pathophysiology of affective disorders involves alterations in central amines arose from observations that antidepressants [tricyclics (TCA) and monoamine oxidase inhibitors (MAOI)] and stimulates activate brain monoamine synapses while drugs that induce depression (e.g., reserpine) reduce monoamine transmission [14,15] (see Tables 2a–c). In its simplest form, the amine hypotheses of affective illness postulate that clinical depression is associated with a functional deficit of one or more CNS monoamines at receptor sites, while mania is related to a functional excess of amine transmission.

A specific biochemical basis for affective disorders has not been established, nor has the exact mechanism by which efficacious medications alleviate symptoms been fully elucidated. Most of these hypotheses focus on a single amine, such as

**Table 2a. Biochemical Studies**

| | Depression | Mania | Anxiety |
|---|---|---|---|
| *Catecholamines* (NE, DA) | MHPG urinary excretion low, normal or high. Either 2 types of depression (A and B) or changes are random. CSF HVA studies inconclusive. | Increased or normal MHPG | All NE metabolites increased in urine. MHPG levels may correlate with anxiety. |
| *Indoleamines* (5-HT) | CSF-5 HIAA reduced | CSF5-HIAA reduced | – |
| *Phenylethylamine* (PEA) | Urinary PAA reduced in many unipolars and bipolars | Urinary PAA increased in most manics but reduced in a subgroup of manics | – |
| *Acetylcholine* (ACh) | – | – | – |

NE, 5-HT or PEA (Table 3), and assume that the clinical problem is due to some abnormality in this amine. Single-disease and two-disease models have been described. The two-disease theories of depression include Maas' Type A (NE type) [16] and Type B (5-HT type) and Sabelli and associates Type I (imipramine responsive) [17] verses Type II (amitriptyline responsive) depression. A "permissive theory" and interactive models have also been proposed. The findings suggest that depression is heterogeneous, but some persons reveal a biochemical vulnerability or susceptibility regarding one amine, while others reveal a similar response to alteration in another amine system.

Changes in amine metabolism in the brain are thought to be reliably reflected in parallel changes in CSF metabolites, as previously reviewed elsewhere [18,19]. Various studies suggest the conclusion that a substantial portion of lumbar 5-hydroxyindoleacetic acid (5-HIAA) and 3-methoxy-4-hydroxyphenylglycol (MHPG) originate in the spinal cord while lumbar homovanillic acid (HVA) comes from the brain [20-22]. Further, while there is an ascending gradient for 5-HIAA, lumbar CSF may reflect the mean metabolite concentrations of more central fluid [23]. CSF 5-HIAA and MHPG may still be clinically and biologically important since many of 5-HT and NE terminals in the spinal cord originate in cell bodies in the brainstem nuclei [19]. Probenecid, a competitive inhibitor of the transport of acid amine metabolites of the neuroamines out of the CSF [24,25], has been used

Table 2b. Effects of Precursors

| | |
|---|---|
| *Catecholamines* (NE, DA) | Dopa fails to ameliorate depression but causes hyperactivity and manic-like symptoms.<br>Dopa may relieve or induce/exacerbate depression (with or without suicidal ideation) in Parkinsonians.<br>Dopa reduces exploration in animals but antagonizes reserpine.<br>Dihydroxyphenylserine (DOPS) induces sedation.<br>Tyrosine ameliorates depression in a small group of patients. |
| *Indoleamines* (5-HT) | L-Tryptophan and 5-HTP exert antidepressant effects in a limited group of patients. |
| *Phenylethylamine* (PEA) | L-Phenylalanine increases exploration, induces amphetamine-like effects and antagonizes reserpine in MAOI-treated animals and exerts stimulant effects in some depressed patients.<br>D-Phenylalanine has similar and stronger effects in animals; antidepressant effects are controversial. |
| *Acetycholine* (ACh) | |

to reduce the potential source of variance arising from CSF outflow of the CNS amine metabolites. These changes cannot be attributed solely to a change in level of probenecid in the CSF between patients and controls [25-28]. This reduction in the transport of acid metabolites of the neuroamines provides a more "dynamic" measure of their turnover. This technique also reduces extraneous variants associated with low lumbar concentrations of metabolites and provides a more integrated measure over time. Probenecid inhibits the system which transports 5-HIAA and HVA out of the CNS [29] but ineffectively blocks MHPG efflux from the CSF [30,31]. Baseline levels of these metabolites are low; probenecid pretreatment allows accumulation of relatively large amounts of 5-HIAA and HVA in CSF and, particularly for 5-HIAA [32], probably makes lumbar CSF more representative of ventricular CSF. However, it has introduced other potential confounding sources of variance, including that associated with progenecid levels themselves.

With the development of an ever-enlarging armamentarium of antidepressants, our task of choice is becoming more complex because of reports of drugs specific for various biochemical subtypes of depression. The purpose of this chapter is to shed some light on further areas of exploration as well as provide a rational basis for pharmacotherapy of the affective disorders. There are a polarity of views. We specifically address the current status of thinking on the biogenic amines and affective disorders.

**Table 2c. Pharmacological Evidence**

| | Amphetamine-like stimulants | Other euphoriants | Antidepressants | | Drugs that may induce depression (reserpine, alphamethyl-dopa, etc.) | Lithium |
|---|---|---|---|---|---|---|
| | | | MAOI | TCA | | |
| *Catecholamines* (NE, DA) | Amphetamines release and mimic NE but methyl-phenidate may not. Amphetamines and methyl-phenidate release and mimic DA. | Marijuana has no significant effects | Increase brain levels | Inhibit NE reuptake but not DA reuptake | Deplete | Increase NE re-uptake |
| *Indolamine* (5-HT) | Amphetamines release 5-HT and stimulate 5-HT and stimulate 5-HT receptors | Marijuana has no significant effects | Increase brain levels | Inhibit 5-HT reup-take in all cases at concentrations greater than those which inhibit NE reuptake | Deplete | Increases 5-HT re-uptake |
| *Phenelethylamine* (PEA) | Amphetamines and methylphenidate release and then enhance levels of PEA | Opioids increase PAA excretion. Marijuana increases PEA levels and decreases PEA disposition | Increase brain levels. Brain MAO (mainly type B) specific for PEA | Increase PEA brain levels and synthesis, and inhibit MAO Type B | Deplete | ? |
| *Acetylcholine* (ACh) | Amphetamines release ACh | Marijuana decreases ACh release (?) | Reduce ACh transmission | Usually block muscarinic re-ceptors and also nicotinic receptors. | Reserpine increases ACh levels | – |

**Table 3. Monoamine Hypotheses of Affective Disorders**

Single-disease hypotheses
- Norepinephrine hypothesis
  - Depression: low norepinephrine
  - Mania: high norepinephrine
- Serotonin hypothesis
  - Depression: low serotonin
  - Mania: high serotonin
- Phenylethylamine hypothesis
  - Depression: low phenylethylamine
  - Mania: high phenylethylamine

Two-disease hypotheses of depression
- Type A versus Type B
  - Type A (norepinephrine type) ·
    - Low norepinephrine
    - Normal serotonin
    - Elevated mood following dextroamphetamine
    - Favorable response to treatment with imipramine or desipramine
    - Failure to respond to amitryptyline
    - Modest increments or no change in norepinephrine (urinary MHPG) following brief trial of dextroamphetamine or following treatment, with imipramine or deispramine
  - Type B (serotonin type)
    - Low serotonin
    - Normal (or high) norepinephrine
    - Lack of mood change during a trial of dextroamphetamine
    - Favorable response to treatment with amitriptyline
    - Failure to respond to imipramine
    - Decrements in norepinephrine (urinary MHPG) following treatment with imipramine, desipramine, or a brief trial of dextroamphetamine
- Type I versus Type II
  - Type I
    - Hypothesized depletion of NE, 5-HT, and/or PEA
    - Responsive to methylphenidate and imipramine-like antidepressants (imipramine, desipramine, chlorimipramine, maprotiline)
  - Type II
    - No evidence for monoamine depletion
    - Nonresponsive to methylphenidate or imipramine-like antidepressants
    - Responsive to amitriptyline and nortriptyline

Permissive hypothesis of bipolar illness
- Depression: low norepinephrine, low serotonin
- Mania: high norepinephrine, low serotonin

## Catecholamine Hypothesis of Affective Disorders

*Norepinephrine and its metabolites.* The CA hypothesis of affective disorders has been developed within a more clinical framework within the past two decades [33-35]. It has been the source of numerous reviews [36-41]. This hypothesis predicts that some if not all depressions are associated with an absolute or relative decrease in CA, particularly the NE available at central adrenergic receptor sites. Certain drugs which alter the affective state in humans also have significant effects on CA disposition and metabolites in the brain. The amount, distribution, or metabolism of NE in the brain may be altered in both depressives and manics. This data has led Schildkraut [33] and Davis and Bunney [34] to propose that some, though probably not all depressive disorders may be associated with an absolute or relative CA deficiency, particularly NE, at functionally important adrenergic receptor sites in brain, while manic disorders may be associated with CA excesses. They further pointed out that this may be a reductionistic over-simplification, and that we need to account for other possible biochemical, physiological, and psychological factors. In fact, the pharmacological studies, which initially gave rise to and suggested this biogenic amine hypothesis [42-48], yielded contradictory reports in further attempts to test the hypothesis, and led to more direct efforts to detect alterations in biogenic amine metabolism in affective disorders.

A direct outgrowth of the CA depletion theory of depression was the measurement of metabolites of NE in depressives in an attempt to demonstrate some disturbance of CA metabolism referable to the CNS [49]. Considerable experimental evidence has accumulated both in support of and at variance with this hypothesis, based primarily on correlations between changes in NE metabolism and affective states. Research has focused on MHPG because a number of these results, particularly thosc of Schildkraut [50-57] and Maas [49,58-62] and their associates, have suggested that MHPG is the major metabolite of brain NE reflecting CNS turnover [49-64], while vanillylmandelic acid (VMA) is the major NE metabolite measured in the urine [65,66]. NE and other metabolites [normetanephrine (NMN), metanephrine (MN)] originate mainly in pools of CA outside the CNS. There are, however, many pitfalls associated with drawing conclusions based on the available data [45]. Research into the proportion of urinary MHPG which represents CNS origin in humans ranges from almost 70% [62] to about 20% [67-69]. The latter investigations have suggested that 40% to 50% of plasma-free MHPG may be converted to VMA [68]. Further, there is a wide range in the content of MHPG reported as normal by different authors, ranging from 900-3500 mcg/24 hours [49, 70-73], indicating that even the chemical methodology may be open to question.

Studies measuring MHPG urinary excretion in depressives have shown abnormally low levels, suggesting decreased turnover rates of NE in the brain and depletion of NE. In an attempt to correct for the fraction of urinary MHPG which derives from the periphery, Schildkraut [74,75] developed a mathematical equation which included the contribution of various urinary CA metabolites of peripheral origin, resulting in a D-type (depression) score:

$$D = C_1\,(MHPG) - C_2\,(VMA) + C_3\,(NE) - C_4\,\frac{(NMN + MN)}{(VMA)} + Co$$

This may provide a further biochemical basis for differentiating the heterogeneous group of depressive disorders. Bipolar depressives, unipolar endogenous depressives, schizophrenia-related depressives and schizoaffective depressives all had D-scores less than 0.5, whereas unipolar depressives of nonendogenous type had D-scores greater than 0.5.

Though it has been demonstrated that MHPG may convert to VMA in the periphery [68], it is not known whether this is stable intra-individually and/or inter-individually, or if it varies over time or among different diagnostic subgroups. There may also be reciprocal influences in noradrenergic systems; stimulation of peripheral nerves can activate central noradrenergic neurons [76,77] and central noradrenergic stimulation can produce a marked increase in plasma MHPG, probably via an alteration of impulse flow in the sympathetic nervous system [78]. Thus, the value of MHPG may lie in aiding our understanding of interactions between central and peripheral events. In any event, MHPG is the only NE metabolite which seems to demonstrate differential change within depressed populations, and pre- and post-treatment [79,80]. However, there is no general consensus as to the exact amount of urinary MHPG that is derived from the brain, nor about its absolute content in urine.

There are some studies showing reduced CSF MHPG in depressives as compared with controls, but other studies have failed to confirm these observations [81-85]. Agren and associates [86] found no differences in CSF MHPG between depressive subgroups, but did not obtain CSF from controls. In a therapeutic trial, Roccatagliata and associates [87] determined CSF MHPG levels pre- and post-imipramine (IMI) in twelve endogenous depressives. The subgroup with higher baseline values had better therapeutic results and a significant decrement in CSF MHPG levels after treatment. These two observatins are exactly opposite to what would be predicted by the CA theory of depression.

While Maas and associates [88] and Agren [86] have found a correlation between urinary and CSF MHPG, other investigators have found a poor correlation. While 24-hour urine collections represent an integrated measure, the physiological significance of data on CSF MHPG remains problematic. CSF MHPG reflects only a single point in time, and thus is more susceptible to variance introduced by alterations in diurnal rhythm. Because MHPG is continuously eliminated through the capillaries within the brain, only a portion of the total MHPG produced ever reaches the CSF.

The usefulness of plasma MHPG is still being determined [89-94]. At present there is no evidence that depressives have lower plasma levels of MHPG, as predicted by the CA theory of depression. Halaris [90] and Halaris and DeMet [91] used this technique serially to follow the effect of lithium and IMI in the treatment of manic and depressed patients, and noted sequential changes in the first four weeks of treatment. Responders eventually returned to baseline values. They also reported that clinical improvement may *precede* normalization of NE metabolism by at least one or two weeks, especially in lithium-treated manics. Jimerson and associates [93] found plasma-free MHPG and total CSF MHPG are significantly correlated in normal humans, and drugs which affect brain MHPG production had produced parallel changes in plasme-free MHPG concentrations [95]. Charney and associates [96,97] studied the effects of acute and chronic desipramine (DMI) on MHPG in plasma and urine in eight endogenous depressives, and found that DMI induced an immediate, continuous, and highly significant reduction in plasma MHPG, which persisted throughout the 30-day active treatment period and was not related to treatment response. This is contradictory to the CA hypothesis of depression. Further, they found that pretreatment levels of urinary MHPG did not relate to treatment response, while the CA theory would have predicted that MHPG should have been lower in responders. Changes in urinary MHPG with treatment related to response. By days 26 to 30 (chronic effects), the responders demonstrated an increase (or no change), while the nonresponders showed a clear decrease. (This effect will be discussed more thoroughly later.)

The relationship between total urinary MHPG and plasma-free MHPG is difficult to interpret in view of questions about the metabolism of free MHPG and the proportion of total urinary MHPG originating in the brain. No relationship was found between plasma and urinary MHPG before or during the DMI treatment, and the effect of DMI on the two measures differed markedly. Further, diurnal variation needs to be accounted for, and Sweeney [92] found the use of plasma MHPG levels presently premature.

The studies of urinary MHPG support the view that a CA deficit plays a role in some but not all forms of depressive illness. In support of this CA hypothesis, a pilot study by Maas and associates [49] demonstrated that urinary MHPG was significantly reduced in a heterogeneous group of depressives, as compared to healthy controls, regardless of sex. A previous review of the literature [72] revealed that depressed individuals as a group tend to excrete 25% less MHPG than healthy controls, but overall, many depressives excrete either normal or greater than normal MHPG. Further, bipolar depressives have consistently been reported to excrete less than normals or unipolar depressives [55,56,80]. There is no difference between endogenous and nonendogenous unipolar depressives, although relatively more of the endogenous subgroup had low MHPG values, i.e., in the range of the bipolars [57,74]. There are contradictory observations regarding the effect of antidepressants upon MHPG excretion. Some investigators have observed increases [70,79], while others, to the contrary, have observed that MHPG levels are reduced by treatment [98] (see later). These contradictory data serve as a warning regarding the interpretation of pretreatment data.

According to the CA hypothesis, an excess in brain NE accounts for mania. There are no data to indicate that, as a group, manic patients excrete more MHPG than normals. Notwithstanding, the data indicate that bipolars excrete significantly more MHPG during euthymia or mania than during depressive episodes [99]. A "switch process," in which change in MHPG excretion precedes affective and behavioral shifts (increase prior to mania and decrease prior to depression) has been described in patients with repeated cycling [99–103]. Further, intermediate levels were reported during euthymic phases [100]. A significant amount of evidence has accumulated suggesting that pharmacological agents may precipitate manic episodes, especially in those with affective disorders [104–106], but also in those with other medical problems [107]. The mode of action of TCA and MAOI is consistent with the hypothesis that high levels of functional monoamine neurotransmitters in the brain are associated with manic symptoms. Brodie and associates [108] gave alpha-methyl-para-tyrosine (AMPT), an inhibitor of tyrosine hydroxylase, the enzyme catalyzing the rate-limiting step in the synthesis of DA and NE, to ten patients (seven manics and three depressed) and noted that five manics became less so, while all the depressives worsened. Further, urinary CA metabolites (MHPG, VMA, DA) were significantly decreased in all patients.

*Dopamine and its metabolites.* Amid controversies involving hypotheses concerning the relevance of NE and 5-HT in the pathogenesis of affective disorders, the catecholamine DA has, by comparison, been neglected. The major metabolites of DA are HVA and dihydroxyphenylacetic acid (DOPAC). HVA, the deaminated o-methylated metabolite of DA, is found in much greater quantity [109]. The percentage of urinary DA metabolite originating centrally is unknwon, and this measurement appears to be of no present practical value. Previous reviews [18,19,110, 111] revealed that baseline CSF HVA has been lower in depressives in some but not all studies. Once again, these studies must be regarded with caution, as the rate of efflux varies in the CSF, and single measures do not reflect rates of production at any given time interval. Probenecid-induced accumulations may be lower in at least some subgroups of depressives, as compared with nonaffectively ill control groups [32,112-117], except in one study [118] involving a diagnostically heterogeneous group of depressives in which the levels were high. In mania, most groups report low or normal baseline and probenecid-induced CSF HVA levels [32,114,115,119-124] except in one study [125]. A concern with these measurements is the potential for activity artifact, especially in manics [126]. The possibility that measurements of CSF HVA may be of value in differentiating various subgroups of depressive disorder (i.e., bipolar depressives versus unipolar depressives) needs further investigation.

Increased rates of DA excretion have been observed during spontaneously developing mania [127–129]. These results suggest that changes in DA metabolism may be implicated in the development of mania and hypomania. The first double-blind study of DL-dopa in depressives was reported by Klerman and associates [130]. In an indirect test of the CA depletion theory of depression, they gave DL-dopa alone and in combination with MAOI (phenelzine). Dopa, a precursor of DA and NE, crosses the blood–brain barrier in animals, and reverses the behavioral and biochemical effects of reserpine-induced depression. These dopa effects are attributed to the synthesis of CA because they are enhanced by MAOI pretreatment. However, they may be direct effects of dopa, because they are enhanced rather than blocked by drugs which inhibit dopa decarboxylation [131]. In this study, neither chronic dopa alone nor in combination led to clinical improvement, but the doses used may have been too low. Goodwin and associates [132] used sustained high doses of L-dopa in 16 patients (bipolar and unipolar depressives, and one schizoaffective). Only 25% of the patients had a consistent improvement in depression. Responders were distinguished by the presence of psychomotor retardation, though some of the nonresponders also had this clinical finding. Further, anger was produced in nonresponders, which may reflect activation of central dopaminergic or noradrenergic pathways. CSF HVA increased significantly in L-dopa-treated patients; 5-HIAA did not. Very large increases in 24-hour urinary excretion of dopa, DA and HVA were noted. MHPG and VMA were measured in two patients. Both levels doubled at doses of 4 to 8 g/day. More interestingly, one had a differential increase in MHPG alone, observed during a brief period of hypomania. These changes provided suggestive evidence that L-dopa altered CA both in brain and in the periphery. Murphy and associates [133] induced a behavioral hypomanic response in seven of eighteen patients (six of seven "bipolars" and one of eleven "unipolars") using doses similar to Goodwin and associates [132]. Similarly, significantly greater amounts of DA and L-dopa were excreted by bipolar depressives who developed hypomania than by unipolar depressives, who did not, during chronic treatment with L-dopa, while HVA urinary levels were much less dissimilar [134]. Further, the differences increased with increasing L-dopa dose. These results were replicated following an acute L-dopa load of 2 g per day in bipolar and unipolar depressives; once again DA excretion was significantly greater in the bipolar depressives, although L-dopa and HVA levels were not.

Randrup and associates [110] have presented, in a detailed review of the literature, evidence for a relationship between brain DA, and mania and depression, based on the antimanic and depressogenic effects of neuroleptics, which are DA receptor blockers. Further, associated with dopaminergic supersensitivity and subsequent acute withdrawal of these drugs, antidepressant response have been noted. This may also be a dose–response relationship, responsible for a direct therapeutic antidepressant effect at low doses, while antimanic or depressogenic at usual antipsychotic doses. These antidepressive effects may also depend upon the particular depressive subtype involved. Van Praag [135] reported a double-blind comparison of chlorimipramine (CMI) and nomifensine in "vital depression" (endogenous depression). The latter drug has a relatve stimulant effect on postsynaptic DA receptors. A reduced predrug post probenecid CSF HVA level was predictive of a significantly better effect in the nomifensine group, but not in the CMI group. Two other studies [136,137] present evidence for a dopaminergic mechanism in mania based on pimozide's efficacy in mania via its relatively specific DA receptor blocking activity. Other pharmacological studies, involving antidepressants and lithium, suggest that a DA deficiency may be associated with depression, while an excess may be associated with mania [138-140].

The induction of hypomania by L-dopa is of special interest in view of the hypothesis of mania representing an excess of brain CA. That L-dopa, in doses large enough to produce hypomania, does not produce a consistent change in or reversal of depressed mood in the majority of patients suggests that the CA deficit hypothesis for depression is an oversimplification and is evidence against the importance of a hypothesized deficit in brain CA, particularly DA, in the majority of depressives. Since brain NE may not be increased by L-dopa, this evidence remains inconclusive. Further, the CA hypothesis for mania as originally stated may only apply strictly to those with a pre-existing abnormally labile affective state. Mania/hypomania was consistently induced in most of the bipolar depressives, suggesting that CA, especially DA, may be directly involved in the genesis or triggering of the behavior in these susceptible individuals. This combination of an activation of hypomania in the absence of a reversal of depression suggests that depression and mania may be separable processes rather than simply the clinical reflections of opposite poles of a single biochemical continuum. Biobehavioral results from the administration of the CA precursor L-dopa may, however, further suggest the presence of distinct subgroups of depression separable on the basis of clinical response to precursors and antidepressants, and subsequent biogenic amine excretion [141].

### Indoleamine Theory of Affective Disorders

The indoleamine hypothesis of affective disorders [142-147] states that functional levels of brain 5-HT are reduced and may directly contribute to or predispose to symptoms of depression, and possibly mania. There have been claims that the neurotransmitter 5-HT rather than NE may better fit the hypothesis of amine depletion based on clinical pharmacological studies and 5-HT precursor and metabolite studies in depressives. For the most part, reserpine and antidepressants affect 5-HT as well as NE in the brain. The IA hypothesis stems from three lines of research [148]: (1) tryptophan metabolism (not be reviewed here; see other reviews for references) [148,149], (2) CSF studies (baseline and post-probenecid-induced accumulations), and (3) postmortem brain studies (see later). Interrelations between 5-HT and hypothalamo-pituitary-adrenal function have also been described [150,151].

In addition to findings of abnormally low blood tryptophan levels, early studies

[145,152–154] demonstrated a decreased urinary excretion of tryptamine in depressives. Tryptamine is possibly a co-transmitter in 5-HT synapses [7]. MAOI increases the brain and urinary levels of tryptamine more than that of 5-HT [155]. We generalize the IA theory of affective disorders to include tryptamine. Consistent with an IA deficit are reviews of the results of 5-HT precursors [tryptophan or 5-hydroxytryptophan (5-HTP)] used in the treatment of depressives, with or without antidepressants [45,142,148,156,157]. These studies demonstrate good precursor therapy response in at least some depressives, especially those with low CSF 5-HIAA, as well as potentiation of the effects of TCA and MAOI. There is some evidence that bipolar depressives are more responsive to L-tryptophan than unipolars, and that some features of the manic behavior may be alleviated by this precursor [158–160]. Brain IA levels are dependent upon tryptophan availability. A significant problem is that the functional state of the brain serotonergic system is not readily assessed in humans. 5-HIAA is the major 5-HT metabolite centrally and peripherally [161]. Measurement of urinary 5-HT, tryptamine, and their metabolites (5-HIAA, indole-3-acetic acid) are not helpful because of the large peripheral contribution. These studies have been reviewed elsewhere [145,161,162]. Further, tryptophan (plasma and CSF) and blood 5-HT levels, as well as 5-HT uptake measurements, are equivocal at best for an IA hypothesis of affective disorders. (Reviews of these studies are available elsewhere [149] and will not be undertaken in this chapter.) CSF 5-HIAA studies, including both baseline levels and probenecid-induced accumulations in depressives, compared with controls, have been reviewed elsewhere [18,19,111,149]. These studies have yielded mixed results. Overall, CSF 5-HIAA has been reported to be reduced in most studies, averaging about 30% less, in at least a subgroup of depressives, compared with controls. No studies have found significantly higher 5-HIAA levels in the patient groups [149]. In a similar review of manics, most groups have reported low or normal baseline and probenecid-induced 5-HIAA accumulations [18,19,149], although, probenecid-induced elevations were less in manics compared with controls or unipolar depressives. A bimodal or bimodal-like distribution, suggesting the existence of a low 5-HIAA subgroup, has been reported [163,164]. However, this may be due to unequal sex distribution; CSF 5-HIAA is reportedly lower in males than in females and there was an over-representation of males in the low 5-HIAA group [149,165]. Kripke [166] suggested the bimodal distribution may be caused by a bimodal distribution in the phases of 24-hour 5-HT rhythms without any alteration in total 24-hour 5-HT turnover. Maas and associates [88] could not find a bimodal distribution. Additional support for the 5-HT theory comes from studies showing patients who received IMI or tranylcypromine may have had their recovery reversed by parachlorophenylalanine (PCPA), a tryptophan hydroxylase inhibitor which decreases 5-HT levels, but not by AMPT, which inhibits NE synthesis [167–169]. PCPA has been administered to several manics without evidence of therapeutic efficacy [149], while mania occurring during tranylcypromine treatment was effectively treated with PCPA [168]. Further, Murphy and associates [149] questioned that the effect may be due to effects of PCPA not mediated by 5-HT origin; PCPA, of course, is metabolized to the parachloro derivative of PEA, an amphetamine-like drug.

Treatment studies provide some data to suggest the possibility of biochemical heterogeneity in depression and support of a 5-HT deficit model. Asberg and associates [163] found, in twenty endogenous depressives treated with nortriptyline (NT), that those with low baseline CSF 5-HIAA did not respond to NT, whereas those with high levels did; yet the 5-HIAA (and indole-3-acetic acid) levels decreased significantly in both groups, indicating the ability of NT to inhibit 5-HT reuptake [170,171] although it has been claimed that NT is a selective NE uptake inhibitor. Van Praag [172] found that depressives responding to NT had higher postprobenecid CSF 5-HIAA levels. Goodwin [165] noted the same with IMI; with amitriptyline (AMI), predrug 5-HIAA demonstrated only a trend toward lower levels in responders. Post and Goodwin [173] found postprobenecid CSF 5-HIAA was reduced during treatment with both AMI and IMI, but the degree of clinical improvement was unrelated to the degree of reduction; HVA was not affected. Bowers [174] found CSF 5-HIAA levels following a probenecid–tryptophan tolerance test in six unipolars before and after successful AMI treatment had decreased despite high CSF L-tryptophan levels, indicating that AMI may decrease central 5-HT turnover by mechanisms not involving central L-tryptophan availability, or that AMI alters tryptophan hydroxylase activity in subsequent 5-HT synthesis. Bertilsson and associates [175] found that in depressives treated with CMI there was a more pronounced affect on 5-HIAA than MHPG, while the latter was evident in those treated with NT; however, MHPG was significantly decreased with both treatments. Thus, pretreatment and treatment levels of these metabolites significantly correlated in both groups. Further, the 5-HIAA reduction with NT treatment was consistent with Asberg's finding [163]. Traskman and associates [176] amplified these findings with the observation that CSF MHPG decrease correlated with plasma desmethyl–CMI concentration. Those depressives with high pretreatment CSF 5-HIAA had a positive correlation between relief from depression and plasma desmethyl-CMI level, as well as between the change in MHPG and decreased depression; thus they benefited from NE uptake blockers. In the low CSF 5-HIAA group, correlation between plasma levels of CMI and its metabolite and improvement were negative, supporting the idea of biochemical heterogeneity of depressives and antidepressant response. Van Praag [135] reported that in thirty endogenous depressives, those with low central 5-HT turnover (decreased CSF 5-HIAA postprobenecid) had better therapeutic response to CMI, and the lower the predrug turnover, the better the response. Eight nonresponders were switched to NT, and five responded. However, there is no demonstrable relationship between predrug CSF MHPG and response to NT (no urinary MHPG was measured, however).

Although it has been accepted that a reduction in CSF 5-HIAA may reflect the hypothesized brain 5-HT reduction, we still do not have a good understanding of the mechanism for this in depressives, i.e., whether the 5-HT deficit is related to a synthesis and/or metabolism dysfunction. The matter is even more confusing in bipolar depressives and manics, who may be representative of a subgroup without a 5-HT deficit state; yet other data support a 5-HT deficiency underlying both mania and depression [159,177]. More information is necessary in order to interpret the data as well as to validate the IA hypothesis. Thus, the data for a single disease theory is mixed and generally unsupportive of the hypothesis, and the data is more suggestive of a two-disease theory.

#### Postmortem Brain Tissue

The findings of various levels of amine metabolites in body fluids described heretofore have been from studies in living humans, truly difficult beings to study because of practical as well as ethical considerations. Here we will provide a brief overview of studies in human brain tissue, which are, of necessity, postmortem studies. Immediate postmortem changes as well as changes associated with preservation of brain tissue and other methodological problems account for a significant amount of artifact and limit the usefulness of this data. This literature has been reviewed elsewhere [18,74,149]. The subjects were suicide victims ("depressed" and "nondepressed"), depressives who died of causes other than suicide, and "controls." In the depressives, antemortem antidepressant use may have also affected the results. Nine studies were reported [178–186]. No abnormalities in NE were reported, and DA was higher in one study [184] and lower in another [185]; however, interpretation of these findings is limited by the lack of control of potential variables. Although some investigators reported reduced IA levels, as reflected in brain 5-HT and 5-HIAA, in general it is not certain whether these reductions are indicative of a subgroup of patients at risk for suicide or of an epiphenomena. Apparently this relationship has not yet been proven. However, support for the relationship is provided by Asberg and associate's report [187] on a subgroup of depressives with disturbed 5-HT turnovers, as determined by low CSF 5-HIAA, in which suicide attempts were significantly more common and of a "more active, determined type," compared with other depressives. Further, in some of these patients, CSF levels had been determined prior to the attempt. With an expanded patient group, Traskman and associates [188] re-examined CSF monoamines in suicide attempters in a follow-up study designed to determine the predictive value of a low CSF 5-HIAA level for future suicide. The attempters had a significantly lower CSF 5-HIAA level than controls, especially those who made more violent attempts, and these differences were even more marked following adjustment for differences in body height and age between the depressives and controls. Further, 5-HIAA was also less than normal in nondepressed suicide attempters, though not significantly so, while HVA was also lower in depressed attempters. Most important was the follow-up result: a 20% mortality by suicide within one year postlumbar puncture in those patients with CSF 5-HIAA levels below the median.

Overall, though it is tempting to draw a conclusion in favor of the IA hypothesis, this conclusion is probably still premature.

### The Phenylethylamine Hypothesis of Affective Behavior: Phenylethylamine and Phenylacetic Acid

2-Phenylethylamine (PEA) is unique among endogenous neuroamines in producing amphetamine-like behavioral and electrophysiological effects [189]. These effects are observed when PEA is administered systemically, because it crosses the blood–brain barrier [190] and, in fact, brain accumulates blood-borne PEA by an active uptake mechanism [191]. Brain PEA levels are highly increased by MAOI because PEA is rapidly metabolized by monoamine oxidase (MAO) type B [192], an enzyme for which PEA is the specific endogenous substrate [193]. The biological actions of PEA are partly mediated by CA release [194] and partly due to other mechanisms [195]. PEA is pharmacologically, structurally, and metabolically related to CA and to amphetamine. Various behavioral studies indicate that amphetamine imitates [189,196] and haloperidol blocks [197] the receptors for PEA in neurons in the brain. Amphetamines initially release and later increase brain PEA [190,196]. All types of antidepressants increase PEA levels in the brain, including not only classical MAOI but also TCA of the IMI type and electroshock [198]. This action is remarkably selective in the case of TCA [199] which do not modify the brain levels of CA or 5-HT. Likewise, tetrahydrocannabinol (the active component of marijuana) selectively enhances brain PEA levels [200]. On the other hand, MAOI [199] and electroshock [201] also increase the brain levels of other amines. Among antipsychotic drugs, chlorpromazine does not alter levels of PEA in the brain, whereas reserpine (which can cause depression in humans) reduces the level of PEA in the brain [202]. Alpha-methyldopa, which can also induce depression, likewise reduces the levels of PEA in the brain [190].

The phenylethylamine hypothesis of affective behavior [201] states that PEA is a neuromodulator responsible for sustaining attention and mood. A deficit in the brain content and/or a decrease in the turnover of endogenous PEA may therefore be a causal factor in certain forms of endogenous depression, whereas an increase in the levels of PEA in the brain or the activation of specific PEA receptors in brain neurons may underlie manic episodes and also contribute to antidepressant and stimulant drug actions.

Using nonspecific methods, several investigators, including ourselves, reported that PEA urinary excretion is reduced in a subgroup of depressed patients [203, 204], but such observations are controversial, because the amounts of PEA excreted are very low and highly variable in both control and depressed subjects.

Using the method of Javaid and co-workers [205] sensitive up to 0.2 mcg/24-hour sample, Fawcett and associates [206] have found that PEA excretion is reduced in many depressed patients in comparison to a control group. Average PEA urinary excretion was 3.1 mcg/24-hour (range of undetectable to 9.0) for 19 control subjects, 1.9 mcg/24-hour (undetectable to 6.6) for 29 unipolar depressives, and 3.34 mcg/24-hour (0–10.5) for 9 bipolar depressives. Excretions below 0.2 mcg/24-hour were observed in 5% of controls, 38% of unipolar, and 33% of bipolar depressives; these differences are statistically significant. Further, the MAOI phenelzine (5 patients) and AMI (7 patients) increased PEA urinary excretion (in some cases over 1500 mcg/24-hour) while amoxapine (4 patients) did not, even when improvement occurred. Manic subjects (N = 6) excreted very variable amounts (from undetectable to 70 mcg/24-hour).

Since PEA is mainly metabolized by MAO type B to form phenylacetate (PAA), we have now studied the 24-hour urinary excretion of this acid in 85 control subjects and 113 patients with unipolar and bipolar affective disorders diagnosed according to DSM-III [207].

Adult control subjects excreted $\bar{X} = 141.1 \pm 10.2$ mg of PAA/24-hour, while elderly subjects excreted less, but in both age groups, PAA excretion ranged between 70 and 175 mg/24-hour in 70% of cases. Both inpatients and outpatients with major depressive disorder, unipolar or bipolar, excreted less: 31 unipolar inpatients, 66.9 ± 5.5 mg/24-hour; 42 unipolar outpatients, 92.1 ± 10.8 mg/24-hours; 8 bipolar inpatients, 67.9 ± 15.3 mg/24-hours; 16 bipolar outpatients, 81.8 ± 11.4 mg/24-hours. A large percentage of depressed patients excreted less than 70 mg/24 hour (from 42% of unipolar outpatients to 71% of bipolar patients). No significant differences in PAA excretion were found between untreated depressed patients (N = 59) and those treated with medications that were not effective (N = 37), while in 13 patients studied longitudinally, effective antidepressant treatment increased PAA excretion. Among 16 manic subjects, PAA excretion was highly variable, but 44% excreted more than 175 mg/24 hour (while this is rare in controls). All these differences were statistically significant. Correlating with the severity of the symptomatology, PAA excretion was lower in inpatients than in outpatients for both the unipolar and the bipolar groups. There were no significant differences in PAA excretion between unipolars and bipolars for both inpatient and outpatient groups. For both unipolar and bipolar patients untreated at admission, the average PAA excretion was lower than that of normal subjects ($p < 0.001$, t test). These results suggest that measurement of PAA urinary excretion may be a valuable diagnostic test in affective disorders. Since PAA is the major metabolite of PEA, the observed differences between control and depressed subjects support the PEA theory of affective behavior.

While depressions were associated with a reduction of PAA in excretion, all the antidepressants tested, including tricyclics, maprotiline, MAOI, and alprazolam increased PAA excretion (as predicted by the PEA theory of affective behavior). In a similar manner, treatment of manic subjects with lithium or antipsychotics was observed to reduce PAA excretion.

The present results support the PEA theory of affect insofar as the excretion of its main metabolite PAA was: (i) reduced in all groups of depressed patients in comparison to control subjects, (ii) increased in a significant number of manic subjects, (iii) increased by antidepressant drugs yet still significantly low in many patients treated unsuccessfully with antidepressants, (iv) reduced by antimanic treatment roughly in parallel with clinical recovery.

Since there were no great differences between untreated depressed inpatients and those treated ineffectively, one may hope that the urinary PAA test might serve in the monitoring of depressive illness regardless of treatment, as blood glucose reflects the diabetic state and measures its control by medication.

The authors are fully aware that relating the PAA urinary excretion to PEA metabolism in the brain implies an assumption not supported by empirical studies. There are actually no data regarding the different proportions in which brain and peripheral tissue contribute to urinary PAA. This question, albeit important, is less significant for PEA metabolites than for other neuroamine products because PEA readily crosses the blood-brain barrier, in fact, brain accumulates blood-borne PEA by a factor of up to 20 [190]. Thus, brain and peripheral concentrations of PEA are, by necessity, in dynamic equilibrium [191].

The measurement of urinary PAA excretion is a simple, reliable and rapid test, because this PEA metabolite is excreted in high (mg) amounts, in contrast to other neuroamine products. PAA excretion seems to be a fairly sensitive test for depressive disorders since the differences noted are so marked that they are reflected not only in average values—as in the case of other neuroamine metabolites—but also in individual cases. Thus, using the 70 mg per 24 hour criterion, there are only 15% false positives among controls, and 29-48% false negatives among depressives requiring hospitalization. Likewise, the test appears to identify about 40% of manic subjects.

The PAA test is nonspecific. Thus, it does not differentiate bipolar vs unipolar depressives nor between other subtypes of depression. Further, low PAA excretion has been observed in a subgroup of manics (Sabelli, unpublished data) and in chronic schizophrenics [208]. There are no normative data concerning other psychiatric or medical disorders. Notwithstanding, the test may be useful to differentiate schizophrenic from manic psychosis (low in schizophrenia, usually high in mania) as well as to identify mild or masked forms of depressive disorders. Thus, many of our depressed "untreated" outpatients had been in psychotherapy for years because their affective symptomatology was mild and had not led them to seek psychiatric diagnosis and pharmacological treatment. We have found that for patients with high PAA urinary excretion who clinically manifest high anxiety levels, insomnia, and active suicidal ideation, and who have a history of depressive disorder and are apparently unresponsive to a wide variety of antidepressants, treatment with either chlorpromazine or simply discontinuing antidepressant medication is helpful.

In summary, we have found the measurement of urinary PAA useful in the following cases: (1) differential diagnosis of manic-like/schizoaffective psychoses (high PAA) which may respond to lithium or carbamazepine, from schizophrenic psychoses (low PAA); and (2) differential diagnosis of depressed mood symptomatic of affective disorders (low PAA) versus depressive mood due to psychological, familial or social conflicts (normal PAA), or anxiety states (high PAA).

These studies have led us to test for the antidepressant effect of the PEA amino acid precursor L-phenylalanine, which we are now using with success alone or in combination with MAOI (Sabelli H, Fawcett J, Gusovsky F, et al: Antidepressant effects of L-phenylalanine. Presented at the II World Conference on Clinical Pharmacology and Therapeutics, Washington, D.C., October 1983).

Further support for a PEA deficit in depressive disorders comes from the work of Sandler and co-workers [209]. They found that PAA levels were lower in the CSF of 24 patients with "primary depressive illness" than in 30 control subjects [209]. Davis and associates [210] have found that depressed patients excrete less urinary p-hydroxymandelic and p-hydroxyphenylacetic acids, the major metabolites of octopamine and tyramine, two "trace amines" probably synthesized in vivo from PEA [211,212]. By way of contrast, these authors have reported elevated PAA blood levels in aggressive psychopaths [213] and elevated PAA CSF levels in schizophrenics [214].

Finally, Karoum and associates [215] have reported on a retrospective study demonstrating that women with brief psychotic episodes and/or bizarre behavior of labile quality (described as "hysterical" or "flakey") associated with a bipolar affective disorder, periodically demonstrated very high urinary PEA excretion rates. Klein and co-workers have postulated the existence of a specific subtype of depression, "hysteroid dysphoria" [216]. They proposed that the disorder may be due to a PEA deficit [216], although no data were presented in support of this view. A recent study by Spitzer and associates [217] has not validated this disease entity. We have seen hysteroid depressed women with low PAA excretion who also demonstrate rapid fluctuations in PAA excretion. Since they also have hypersomnia and high impulsivity ratings on the KDS-3A [218,219], we suspect that these are minor forms of bipolar illness.

### Central Cholinergic Factors

Several investigators [220-222] have proposed that alterations in the activity of central cholinergic synapses play a role in the pathogenesis of affective disorders, with depression representing a cholinergic overactivity and mania a hypofunction. This concept has been related to the notion of cholinergic–adrenergic balance [220, 222], a hypothesis derived from the traditional picture of the autonomic system.

Even in the autonomic system, such a picture is oversimplified. ACh and CA are often synergic in peripheral effectors (e.g., skeletal muscles) ACh is the physiological mediator in sympathetic ganglia, causing release of CA from the adrenal gland and from sympathetic nerve endings, etc. Further, most organs are *not* doubly innervated (e.g., only CA regulate the vascular system). The situation is even more complex in the CNS, where there are a multiplicity of neurotransmitters.

Evidence for cholinergic disturbance in affective disorders includes the fact that (1) many antidepressants block muscarinic receptors [223] (but so do many antipsychotics, while some antidepressants do not); (2) atropinic drugs can cause manic-like psychosis and increased activity [224] and potentiate amphetamine [224] as antidepressants do; (3) physostigmine can produce a depressive state; [224] and (4) some TCA, but not antipsychotics, block nicotinic responses in peripheral nerves and in cerebral evoked potentials [12,225]. Unfortunately, there is no central metabolite of ACh which we can measure. The studies involving Ach have involved the administration of physostigmine, arecholine, or atropine, or other atropine-like drugs, or ACh precursors. These challenge studies have indirectly and qualitatively measured neurotransmitter interactions by measurements made in other systems (e.g., neuroendocrine responses and sleep studies).

## The Two-Disease Theory of Depression

It is highly unlikely that a depressive process, which involves so many different brain functions, would involve only one neuroamine transmitter. Unipolar and bipolar depressives do not differ only in the presence or absence of hypomanic or manic periods but often also in the symptomatology of the depressive phase. Thus, unipolar depressives are characterized by insomnia and trait anxiety (as measured by the KDS-3A) [219] while bipolar depressives often show hypersomnia [226,227] and trait impulsivity (as measured by the KDS-3A) [219]. A considerable number of bipolar patients have a history of attentional deficit disorder, which may also be a neuroamine disorder [228,229]. There are also distinctions between depressed patients with anorexia and those with increased appetite and those with anxiety and those without, etc. The underlying hypothesis that neuroamines regulate brain functions including sleep, appetite, anxiety, and impulsivity requires that such heterogeneous symptomatology be reflected in biochemical heterogeneity. As we have discussed in "Catecholamine hypothesis of affective disorders," there is evidence that urinary MHPG levels may be low, normal or high in depression. Such data is thus at variance with the theory that all depressions are due to CA defects. MHPG measurements may have some value in the subtyping of depression (16,54, 57,73,80,230,231]. The differences observed, however, are so small, that it is doubtful that they can be useful in predicting response to treatment in individual patients. In fact, we do not use MHPG measurements in our clinical practice.

Maas [16] suggested that there are two distinct subtypes of depression separable biochemically and on the basis of response to pharmacological intervention, of which only one is due to a CA deficit. Maas' two-disease theory suggests that some depressives have low NE and normal 5-HT while others have low 5-HT and normal NE. This distinction may have implications for treatment, based on (relatively) selective inhibition of uptake of biogenic amines by various antidepressants in clinical use, providing a theoretical rationale for trying a second antidepressant if the patient is a nonresponder to the first. Thus, Type A depression has a (1) low pretreatment urinary MHPG; (2) favorable clinical response to IMI or DMI; (3) clinical response that is predictable by a brightening of mood following a brief trial of dextroamphetamine; (4) modest increment or no change in MHPG following any of these three drugs, and (5) failure to respond to AMI. On the other hand, Type B depression is characterized by (1) a normal or high MHPG; (2) a favorable response to AMI; (3) a lack of mood change following dextroamphetamine; (4) a failure to respond to IMI or DMI; and (5) a decrement in MHPG following any of the latter three drugs. Maas speculated that Type B depression probably reflects a disorder of the 5-HT system. He further suggested that the CA involved in Type A depression is NE, not DA, but added that the latter CA may be involved in mania, which is not explained by this two-disease model.

Overwhelming clinical experience as well as a few careful studies indicate that many depressed patients who failed to respond to one antidepressant will respond to another. This pharmacological evidence supports the view that depression is a syndrome which reflects many different biochemical disturbances. According to the single-disease theories, all TCA have the same basic pharmacologic reaction, the inhibition of biogenic amine reuptake. Thus, if a patient failed to respond to an adequate dose of one TCA, one would expect a similar lack of response to another. In support of this view (but against most others) Klein and associates believes that all TCA have approximately equal effectiveness when used in appropriate dose [232]. On the basis of our own study of TCA responses and their prediction by the Stimulant Challenge Test [17], we have concluded that there are at least two types of depression: Type I, associated with a deficit in various amine systems and responsive to IMI-like antidepressants, and Type II, at times associated with a deficit in PEA but not in NE, and responsive to AMI and NT (see Chapter 9).

What are the data from the clinical trials designed to test this model of amine metabolites as biological predictors of drug response? Fawcett and associates [70] reported that low MHPG excretion correlated with therapeutic response to IMI and DMI. Maas and associated [79] reported similar low predrug MHPG excretion as a harbinger of response to the same drugs, but they claimed that the significant feature was the treatment to pretreatment MHPG ratio rather than the absolute excretion value per se. Thus, MHPG levels increased or remained stable after four weeks of treatment in responders, while showing a marked decrement in treated nonresponders. Note, however, that these changes were not confirmed by other investigators (see below). Schildkraut [233] and Modai and associates [234] observed that patients with higher pretreatment MHPG responded to AMI. MHPG rose significantly during treatment with AMI, though this rise was statistically lower in responders [234]. Sacchetti and associates [235] concluded that CMI and AMI, although with a lesser degree of specificity, were indicated in the treatment of depressives with normal or high MHPG urinary excretion. Beckmann and Goodwin [98] studied unequivocal responders to both IMI and AMI in primary unipolar depressives [236] and found that IMI responders had significantly lower MHPG levels when compared with nonresponders. However, closer review of these data showed evidence of overlap: Only one-third of the patients were clearly distinguished as responders to either drug. Further, their results differ from Maas' and Fawcett's in that a decrement was associated with treatment in both groups, and was independent of clinical response. In another study, Beckmann and associates [237] replicated the findings of Greenspan and associates [238], who noted increased urinary MHPG excretion during response to chronic lithium treatment in their agitated depressives. Additionally, Beckmann and associates [98,237] found MHPG levels reduced in nonresponders.

In a study involving depressives randomly treated (treatment not described), Pickar and associates [239] found improvement was associated with a significant increase in MHPG excretion, while ill patients continued to excrete less MHPG than both a normal comparison group and the recovered patients. Cobbin and associates [240] measured pretreatment MHPG in depressives allowed a variety of antidepressant pharmacotherapies. The low MHPG experimental group, treated with IMI, DMI, and NT, and the normal-high experimental group, treated with AMI, had more significant improvement than a comparison group treated with all available antidepressants, including protriptyline and doxepin. High pretreatment MHPG predicted response to AMI-like TCA, while low pretreatment MHPG predicted response to IMI-like TCA in both male and female patients. Hollister and associates [241] also demonstrated differential response to NT, the secondary amine metabolite of AMI. The six lowest excreters improved significantly more than the six highest (N = 17), although the Hamilton Depression Rating Scale score was not reduced significantly among the nine low versus eight normal-high excreters overall.

Gaertner and associates [242] treated twenty-nine inpatients with primary affective disorder with AMI and measured pretreatment MHPG and AMI + NT blood levels during treatment. They found that AMI responders had significantly higher pretreatment MHPG excretion than the nonresponders, although the relationship was only weak. There was also a trend toward lower plasma levels of drug in the reponders.

Other data demonstrate no consistent relationship between CA and treatment response [243]. Prange [244] found IMI produced a fall in MHPG excretion in both normal and depressed females, and failed to confirm that good responders had initially lower MHPG. They also found that the important chemical changes tended to occur later than the important clinical changes. Shopsin and associates [245] reported on three depressed females with normal MHPG who responded to IMI. Sacchetti [246], Coppen [247], Steiner [248], and Spiker [249], and their associates found no correlation between pretreatment MHPG and response to AMI. The latter group also measured AMI and NT levels, probably the only group to do so other than Gaertner and associates [242]. Veith and associates [250] concluded that measurement of pretreatment MHPG alone is not adequate to predict treatment response or dictate TCA selection for unipolar depressives, and that the effects of DMI and AMI on urinary MHPG excretion indicates that TCA response may be mediated through effects other than alterations of NE alone. Further, Beckmann and Murphy [251] found baseline MHPG correlated with monoamine oxidase (MAO) activity, but neither pretreatment MHPG nor phenelzine-induced decrements distinguished responders from nonresponders, nor predicted responsiveness.

How can we interpret this data relating MHPG, treatment response, and the biogenic amine theories of depression? Are lowered MHPG values related to the depression per se, or do they constitute a characteristic of the depressed population? Blackwell [252] has called this potential biological marker of depression the "*M*yth of *H*eterogeneous *P*sychiatric *G*roups" in depression. Hollister and associates [71] found wide intraindividual variation in urinary MHPG excretion within normal control volunteers (900–3500 mcg per day) whereas Sweeney and associates [92] found that the stability of plasma free MHPG within affective disorder patients contrasted with lability in normal male volunteers. Hollister [71] suggested that these excretory patterns are neither states nor traits, but despite the fact that substantial changes in MHPG may occur in normals without any accompanying change in affect, conceded that MHPG may yet prove useful for categorizing depressives and predicting response to treatment. Beckmann and Goodwin [253] agreed that the concept of biological heterogeneity among major depressive disorders is supported by the data, but that the relationship between MHPG and various psychological and physiological parameters is not as clear cut when applied to attempts to relate differential levels of MHPG to the prediction of differential antidepressant response. Further, as reported by Hollister, total urinary MHPG excretion is not significantly different between depressed and normal individuals.

A modification of the CA hypothesis has been proposed by Schildkraut and associates [73,230,254], who suggest that the data support the biochemical heterogeneity of unipolar depressive disorder, and indicate that there may be at least three subgroups. Each of these subgroups may be differentially responsive to TCA therapy.

Rosenbaum and Schatzberg and their associates [73,254,255] observed that low pretreatment urinary MHPG predicted more favorable responses to IMI and maprotiline (both more rapidly and at lower doses). However, they further noted that a subgroup of patients who were "high" excreters (greater than 2500 mcg per day) also improved, provided they were treated with higher doses and achieved higher blood levels of maprotiline, while only one patient with intermediate excretion (1950 to 2500 mcg per day) responded. Schatzberg and associates [73] reported that depressives with low pretreatment urinary MHPG were more sensitive to and responded more rapidly to treatment with maprotiline than patients with high pretreatment urinary MHPG. Further analysis of their data indicated that patients with high MHPG (greater than 1950 mcg per day) who responded favorably to maprotiline, predominantly a potent NE reuptake blocker with little effect on 5-HT uptake [256,257], required not only higher doses but also higher blood levels of maprotiline than did low MHPG responders, and the responses occurred later in treatment. In fact, five of six patients with high MHPG had levels greater than 2500 mcg per day, leadint to the suggestion that unipolar depressive disorders with urinary MHPG between 1950 and 2500 mcg per day may be a third subgroup ("intermediate" MHPG excreters) that has a neurochemical abnormality which is unrelated to noradrenergic neuronal systems, and is not affected by maprotiline treatment. These data also correlate with Schildkraut's hypothesis [57, 230] of biologically discrete subgroups of unipolar depression with markedly elevated urinary MHPG levels. Schildkraut explained the wide variation of MHPG excretion (700 to 3400 mcg per day) in his study population as the basis for his "trinity" of high, intermediate, and low excreters among depressive subtypes. Related to this, Maas [258] proposed that chronic antidepressive pharmacotherapy (seven or more days of treatment) is associated with an increase in brain MHPG. This provides further evidence of increased brain NE turnover with chronic drug administration. Maas added that other studies, using other methods, have produced contradictory findings (e.g., Charney et al. [96,97] see earlier). These studies by Rosenbaum and Schatzberg [73,254,255] do not report on post-treatment MHPG levels. Schildkraut [230] in fact does leave open the possibility of an interaction with 5-HT and ACh in his intermediate and high MHPG subgroups, respectively. As both Schildkraut [259] and Blombery [68] and their associates suggest, even if the majority of urinary MHPG is peripheral in origin, the levels could be clinically useful as a predictor of therapeutic response or in subclassifying depressive disorders.

### Permissive Theory and Interactive Models

A major drawback to the interpretation of drug-response and amine metabolite correlation studies is that each study had a different patient population (i.e., differences in inclusion and exclusion diagnostic criteria used) and did not report both 5-HIAA and MHPG in the same patient population [19,165].

The observation that 5-HIAA levels in the CSF of depressives, both unipolar and bipolar, remain low even after recovery suggested the potential importance of 5-HT and led to a theory relating 5-HT and NE in depression—the "permissive theory" [159]. Thus, a chronic 5-HT deficit state interacts with changes in CA, rendering these individuals chemically vulnerable to depression or mania, depending upon the relative amount of CA available in relation to the low 5-HT levels; i.e., low 5-HT "permits" these affective swings, and must be present for the expression of one's vulnerability to affective disorder. Acute mood changes therefore represent changes in CA levels. IA changes in the same direction (decrease) in both mania and depression, while CA levels vary [159,260,261]. A study by Ridges and associates [262] further illustrates this theory in the treatment response of depressives. They studied simultaneous urinary excretion of 5-HIAA and MHPG in twenty endogenous depressives kept on a rigid diet for three days prior to urine collections, and who subsequently were treated with either maprotiline or CMI (ten patients on each) for twenty-eight days. Changes in the amine levels were not consistent with the known preferences of the two drugs for single amine systems. However, low pretreatment 5-HIAA was found to predict responsiveness to both drugs, though significantly only for CMI. High 5-HIAA predicted poor drug response. However, blood levels, especially desmethyl-CMI levels, were not measured or correlated with amine excretion.

This hypothesis is basically a merger of the 5-HT deficit theory and the CA hypothesis of affective disorders. A deficit or other functional disturbance of the transmitter agent of both NE and 5-HT systems causes mania and depression. As reviewed by Murphy and associats [149], it is supported by probenecid-5-HIAA data as well as by L-tryptophan and fenfluramine antidepressant studies, and by PCPA effects in humans. As demonstrated by Prange [159] L-tryptophan may be efficacious in treating mania. Fenfluramine may be effective in mania also [263–265].

Tissot [266] presented a novel theory based on the fact that manic-depressives show an increased uptake of exogenous L-5-hydroxytroptophan when depressed and of L-dopa when manic; he proposed that increased tryptophan uptake causes alterations in the balance of monoaminergic system activity. Thus, depression is a hyperserotoninergic and relative hypocatecholaminergic state, while the converse explains mania. An oscillation in these two systems is thus responsible for this cyclical illness.

Thus it remains to be seen whether subgroups with reciprocal relationships (ie.., high MHPG–low 5-HIAA, and high 5-HIAA–low MHPG) or other correlations could be found. A few of these comparative studies were reported earlier in the section on 5-HT. Goodwin and associates [165] studied a series of depressives in an attempt to delineate this pattern. The low CSF 5-HIAA subgroup did have a significantly higher urinary MHPG level. This did not appear to be an artifact of age, sex, or polarity of illness. More recently, Maas and associates [88] reported on eighty-seven depressives from the NIMH Collaborative Study on the Psychobiology of Depression, relating pretreatment CSF 5-HIAA, MHPG, and HVA levels and urinary MHPG to response to IMI and AMI. Although no significant differences were found between the two drugs in antidepressant efficacy, low CSF and urinary

MHPG and low CSF 5-HIAA were both significantly associated with favorable response to IMI (statistically significant only for urinary MHPG and CSF 5-HIAA), while high levels of either MHPG or 5-HIAA predicted neither success nor failure. Pretreatment CSF HVA was not related in any way to IMI responsiveness. The MHPG (urine and CSF)–5-HIAA correlations were positive and statistically significant for females but not for males (for whom only CSF and urine MHPG were statistically significantly correlated), and they were not inversely related to each other. None of the amine values were correlated significantly with AMI responsiveness except for a trend for high HVA to be associated with a favorable response. The 5-HIAA distribution was not bimodal. Thus, the existence of a subtype characterized by low MHPG and/or low CSF 5-HIAA, responsive to IMI, is postulated. This monoamine relationship could imply either independent change in neuronal system function or an interactive relationship between the two systems.

But we still need to define which measures are most useful. Another study questioning the value of urinary MHPG in distinguishing these groups was done by Potter and associates [267,268], comparing the effects of a specific 5-HT uptake inhibitor (zimelidine) [269] with the specific NE uptake inhibitor DMI. Further, norzimelidine, the demethylated metabolite, is an even more specific 5-HT inhibitor [269]. The same patients were studied with each drug. DMI produced a dramatic decrease in CSF as well as urinary MHPG but did not reduce CSF 5-HIAA, while zimelidine produced the opposite effect in CSF but also significantly reduced urinary MHPG. Further, the DMI effect on urinary MHPG did not correlate with the reduction of this metabolite in CSF. The urinary MHPG decrement did not correlate well with concentrations of parent drug or metabolite of either drug. This demonstrates a dissociation of MHPG changes in the CSF and urine despite the use of drugs with specific effects, which may indicate that urinary changes do not reflect CNS events. Thus, in order to assess biochemical specificity of drug action, urinary MHPG may not be adequate, though still useful for subtyping patients, as described earlier.

### Functional Amine Hypothesis

Since depression and mania are disease states characterized by alterations in affect, energy, and sleep, and since amines appear to be involved in these functions, this association is considered to provide additional supportive evidence for relating amines to these two disease states. Since mania and depression are two phases of the same bipolar illness, which usually alternate, but that may also co-exist ("mixed affective states"), it is likely that a common biochemical abnormality underlies both. Because mania and depression represent opposite states regarding mood, sleep, and energy, one can also expect other synaptic abnormalities to be opposite. There is some evidence for a deficit in serotonergic transmission in both phases of bipolar illness, with high adrenergic amines (CA and PEA) in mania and low adrenergic amines in depression. In the case of the IA, the "too much–too little" hypothesis is challenged by Prange and Coppen and their associates [159,177,270], who report a 5-HIAA decrement in both mania and depression.

### Conclusions

Thus, information on the mode of action, including biochemical specificity of drug action, of TCA and MAOI, reserpine, amphetamine, and other drugs altering monoamine metabolism and disposition has provided pharmacological support for the monoamine hypotheses of depression, but has not distinguished the relative importance of CA, IA, or PEA. One drawback is that it is difficult to pharmacologically intervene in one of these systems without affecting the other. Despite claims that patients who respond to TCA which have a main effect of NE uptake will not respond to drugs with a major effect on 5-HT uptake, and vice versa, the literature cited above has demonstrated otherwise. In fact, most antidepressants affect PEA levels and CA reuptake much more, affecting 5-HT reuptake only at very high concentrations. This overlap has been suggested by the plasma level findings [271, 272]. Other drawbacks are related to the multiple possible interactions among neurotransmitter systems, all of which may be affected by these different drugs, as well as potential interactions of neurotransmitters with neuroendocrine systems, and vice versa [273,274]. Further, the validity of these biologic biogenic amine theories have also been challenged by the efficacy of various "atypical" antidepressants, such as mianserin and prindole [275]. Although these hypotheses are attractive, there is a definite polarity of views which has not been resolved. These data are of heuristic value until a more advanced understanding of basic functional neurochemistry and neurophysiology of the CNS is forthcoming. Abnormalities of the metabolism of any one amine probably do not account for all the diverse clinical and biological phenomena of affective disorders [88,276–279]. Further, biochemical differences might be related to differences in clinical phenomena and subtypes of these disorders. In this respect, the fact that the urinary excretion of PAA is low in most depressives indicates that PEA deficit may be a major factor in this illness but that it does not account for all of its multifaceted symptomatology. Certainly, clinical observations of treatment response constitute a major source of evidence supporting these various biochemical hypotheses, which originally arose from observations of the effects of drugs on biochemical variables. Despite the negative studies, there are enough positive data suggesting that continued investigation of monoamine profiles in affective disorders have considerable potential for expanding our knowledge and understanding of the biological mechanisms underlying these disorders and for planning rational pharmacologic intervention. Certainly, the data suggest more work addressing specific problems before these monoamine profiles can be of practical clinical use.

## ANXIETY DISORDERS (Table 2a)

There is a paucity of studies of biogenic amines and anxiety. This is especially unfortunate because anxiety complicates the evaluation of depression and its biological correlates in a number of ways. As regards clinical practice, the symptoms of anxiety may be crucial to differentiate subtypes of depression and to determine the effectiveness of particular agents. Clinically, depression and anxiety often occurs together and in fact, TCA responders often have an anxiety-prone personality, in contrast to lithium responders, who tend to be impulsive [219]. At the psychological level, the association of depression with anxiety and irritability, or even overt anger, may be understood in terms of the "conflict theory of depression": anxiety (fight), fear (flight), and surrender and defeat (depression) are three alternative but often combined responses to conflict (Sabelli, manuscript in preparation). On a biochemical level, anxiety as well as depression affect the metabolism of CA, as well as cortisol levels. Thus the clinical investigation of CNS CA turnover by measuring peripheral MHPG needs to take into account not only quantification of the severity of depression but also the intensity of anxiety.

Two hypotheses regarding the role of CA in affective symptomatology are potentially contradictory. Although depression and anxiety often coexist clinically, CA are assumed to be decreased in depression [33,34] and increased in anxiety [280,281]. The CA theory of affect dates from the studies of Cannon [282,283] demonstrating the peripheral release of these amines in fight-or-flight reactions and, by implication, in the pathogenesis of anxiety. Based on clinical experiments, Toman and associates [284] formally posited the view that brain CA release mediates anxiety, a view considered as the first formulation of this CA theory of affect [285]. Supporting this view, there are reports of a significant correlation between changes in urinary MHPG and anxiety ratings [286,287]. Post and associates reported positive correlations between CSF NE and anxiety in depressives [288]. Beta-adrenergic blockers, such as propranolol, and antipsychotics (which block DA and alpha-adrenergic NE receptors) have been shown to decrease specific forms of anxiety [289-298].

On the other hand, both TCA and MAOI are effective in treating cases with mixed anxiety and depression and can selectively reduce anxiety, for instance, in phobic and panic disorders [299-302]. These observations may seem contradictory to the view of anxiety as NE-mediated fear, if antidepressants would act by increasing central NE function. Alternatively, recent animal models of TCA effects suggest that TCA can act by *down*-modulating CA system receptors [303-305]. This will be compatible with emerging evidence that TCA might work by inhibiting noradrenergic activity [306] to produce receptor subsensitivity [303,307]. Similarly, MAOI, by preferentially raising the brain levels of nonhydroxylated amines (PEA, tyramine, etc.), may produce a relative deficit in brain NE. A measure of the metabolism of nonhydroxylated adrenergic amines may assist in the understanding of central adrenergic activity in anxiety and depression, and the therapeutic effects of TCA and MAOI. This problem can be examined by studying the relative excretion of NE versus PEA urinary products.

## SCHIZOPHRENIA

### Introduction

Almost since schizophrenia was first defined as a clinical syndrome, speculations on possible biochemical factors in the disease have been made. One disturbing issue, still to be definitively resolved, is whether schizophrenia is a single entity or a group of more or less distinctive illnesses, the schizophrenias, each with its own biologic basis. To date, no biochemical lesion has yet been definitively established beyond doubt to be linked to schizophrenia. Two major hypotheses have dominated the search for the biological basis of schizophrenia. The earlier hypothesis suggested that the schizophrenic symptoms have their origins in the endogenous production or abnormal accumulation of a methylated psychotogen. The other, and more currently held hypothesis, holds that the illness results from a functional hyperactivity of one or more cerebral dopaminergic systems. Despite a large number of reported abnormal biochemical findings, few have been independently confirmed. There is certainly no evidence for any common etiology or pathogenesis.

### The Transmethylation Hypothesis

The similarities between the psychotomimetic effects of some hallucinogenic drugs and some forms of schizophrenia are so striking that it has long been suspected that this illness may result from the formation of a psychotoxic metabolite. Earlier in the century, abnormal indoles were found in the urine of schizophrenics, and it was speculated that schizophrenia resulted from gastrointestinal abnormalities. Modern theories start with the observations that adrenochrome, the oxidation product of epinephrine, has psychomimetic effects, but earlier reports on the excessive formation of adrenochrome in schizophrenia were refuted.

Based on the similarities between mescaline psychosis and schizophrenia, Osmond and Smythies [308] suggested that excessive methylation of brain amines might play an etiological role in schizophrenia. Thus, in addition to N-methylation of NE, resulting in the synthesis of epinephrine, O-methylation occurred and resulted in the formation of a "mescaline-like" substance such as dimethoxyphenylethylamine (DMPEA) [308]. In 1962, Friedhoff and Van Winkle [309] reported the presence of DMPEA, called the "pink spot" because of its color on staining, in the urine of fifteen of nineteem schizophrenics but in none of fourteen normal urines. Since then, a large number of groups have failed to confirm these observations. DMPEA is found in the urine of normals [310] and no consistent differences between schizophrenic and normal controls have been found [311].

The discovery of 5-HT in mammalian brain and the fact that LSD, a psychedelic drug, interferes with serotonergic neuronal systems expanded the original methylation hypothesis. These findings, as well as previous findings of intensification of psychosis in schizophrenics by L-methionine or betaine, the increase in S-adenosylmethionine in rat brain and liver by methionine feeding, and the existence of at least one enzyme capable of transmethylating normal metabolites to psychotomimetic compounds [312-314], led to the formulation of the "transmethylation hypothesis of schizophrenia" [315]. This hypothesis postulates that schizophrenia arises from the abnormal accumulation and persistence of excessive amounts of psychotogenic N- or O-methylated biogenic amine derivative(s) [316] of normal metabolites. These derivatives are capable of inducing some of the symptoms of schizophrenia.

Bumpus and Page [317] proposed that schizophrenia may result from the metabolism of endogenous 5-HT to its psychomimetic derivative N,N-dimethylserotonin (bufotenine). Such reaction can occur in normals since the enzyme required exists in a variety of tissue [318,319]. Fischer and co-workers [320-324] identified a bufotenine-like substance in the urine of schizophrenics. Several authors confirmed these findings [325-327], while others did not [328]. More recently, it has been demonstrated that N,N-dimethyltryptamine (N,N-DMT) is excreted in excessive amounts in schizophrenics as well as in normals under stress [329]. While those who search for a unique and specific metabolic disorder in schizophrenia have considered these observations as refuting the role of N-methylated IA in the pathogenesis of schizophrenia, we consider that these results indicate that the excessive formation of N-methylated IA, as well as other metabolites whose production is enhanced by stress, may indicate some common processes in both conditions. Obviously schizophrenics suffer from much endogenous anxiety and exogenous stress. Of course, there is more to schizophrenia than stress, but the role of N-methylated IA cannot be disregarded. Thus loading experiments with methyl donors, tryptophan and MAOI show that such combination can produce florid psychosis in chronic schizophrenics [326,330-334].

Over two decades have passed since the introduction of the transmethylation hypothesis. Still no conclusions are available regarding its involvement in or even its relevance to schizophrenia.

### CNS Amines and Schizophrenia: Catecholamine and Indoleamine Hypotheses (Table 4)

The possible role of CA on the pathophysiology of schizophrenia has been a major focus of speculation. This is particularly true for the role of DA in producing the functional hyperactivity/overactivity [335] of specific DA neurons, especially

**Table 4. Neuroamine Changes in Schizophrenia**

| | Dopamine | Norepinephrine | Serotonin | Phenylethylamine |
|---|---|---|---|---|
| Current theories (amine theories) | ↑ | ↓ | ↑ Psychotoxic methylated metabolites | ↑ |
| Supporting evidence | Antipsychotics block DA receptors | Anhedonia, decreased drive, withdrawal | Methylated indole ethylamines in acutely psychotic schizophrenics | Increased urinary PEA |
| Contradictory evidence | Decreased metabolites in CSF | Increased metabolites in urine, blood, CSF | Decreased urinary metabolite | Anhedonia, decreased drive, withdrawal. Decreased PAA |
| Conflict/stress multiple amine model (this paper) | Receptor hypersensitivity ? | ↑ Reflecting anxiety and stress | ↑ Methylated indole ethylamines 2° to stress in acute cases only | ↓ As inhibition of drives to reduce conflicts |

in the mesocorticolimbic system, thereby producing psychotic symptoms. DA release may be enhanced, or there may be an increased number and/or sensitivity of DA postsynaptic receptors, or a decreased number of presynaptic DA receptors [336]. Compared with affective disorders, there is a paucity of metabolite data available in schizophrenia, particularly chronic schizophrenia [18]. A variety of direct and indirect approaches have been attempted in order to detect a defect in cerebral activity.

The DA hypothesis of schizophrenia [337–340] postulates that schizophrenic symptoms result from abnormal cerebral dopaminergic activity, and rests almost entirely upon pharmacologic evidence. Drugs which increase dopaminergic activity, such as amphetamines, [341–344] methylphenidate [345–347], cocaine [348, 349], and L-dopa [350,351] can precipitate or exacerbate schizophreniform symptomatology. Neuroleptic antipsychotics act by decreasing central dopaminergic transmission and cause parkinsonian side effects in humans, while in animal studies they block DA receptors, increase DA turnover, block DA-mediated increases in cAMP and reverse amphetamine-induced suppression of single nerve-cell firing in relative proportion to their antipsychotic efficacy. However, the amphetamine and cocaine models for these psychoses may also be consistent with roles for PEA, NE, 5-HT, or ACh. There are thus overlapping spectra of pharmacologic efficacy, with effects varying between acute and chronic states. It should also be noted that antiparkinsonian agents such as amantadine which facilitate dopaminergic transmission, ameliorate the parkinsonian side effects of antischizophrenic drugs without decreasing their antipsychotic effect [352].

In studies of CSF amine metabolites in schizophrenia, the most consistent finding has been a reduction in the postprobenecid accumulation of the DA metabolite HVA. Baseline levels of HVA, DOPAC, 5-HIAA and MHPG, as well as postprobenecid CSF 5-HIAA accumulation, generally show no significant difference. Rather than the predicted increases in DA turnover being demonstrable in schizophrenics, clinical studies [18,121,144,353,354] have demonstrated that during or following the acute episode, DA turnover may be reduced, especially in Schneiderian-positive, "process" or poor prognosis schizophrenics. These data are not consistent with the hyopthesis that there is an increased release of DA at central synapses, but it does not rule out hyperactivity at dopaminergic synapses due exclusively to an excess in DA receptors. The analysis of the data, however, may be complicated by the possible alterations in the metabolism of released DA. For instance, it has been speculated that schizophrenics may suffer from a relative deficit in brain MAO.

Bowers [355] found that CSF 5-HIAA and HVA accumulated less after probenecid in chronic schizophrenics compared with acute schizophrenics and bipolar affective disorders. He interpreted the data as consistent with the hypothesis that a central MAO-B deficiency may be associated with chronic schizophrenia, although relatively low values for both metabolites were also found in bipolar depressives.

Neuroleptics have been found to have a relatively selective effect on CSF HVA in schizophrenics, consistent with animal data indicating that these drugs increase brain DA turnover [356]. In schizophrenics, CSF HVA accumulation is increased pre- and postprobenecid following acute and subacute phenothiazine and butyrophenone treatment. Following recovery, with or without neuroleptics, repeat CSF studies after a two-week or more drug washout period reveal significantly lower HVA accumulations. This represents evidence of reduced DA turnover in patients recovered from acute schizophrenic episodes. The data demonstrating decreases in HVA accumulation during recovery are more compatible with the hypothesis that alterations in DA metabolism may reflect an underlying predisposition to the acute illness [357]. During the acute episode HVA may increase from this low level. There may be a differential effect of neuroleptic treatment on CSF HVA. the magnitude depends on the duration of drug treatment. Acute treatment (less than three weeks) with chlorpromazine or thioridazine has produced a substantial increase in probenecid-induced HVA accumulation, whereas following more chronic treatment a difference from baseline was no longer demonstrable. Studies with pimozide, a more specific selective DA receptor blocker, suggests individual differences in the relationship between duration of treatment and HVA changes. Some patients maintain a substantial HVA effect even after receiving the drug for more than three weeks.

The crux of the issue of specificity is the interaction between underlying biological/biochemical disturbance and superimposed dysfunction. Certainly, clinical phenomenology as well as historical features of the illness may also be involved.

Since direct evidence for dopaminergic system overactivity in schizophrenia has not been forthcoming, other CNS amine metabolites have been examined. Stein and Wise [358] proposed, from a self-stimulation model, that a deficit in noradrenergic function accounts for the anhedonia, lack of motivation and social withdrawal of chronic schizophrenics. Goodwin and Post [18] studied acute schizophrenics and did not find decreased CSF MHPG, but instead found it tended to be higher in most acutely psychotic patients. This is consistent with findings of high-normal levels of CSF VMA in both acute and recovered schizophrenics [359]. Further, Lake and associates [360] found higher CSF NE concentrations in schizophrenics, especially those with paranoid features, compared to age-matched normal controls. Kemali and associates [361] confirmed the previous reports of increased plasma and CSF NE levels, but not DA or epinephrine levels in drug-free schizophrenics, compared with controls; there were no significant urinary metabolite findings. This central NE increase may reflect central noradrenergic overactivity of questionable pathophysiological significance; the peripheral increase may reflect higher nonspecific arousal levels. Autopsy studies reported may lend some support to the hypothesis that NE is inceased in schizophrenia. However, it is hard to know in all cases whether the changes in NE levels are due to schizophrenia or to neuroleptic treatment.

Decreased MHPG excretion has been reported in schizophrenia-related depressions [362,363]. We were unable to find any comprehensive studies regarding urinary MHPG excretion in schizophrenic syndromes.

Alterations in 5-HT metabolism have been proposed to be involved in at least some forms of schizophrenia on the basis of the interference produced by LSD and related hallucinogens of this amine and the serotonergic neuronal system [364, 365], but generally CSF 5-HIAA levels in schizophrenics do not differ significantly from normal or neurologic controls. MacKay and associates [366] reported that 5-HIAA distribution in the human brain parallels that of 5-HT, but the relative contribution of cerebral 5-HIAA to lumbar CSF 5-HIAA concentration is unclear. That 5-HT metabolism may be relevant to at least a subgroup of schizophrenics was suggested by Post and associates' findings of low 5-HIAA in those with the most subjective distress and in those with prominent hallucinations [357]. Bowers [367] reported a significant decrease in probenecid-5-HIAA during psychedelic drug-induced psychoses. Sedvall and Wade-Helgodt [368] divided schizophrenics into those with and those without a family history of schizophrenia; those with such a history had more aberrant CSF 5-HIAA accumulations than those without. Potkin and associates [369] found decreased CSF 5-HIAA levels in a subgroup of schizophrenics with enlarged ventricles compared with those with normal-size ventricles (but not different from neurological controls) and ventricular size correlated inversely with 5-HIAA concentrations. There were no differences between medication-free and neuroleptic-treated schizophrenics.

In studies of biogenic amines and CA-related enzymes in autopsied brains of schizophrenics [370,371], the only changes found consistently were an increase in the number of DA receptors [372], increased DA receptor sensitivity in the basal ganglia [372,373], and enhanced DA concentrations [374]. Although DA has been found elevated in the nucelus accumbens [375], especially in chronic paranoid schizophrenics [363], this has not been a consistent finding [371,376]. DA concentrations have also been found elevated in the caudate and putamen [377]. The significance of these findings is unclear [378]. Elevated NE concentrations have also been found, especially in NE-rich areas of the limbic forebrain and related structures, the hypothesized site of dysfunction in schizophrenia [371,376,377, 379, 380].

Tissot [266] suggested that decreased tryptophan transport and uptake represents the central pathophysiological factors in schizophrenia; increased tyrosine uptake could lead to augmented dopaminergic activity potentially due to enhanced tyrosine hydroxylation and CA formation. If DA activity is sufficiently enhanced, a DA hypoactivity would result, possibly due to dopamine-beta-hydroxylase blockade and/or NE displacement by DA. Diminished 5-HT system activity could facilitate this mechanism. Thus he describes a hyposerotonergic-hyperdopaminergic biochemical model of schizophrenia, with or without noradrenergic insufficiency.

**Phenylethylamine and Schizophrenia (Table 4)**

In early studies, Fischer [203,381] reported elevated urinary PEA in schizophrenics and thought it may have etiological importance. This association is further considered in reviews by Wyatt and associates [382] and by Sandler and Reynolds [383]. Wyatt and associates [208,384–386] examined the potential role of PEA and its major metabolite, PAA, in the pathophysiology of schizophrenia. They found increased PEA and decreased PAA urinary excretion in schizophrenics (primarily paranoid) when compared with normals. This may parallel changes found in platelet MAO activity (reduced MAO-B activity in chronic schizophrenics [387]). The altered PEA excretion found in schizophrenics suggests that PEA may be a major mediator of the schizophrenic process. Borison and associates [388] have in fact speculated that PEA-induced stereotypies, which are more selectively antagonized by neuroleptics, may be a better model of schizophrenia than the currently used D-amphetamine-induced stereotypies.

While these data are interesting, especially in light of the role of amphetamines in producing psychotic states, these results must be viewed with caution and the findings need to be replicated. There are many potential sources of variances in the methods of collection and measurement, and although PEA crosses the blood brain barrier, the relationship of urinary (peripheral) PEA to circulating brain levels is unknown. The relationship between clinical state and urinary PEA (and PAA) excretion also needs to be determined. Finally, the potential psychotomimetic effects of PEA in humans need to be explored. In our view, the measurement of urinary PEA is a poor indicator of its central metabolism because most PEA is rapidly metabolized to PAA.

Schizophrenics as a group excrete very low amounts of PAA (78.6 mg/24 hr, in contrast to 156.2 mg/24 hr in controls) [208]. In contrast, the urinary excretion of PAA is very high in most of the schizoaffectives we have studied (200–700 mg/24 hr). Our conclusion is that brain PEA is reduced in schizophrenia as well as in depression, in line with their common clinical symptomatology (anhedonia; lack of motivation, interests and energy; difficulty in concentration; trouble sleeping; continuous worrying; depressed mood and crying; anxiety; low self-esteem; and vulnerability to rejection).

In our view, illnesses such as those grouped as schizophrenia, which affect so many different brain functions, must by necessity alter the release and metabolism of a wide variety of synaptic transmitters. This will result not only in quantitative alterations in the formation of the metabolites of the hormones that mediate transmission at synapses which function more or less than usual, but also in the increased production of otherwise minor metabolites (which may be potentially psychotoxic) as a result of such differential alteration in various metabolic pathways. It is conceivable, for instance, that when 5-HT synapses are hyperactive, more tryptamine is released and more is converted to N,N-DMT. Althouth it is in principle possible to interpret schizophrenia as a genetically determined toxic psychosis produced by such endogenous metabolites, there is also the possibility that at least some form of schizophrenia may be in part the result of exogenous or endogenous stresses. In our view, one could make an argument to correlate some of the symptoms of schizophrenia with some of the biochemical changes believed to occur in this illness. One may speculate that psychoses are psychological defense mechanisms, which through avoidance of logical reasoning protect the individual from facing painful contradictions and conflicts. Such avoidance of logic may be driven by excessive anxiety, either NE-mediated as in manic psychosis (and possibly also in schizophrenia), or DA-mediated as in schizophrenia. Further avoidance of painful conflict occurs via the inhibition of pleasure-seeking; such anhedonia and lack of motivation would be reflected by a profound PEA deficit, evidenced by the observed reduction in urinary PAA. Further, stress itself, as Corbett demonstrated [329], may enhance the production of psychotoxic metabolites. While such speculative hypotheses did nothing to the factual description of what biochemical changes occur in schizophrenias, explanations are helpful to introduce order into our description as well as to suggest further experimentation.

## CONCLUSIONS

Current research findings of multiple biochemical alterations in schizophrenia and affective disorders are leading most investigators away from the one amine-one illness model, to consideration of multiple transmitter, multiple modulator mechanisms. Mood and related CNS functions appear to be regulated by a multiplicity of amines, including but not exclusively, CA, ACh, 5-HT and PEA. Depression may result from the failure of one or more of these chemical regulatory mechanisms, whereas schizophrenic processes are accompanied by a disruption of DA, NE, PEA, indoleamines and possibly other modulators. The CA and the 5-HT theories of psychiatric disorders have proven of great value in the development of new therapies, while the measurement of the PEA metabolism appears to be a useful approach to the diagnosis of affective disorders and particularly the differential diagnosis between schizophrenic and some schizoaffective syndromes.

Experimental evidence for a role of each of the neuroamine systems suspected has been found in various psychiatric disorders. This evidence is at variance with the view that a single neuroamine mechanism is involved. Likewise, all drugs capable of exerting powerful and relatively selective effects on emotional behavior appear to simultaneously affect many if not all neuroamine mechanisms.

We have, therefore, proposed [276] that psychiatric disorders as well as their alterations by most (if not all) psychotropic drugs result from and require the simultaneous modification of many modulator mechanisms. Thus, schizophrenic illnesses may require the simultaneous overactivity of several neuroamine systems, and antischizophrenic effects may be attributable to the depletion or blockade of several neuroamine receptors. In contrast, the effect of psychotomimetics (e.g., LSD) may in turn result from concomitant activation of several modulator mechanisms (ACh, neuroamines, etc.). Since several amines seem to sustain mood, the occurrence of depression may require the simultaneous failure of several of these neuroamine systems, whereas antidepressant action requires instead (direct or indirect) activation of receptors for hydroxylated and nonhydroxylated monoamines without concomitant stimulation (or with blockade) of cholinergic systems. In addition, nicotinic cholinergic receptors seem to be essential in the modulation of behavior, because interactions with nicotine allow us to differentiate IMI-like antidepressants from phenothiazine tranquilizers in peripheral nerve [12], evoked potentials [389], and spontaneous EEG [390].

The involvement of several amine systems in psychiatric illness, as well as the multiplicity of actions of psychotropic drugs is probably not accidental. The neural structures underlying complex behavioral functions certainly do not resemble the simple linear pathways of the peripheral autonomic systems or the spinal reflex arcs. Thus, only the simultaneous alteration of several chemical modulator mechanisms allow us to modify the function of networks essentially characterized by parallel pathways ("redundancy") and feedback circuits. Jouvet [391] has pointed out that the need for the activation of three different modulator mechanisms (indolethylamine, catecholamine, and ACh) to trigger REM sleep may represent a safeguard (developed through evolution) which protects against the projection of oneiric activity into the stream of consciousness.

The view that behavioral changes should not be thought of as an alteration of a specific amine but rather as an imbalance of several modulator systems has often been formulated in terms of a balance between a pair of antagonistic mediators (5-HT versus catecholamines, ACh versus catecholamines, etc.). This formulation is rooted in the notion of an antagonism between sympathetic and parasympathetic mediators, although such antagonism is not observed even in most peripheral organs. For example, two modulators may be functionally synergistic for some central functions and antagonistic for others. In our view, cholinesters, catecholamines, and tryptamines modulate synaptic transmission in the neural networks subserving patterns of sedation and sleep as well as in mechanisms for arousal and wakefulness. For instance, ACh plays an important role in EEG arousal (and by implication on the reticular activating mechanisms [392]) as well as in REM sleep [391,393]. In the same manner, catecholamines appear to be involved in the mechanisms for arousal [392] as well as those for REM sleep [391]. The ability of the major psychotropic drugs to interact with a whole spectrum of neuroamines in the CNS has led Toman and Sabelli [276] to conclude that the search for more effective drug therapy must be directed to finding agents with multiple receptor effects rather than agents with a single specific receptor action.

On the other hand, depressive and anxious moods do not occur only as a result of genetically determined illnesses but also in a variety of circumstances. It would be fruitful to attempt to link these biochemical and psychological processes. While at this point such attempts can be only speculative, we have found the following formulation intriguing.

Current psychopharmacological studies regarding the modulation of the genetically inherited pathways of behavior studied by ethology suggest that each of these different brain programs (respiration, sleep, sex, etc.) consist of an appetitive sequence of interactions with other individuals, followed by a pleasurable consummatory act. Whereas the appetitive sequence is modulated by specific neurotransmitters, catecholamines [394] and possibly other phenylethylamines mediate consummatory pleasure. When a person conflicts with others or with the environment, or even with himself, the pursuit of such appetitive drives toward consummation is inhibited, and instead behavior is channeled through three major defense pathways: (i) anger and defense; (ii) fear (anxiety and escape); and (iii) depression and surrender. Thus, depression, anxiety and anger are often combined. Catecholamines and related messengers do not only mediate pleasure but they may also support fight-or-flight reactions, while their deficit may favor depression. Thus, PEA deficit and the corresponding inhibition of pleasure-seeking or consummation would be characteristic of depressive illness, while catecholamines may be high (anxious depression) or low. We further speculate that an extreme conflict, such as that experienced by individuals with a genetically determined predisposition to schizophrenia, would lead to high CA release, inhibition of PEA mechanisms and formation of psychotoxic metabolites.

Anxiety seems to be mediated by catecholamines (central and peripheral) and by corticosteroids (which are produced peripherally but readily cross the blood brain barrier). Thus, anxious patients show high MHPG urinary excretion and high plasma cortisol levels, while anxiety is reduced by both NE and DA blockers. The biochemistry of anger, which can be prominent in mania, is less understood, but animal studies suggest that an excess of DA or ACh can trigger rage. As manifestations of conflict, depressions are often accompanied by anger and fear (anxiety) mediated by NE (high MHPG excretion). In more profound depressions all efforts are abandoned, and this surrender syndrome represents NE depletion. Depressions, thus, are heterogeneous: there are high NE anxious depressives and low NE defeated (giving-up) depressives, and high DA hyperactive (agitated) depressives and low DA retarded depressives, as well as other depressions which appear to involve a deficit in brain PEA (detectable as a low excretion of PAA by urine). We interpret those relatively rare cases of depressive mood in the presence of high PAA excretion as a compensatory increase in PEA to defend against depression of other origin.

## ACKNOWLEDGEMENTS

Our grateful thanks and appreciation to June Ascareggi, for without her assistance and technical skills this manuscript could not have become a reality.

Our phenylethylamine research was supported in part by the Retirement Research Foundation and a gift from the Illinois Capacitor Foundation.


## REFERENCES


1. Sabelli HC, Giardina WJ: Amine modulation of affective behavior. In Sabelli HC (ed): Chemical Modulations of Brain Function. New York, Raven Press, 1973
2. Udenfriend S: Molecular biology of the sympathetic nervous system. Pharmacol Rev 24:165–166, 1972
3. Zeller EA: Comparative physiochemistry of phenylethylamine targets. In Mosnaim AD, Wolf ME (eds): Noncatecholic Phenylethylamines: Biological Mechanisms and Clinical Aspects. New York, Marcel Dekker, 1978
4. Molinoff PB, Axelrod J: Distribution and turnover of octopamine in tissues. J. Neurochem. 19:157–163, 1972.
5. Cajal SR: Neuron Theory or Reticular Theory? Objective Evidence of the Anatomical Unity of Nerve Cells. (Purkiss MU, Fox, CA (trans)). Madrid, Conseju Superior de Investigaciones Cientificas Instituto Ramon Y Cajal, 1954
6. Dale HH: Pharmacology and nerve endings. Proc R Soc Med 28:319–332, 1935
7. Sabelli HC, Mosnaim AD, Vasquez AJ, et al: Biochemical plasticity of synaptic transmission: A critical review of Dale's Principle. Biol Psychiatry 11: 481–524, 1976
8. Nachmanson D: Chemical and Molecular Basis of Nerve Activity. New York, Academic Press, 1959
9. Armett CJ, Ritchie JM: The action of acetylcholine and some related substances on conduction in mammalian non-myelinated nerve fibers. J Physiol 155:372–384, 1961
10. Toman JEP, Sabelli HC: Neuropharmacology of earthworm giant fibers. Int J Neuropharmacology 7:543–556, 1968
11. Kosterlitz HW, Lees GM, Wallis DI: Resting and acitve potentials recorded by the sucrose-gap method in the superior cervical ganglion of the rabbit. J Physiol 195:39–53, 1968
12. Sabelli HC, Gorosito M: Evidence for biogenic amine receptors in toad sciatic nerves. Int J Neuropharmacology 8:495–513, 1969
13. Barany E, Nordqvist, P: Influence of histamine on nerve block due to antihistaminics. Nature 164:701, 1949
14. Brodie BB, Shore PA: A concept for a role of serotonin and norepinephrine as chemical mediators in the brain. Ann NY Acad Sci 66:631–642, 1957
15. Brodie BB, Costa E: Some current views on brain monoamines. Psychopharmacology Service Center Bulletin 2:1–25, 1962

16. Maas JW: Biogenic amines and depression: Biochemical and pharmacological separation of two types of depression. Arch Gen Psychiatry 32:1357–1361, 1975
17. Sabelli HC, Fawcett J, Javaid JI, et al: The methylphenidate test for differentiating desipramine-responsive from nortriptyline-responsive depression. Am J Psychiatry 140:212–214, 1983
18. Goodwin FK, Post RM: Studies of amine metabolites in affective illness and in schizophrenia: A comparative analysis. In Freedman DX (ed): Biology of the Major Psychoses. New York, Raven Press, 1975
19. Zis, AP, Goodwin FK: The amine hypothesis. In Paykel ES (ed): Handbook of Affective Disorders. New York, Guilford Press, 1982
20. Garelis R, Young SN, Lal S, et al: Monoamine metabolites in lumbar CSF. The question of their origin in relation to clinical studies. Brain Res 79:1–8, 1974
21. Goodwin FK, Post RM: Catecholamine metabolite studies in the affective disorders: Issues of specificity and significance. In Usdin E, Hamburg DA, Barchas JD (eds): Neuroregulators and Psychiatric Disorders. New York, Oxford University Press, 1977
22. Post RM, Goodwin FK: Approaches to brain amines in psychiatric patients: A reevaluation of cerebrospinal fluid studies. In Iversen LI, Iversen SD, Snyder SH (eds): Handbook of Psychopharmacology, Vol. 13. Biology of Mood and Antianxiety Drugs. New York, Plenum Press, 1978
23. Banki CM, Molnar G: Cerebrospinal fluid 5-hydroxyindoleacetic acid as an index of central serotonergic processes. Psychiatry Res 5:23–32, 1981
24. Neff TH, Tozer TN, Brodie BB: Application of steady-state kinetics to studies of the transfer of 5-hydroxyindoleacetic acid from brain to plasma. J Pharmacol Exp Ther 158:214–218, 1967
25. Van Praag HM, Korf J, Schut D: Cerebral monoamines and depression: An investigation with the probenecid technique. Arch Gen Psychiatry 28:827–833, 1973
26. Van Praag HM, Korf J, Dols LCW, et al: A pilot study of the predictive value of the probenecid test in the application of 5-hydroxytryptophan as an antidepressant. Psychopharmacologia 25:14–21, 1972
27. Sjostrom R: Steady-state levels of probenecid and their relation to acid monoamine metabolites in human cerebrospinal fluid. Psychopharmacologia 25:96–100, 1972
28. Sjostrom R, Roos B–E: 5-hydroxyindoleacetic acid and homovanillic acid in cerebrospinal fluid in manic-depressive psychosis. Eur J Clin Pharmacol 4: 170–176, 1972
29. Moir ATB, Ashcroft GW, Crawford TBB, et al: Central metabolites in cerebrospinal fluid as a biochemical approach to the brain. Brain 93:357–368, 1970
30. Gordon EK, Oliver J: 3-methoxy-4-hydroxyphenylethyleneglycol in human cerebrospinal fluid. Clin Chem Acta 35:145–150, 1971
31. Gordon EK, Oliver J, Goodwin FK, et al: Effect of probenecid on free 3-methoxy-4-hydroxyphenylethyleneglycol (MHPG) and its sulfate in human cerebrospinal fluid. Neuropharmacology 12:391–396, 1973
32. Goodwin FK, Post RM, Dunner DL, et al: Cerebrospinal fluid amine metabolites in affective illness: The probenecid technique. Am J Psychiatry 130: 73–79, 1973

33. Schildkraut JJ: The catecholamine hypothesis of affective disorders: A review of supporting evidence. Am J Psychiatry 122:509–522, 1965
34. Bunney WE, Davis JM: Norepinephrine in depressive reactions: A review. Arch Gen Psychiatry 13:483–494, 1965
35. Schildkraut JJ, Kety SS: Biogenic amines and function. Science 156:21–30, 1967
36. Prange AJ: The pharmacology and biochemistry of depression. Dis Nerv Syst 25:217–221, 1964
37. Schildkraut JJ: Neuropharmacology and the affective disorders. N Engl J Med 28:197–201, 248–255, 302–308, 1969
38. Shopsin B, Wilk S, Sathananthan G, et al: Catecholamines and affective disorders revisited: A critical assessment. J Nerv Ment Dis 158:369–383, 1974
39. Baldessarini RJ: The basis for amine hypothesis in affective disorders: A critical evaluation. Arch Gen Psychiatry 32:1087–1093, 1975
40. Davis JM: Central biogenic amines and theories of depression and mania. In Fann WE, Karacan I, Pokorny AD, et al (eds): Phenomenology and Treatment of Depression. New York, Spectrum Publications, Inc., 1977
41. Garver DL, Davis JM: Mini review: Biogenic amine hypothesis of affective disorders. Life Sci 24:383–394, 1979
42. Kuhn R: Uber die behandlung depressive zustande mit einem iminodibenzylderivat (G22355). Schweiz Med Wochenschr 87:1135, 1957
43. Kuhn R: The treatment of depressive states with G22355 (imipramine hydrochloride). Am J Psychiatry 115:459–464, 1958
44. Everett GM, Toman JEP: Mode of action of Rauwolfia alkaloids and motor activity. In Masserman J (ed): Biological Psychiatry. New York, Grune and Stratton , 1959
45. Davis JM: Theories of biological etiology of affective disorders. Internat Rev Neurobiol 12:145–175, 1970
46. Goodwin FK, Bunney WE: Depression following reserpine: A reevaluation. Seminars in Psychiatry 3:435–448, 1971
47. Mendels J, Frazer A: Brain biogenic amine depletion and mood. Arch Gen Psychiatry 30:447–451, 1974
48. Charney DS, Menkes DB, Heninger GR: Receptor sensitivity and the mechanism of action of antidepressant treatment: Implications for the etiology and therapy of depression. Arch Gen Psychiatry 38:1160–1180, 1981
49. Maas JW, Fawcett JA, Dekirmenjian H: 3-methoxy-4-hydroxyphenylglycol (MHPG) excretion in depressive states: A pilot study. Arch Gen Psychiatry 19:129–134, 1968
50. Schildkraut JJ, Green R, Gordon EK, et al: Normetanephrine excretion and affective states in depressed patients treated with imipramine. Am J Psychiatry 123:690–700, 1966
51. Schanberg SM, Schildkraut JJ, Breese GR, et al: Metabolism of normetanephrine $H^3$ in rat brain—Identification of conjugated 3-methoxy-4-hydroxyphenylglycol as major metabolite. Biochem Pharmacol 11:247–254, 1968
52. Schanberg SM, Breese, GR, Schildkraut JJ, et al: 3-methoxy-4-hydroxyphenylglycol sulfate in brain and cerebrospinal fluid. Biochem Pharmacol 17: 2006–2008, 1968
53. Schildkraut JJ, Watson R, Draskoczy PR, et al: Amphetamine withdrawal: Depression and MHPG excretion. Lancet 2:485–486, 1971
54. Schildkraut JJ: Catechloamine metabolism and affective disorders: Studies of

MHPG excretion. In Usdin E, Snyder S (eds): Frontiers in Catecholamine Research—Third International Catecholamine Symposium. New York, Pergamon Press, 1973
55. Schildkraut JJ, Keeler BA, Grab EL, et al: MHPG excretion and clinical classification of depressive disorders. Lancet 1:1251–1252, 1973
56. Schildkraut JJ, Keeler BA, Paporisek M, et al: MHPG excretion in depressive disorders: Relation to clinical subtypes and desyncrhonized sleep. Science 181:762–764, 1973
57. Schildkraut JJ, Orsulak PJ, Schatzberg AF, et al: Toward a biochemical classification of depressive disorders: I: Differences in urinary excretion of MHPG and other catecholamine metabolites in clinically defined subtypes of depression. Arch Gen Psychiatry 35:1427–1433, 1978
58. Maas JW, Landis DH: In vivo studies of the metabolism of norepinephrine in the central nervous system. J Pharmacol Exp Ther 163:147–162, 1965
59. Dekirmenjian H, Maas JW: An improved procedure of 3-methoxy-4-hydroxyphenylethylene glycol determination by gas-liquid chromatography. Anal Biochem 35:113–122, 1970
60. Maas JW, Landis DH: The metabolism of circulating norepinephrine in human subjects. J Pharmacol Exp Ther 177:600–612, 1971
61. Maas JW, Dekirmenjain H, Jones F: The identification of depressed patients who have a disorder of norepinephrine metabolism and /or disposition. In Usdin E, Snyder S (eds): Frontiers in Catecholamine Research—Third International Catecholamine Symposium. New York, Pergamon Press, 1973
62. Maas JW, Hattox SE, Greene NM, et al: 3-methoxy-4-hydroxyphenylglycol production by human brain in vivo. Science 205:1025–1027, 1979
63. Axelrod J, Kopin IJ, Mann JD: 3-methoxy-4-hydroxyphenylglycol sulfate: A new metabolite of epinephrine and norepinephrine. Biochem Biophys Acta 36:576–577, 1959
64. Gitlow SE, Mendlowitz M, Bertani LM, et al: Human norepinephrine metabolism—its evaluation by administrtation of tritiated norepinephrine. J Clin Invest 50:859–865, 1971
65. Goodall McC, Rosen L: Urinary excretion of noradrenalin and its metabolites at ten-minute intervals after intravenous injection of dl-noradrenalin-2-$C^{14}$. J Clin Invest 42:1578–1588, 1963
66. Ebert MH, Kopin IJ: Differential labelling of origins of urinary catecholamine metabolites by dopamine-$C^{14}$. Transactions of the Association of American Physicians LXXXVIII:256–264, 1975
67. Kopin IJ: Measuring turnover of neurotransmitters in human brain. In Lipton MA, DiMascio A, Killam KF (eds): Psychophramacology: A Generation of Progress. New York, Raven Press, 1978
68. Blombery PA, Kopin IJ, Gordon EK, et al: Conversion of MHPG to vanillylmandelic acid. Arch Gen Psychiatry 37:1095–1098, 1980
69. Mardh G, Sjoquist B, Anggard E: Norepinephrine metabolism in man using deuterium labelling: The conversion of 4-hydroxy-3-methoxyphenylglycol to 4-hydroxy-3-methoxymandelic acid. J Neurochem 36:1181–1185, 1981
70. Fawcett J, Maas J, Dekirmenjian H: Depression and MHPG excretion: Response to dextroamphetamine and tricyclic antidepressants. Arch Gen Psychiatry 26:246–251, 1972
71. Hollister LE, Davis KL, Overall LE, et al: Evaluation of MHPG in normal subjects. Arch Gen Psychiatry 35:1410–1415, 1978

72. Goodwin FK, Potter WZ: Norepinephrine metabolite studies in affective illness. In Usdin E, Kopin IJ, Barchas J (eds): Catecholamines: Basic and Clinical Frontiers, Vol. 2. Proceedings of the Fourth International Catecholamine Symposium. New York, Pergamon Press, 1979
73. Schatzberg AF, Rosenbaum AH, Orsulak PJ, et al: Toward a biochemical classification of depressive disorders. III. Pretreatment urinary MHPG levels as predictors of response to treatment with maprotiline. Psychopharmacology 75:34–38, 1981
74. Schildkraut JJ: Current status of the catecholamine hypothesis of affective disorders. In Lipton MA, DiMascio A, Killam KF (eds): Psychopharmacology: A Generation of Progress. New York, Raven Press, 1978
75. Schildkraut JJ, Orsulak PJ, LaBrie RA, et al: Toward a biochemical classification of depressive disorders: II. Application of multivariate discriminate function analysis to data on urinary catecholamines and metabolites. Arch Gen Psychiatry 35:1436–1439, 1978
76. Cedarbaum JM, Aghajanian GK: Activation of locus coeruleus noradrenergic neurons by peripheral nerve stimulation. Presented at the 7th Annual Meeting for Society of Neuroscience, Anaheim, California, 1977
77. Aghajanian GK, Cedarbaum JM, Wang RY: Evidence fo norepinephrine-mediated collateral inhibition of locus coeruleus neurons. Brain Res 136:570–577, 1977
78. Crawley JN, Hattox SE, Maas JW, et al: 3-methoxy-4-hydroxy-phenyl ethylene glycol increase in plasma after stimulation of the nucleus locus coeruleus. Brain Res 141:380–384, 1978
79. Maas JW, Fawcett JA, Dekirmenjian H: Catecholamine metabolism, depressive illness, and drug response. Arch Gen Psychiatry 26:252–262, 1972
80. DeLeon-Jones F, Maas JW, Dekirmenjian H, et al: Diagnostic subtypes of affective disorders and their urinary excretion of catecholamine metabolites. Am J Psychiatry 132:1141–1148, 1975
81. Wilk S, Shopsin B, Gershon S, et al: Cerebrospinal fluid levels of MHPG in affective disorders. Nature 235:440–441, 1972
82. Shopsin B, Wilk S, Gerhson S, et al: Cerebrospinal fluid MHPG: An assessment of norepinephrine metabolism in affective disorders. Arch Gen Psychiatry 28: 230–233, 1973
83. Post RM, Gordon EK, Goodwin FK, et al: Central norepinephrine metabolism in affective illness: MHPG in the cerebrospinal fluid. Science 179:1002–1003, 1973
84. Shaw DM. O'Keefe R, Mac Sweeney DA, et al: 3-methoxy-4-hydroxyphenylglycol in depression. Psychol Med 3:333–336, 1973
85. Subrahmanyan S: Role of biogenic amines in certain pathological conditions. Brain Res 87:355–362, 1975
86. Agren H: Depressive symptom patterns and urinary MHPG excretion. Psychiatry Res 6:185–196, 1982
87. Roccatagliata G, Albano C, Abbruzzese G: CSF-MHPG in depressive syndromes: Basal values and imipramine-induced modifications. Neuropsychobiology 7:169–171, 1981
88. Maas JW, Kocsis JH, Bowden CL, et al: Pretreatment neurotransmitter metabolites and response to imipramine or amitriptyline treatment. Psychol Med 12:37–43, 1982
89. Markianos E, Beckmann H: Diurnal changes in dopamine-B-hydroxylase,

homovanillic acid and 3-methoxy-4-hydroxyphenylglycol in serum of man. J Neural Transm 39:79–93, 1976
90. Halaris AE: Plasma 3-methoxy-4-hydroxyphenylglycol in manic psychosis. Am J Psychiatry 135:493–494, 1978
91. Halaris AE, DeMet EM: Studies of norepinephrine metabolism in manic and depressive states. In Usdin E, Kopin IJ, Barchas J (eds): Catecholamines: Basic and Clinical Frontiers, Vol 2. Proceedings of the Fourth International Catecholamine Symposium. New York, Pergamon Press, 1979
92. Sweeney DR, Leckman JF, Maas JW, et al: Plasma free and conjugated MHPG in psychiatric patients: A pilot study. Arch Gen Psychiatry 37:1100–1103, 1980
93. Jimerson DC, Ballenger JC, Lake CR, et al: Plasma and CSF MHPG in normals. Psychopharmacol Bull 17:86–87, 1981
94. Kopin IJ, Gordon EK, Jimerson DC, et al: Relation between plasma and cerebrospinal fluid levels of 3-methoxy-4-hydroxyphenylglycol. Science 219: 73–75, 1983
95. Leckman JF, Maas JW, Redmond DE, et al: Effects of oral clonidine on plasma 3-methoxy-4-hydroxyphenylglycol (MHPG) in man: Preliminary report. Life Sci 26:2179–2185, 1980
96. Charney DS, Heninger GR, Sternberg DE, et al: Plasma MPHG in depression: Effects of acute and chronic desipramine treatment. Psychiatry Res 5:217–229, 1981
97. Charney DS, Heninger GR, Sternberg DE, et al: Presynaptic adrenergic receptor sensitivity in depression: The effect of long-term desipramine treatment. Arch Gen Psychiatry 38:1334–1340, 1981
98. Beckmann H, Goodwin FK: Antidepressant response to tricyclics and urinary MHPG in unipolar patients: Clinical response to imipramine or amitriptyline. Arch Gen Psychiatry 32:17–21, 1975
99. Jones FD, Maas JW, Dekirmenjian H, et al: Urine catecholamine metabolites during behavioral changes in a patient with manic-depressive cycles. Science 179:300–302, 1973
100. Bond PA, Jenner FA, Sampson GA: Daily variations of the urine content of 3-methoxy-4-hydroxyphenylglycol in two manic-depressive patients. Psychol Med 2:81–85, 1972
101. Bunney WE, Goodwin FK, Murphy DL, et al: The "switch process" in manic-depressive illness. II. Relationship to catecholamines, REM sleep, and drugs. Arch Gen Psychiatry 27:304–309, 1972
102. Post RM, Stoddard FJ, Gillin JC, et al: Alterations in motor activity, sleep, and biochemistry in a cycling manic-depressive patient. Arch Gen Psychiatry 34:470–477, 1977
103. Wehr TA, Muscettola G, Goodwin FK: Urinary 3-methoxy-4-hydroxyphenylglycol circadian rhythm: Early timing (phase-advance) in manic-depressives compared with normal subjects. Arch Gen Psychiatry 37:257–263, 1980
104. Zis AP, Cowdry RW, Wehr TA, et al: Tricyclic-induced mania and MHPG excretion. Psychiatry Res 1:93–99, 1979
105. Lewis JL, Winokur G: The induction of mania: A natural history study with controls. Arch Gen Psychiatry 39:303–306, 1982
106. Nasrallah HA, Lyskowski J, Schroeder D: TCA-induced mania: Differences between switchers and nonswitchers. Biol Psychiatry 17:271–274, 1982
107. Krauthammer C, Klerman GL: Secondary mania: Manic syndromes associated with antecedent physical illness or drugs. Arch Gen Psychiatry 35:1333–1339, 1978

108. Brodie HKH, Murphy DL, Goodwin FK, et al: Catecholamines and mania: The effect alpha-methyl-para-tyrosine on manic behavior and catecholamine metabolism. Clin Pharmacol Ther 12:218-224, 1971
109. Goodall McC, Alton H: Metabolism of 3-hydroxytryptamine (dopamine) in human subjects. Biochem Pharmacol 17:905–914, 1968
110. Randrup A, Munkvad I, Fog R, et al: Mania, depression, and brain dopamine. In Essman WB, Valzelli L (eds): Current Developments in Psychopharmacology, Vol 2. New York, Spectrum Publications, Inc., 1975
111. DeLeon-Jones FA: Biochemical aspects of affective disorders. In Val ER, Gaviria FM, Flaherty JA (eds): Affective Disorders: Psychopathology and Treatment. Chicago, Year Book Medical Publishers, Inc., 1982
112. Van Praag HM, Korf J, Puite J: 5-hydroxyindoleacetic acid levels in the cerebrospinal fluid of depressive patients treated with probenecid. Nature 225:1259–1260, 1970
113. Korf J, Van Praag HM: Amine metabolism in human brain: Further evaluation of the probenecid test. Brain Res 35:221–230, 1971
114. Sjostrom R: 5-hydroxyindoleacetic acid and homovanillic acid in cerebrospinal fluid in manic-depressive psychosis and the effect of probenecid treatment. Eur J Clin Pharmacol 6:75–80, 1973
115. Bowers MB: Lumbar CSF 5-hydroxyindoleacetic acid and homovanillic acid in affective syndromes. J Nerv Ment Dis 158:325–330, 1974
116. Van Praag HM, Korf J: Neuroleptics, catecholamines, and psychoses: A study of their interrelations. Am J Psychiatry 132:593–597, 1975
117. Berger PA, Faull KF, Kilkowski J, et al: CSF monoamine metabolites in depression and schizophrenia. Am J Psychiatry 137:174–180, 1980
118. Bowers M: Cerebrospinal fluid 5-hydroxyindoleacetic acid (5HIAA) and homovanillic acid (HVA) following probenecid in unipolar depressives treated with amitriptyline. Psychopharmacologia 23:26–33, 1972
119. Dencker SJ, Malm V, Roos B–E, et al: Acid monoamine metabolites of cerebrospinal fluid in mental depression and mania. J Neurochem 13:1545–1548, 1966
120. Roos B-E, Sjostrom R: 5-hydroxyindoleacctic acid (and homovanillic acid) levels in in the CSF after probenecid application in patients with manic depressive psychosis. Pharmacologica Clinica 1:153–155, 1969
121. Bowers MB, Heninger GR, Gerbode FA: Cerebrospinal fluid 5-hydroxyindoleacetic acid and homovanillic acid in psychiatric patients. Int J Neuropharmacol 8:255–262, 1969
122. Papeschi R, McClure DJ: Homovanillic and 5-hydroxyindoleacetic acid in cerebrospinal fluid of depressed patients. Arch Gen Psychiatry 25:354–358, 1971
123. Sjostrom R: Cerebrospinal fluid content of 5-hydroxyindoleacetic acid and homovanillic acid in manic-depressive psychosis. Acta Universitatis Upsaliensis 154:16–17, 1973
124. Banki CM: Correlation between cerebrospinal fluid amine metabolites and psychomotor activity in affective disorders. J Neurochem 29:255–257, 1977
125. Sjostrom R, Roos B-E: 5-hydroxyindoleacetic acid and homovanillic acid in cerebrospinal fluid in manic-depressive psychosis. Eur J Clin Pharmacol 4:170–176, 1972
126. Post RM, Kotin J, Goodwin FK, et al: Psychomotor activity and cerebrospinal fluid amine metabolites in affective illness. Am J Psychiatry 130:67–72, 1973

127. Strom-Olsen R, Weil-Malherbe H: Humoral changes in manic-depressive psychosis with particular reference to excretion of catecholamines in urine. J Ment Sci 104:696–704, 1958
128. Sloane RB, Hughes W, Haust HL: Catecholamine excretion in manic-depressive and schizophrenic psychosis and its relationship to symptomatology. Can Psychiat Assoc J 11:6–19, 1966
129. Messiha F, Agallianos D, Clower C: Dopamine excretion in affective states and following $Li_2CO_3$ therapy. Nature 225:868–869, 1970
130. Klerman GL, Schildkraut JJ, Hasenbush LL, et al: Clinical experience with dihydroxyphenylalanine (DOPA) in depression. J Psychiat Res 1:289–297, 1963
131. Vasquez AJ, Sabelli HC: Potentiation of the central nervous system effects of DOPA by decarboxylase inhibition: Possible direct role of this neuroamino acid in brain mechanisms. Experimental Neurology 46:44–56, 1975
132. Goodwin FK, Murphy DL, Brodie HKH, et al: L-dopa, catecholamines, and behavior: A clinical and biochemical study in depressed patients. Biol Psychiatry 2:341–366, 1970
133. Murphy DL, Brodie HKH, Goodwin FK, et al: Regular induction of hypomania by L-dopa in "bipolar" manic-depressive patients. Nature 229:135–136, 1971
134. Murphy DL, Goodwin FK, Brodie HKH, et al: L-dopa, dopamine, and hypomania. Am J Psychiatry 130:79–82, 1973
135. Van Praag HM: Significance of biochemical parameters in the diagnosis, treatment and prevention of depressive disorders. Biol Psychiatry 12:101–131, 1977
136. Gerner RH, Post RM, Bunney WE: A dopaminergic mechanism in mania. Am J Psychiatry 133:1177–1180, 1976
137. Post RM, Jimerson DC, Bunney WE, et al: Dopamine and mania: Behavioral and biochemical effects of the dopamine receptor blocker pimozide. Psychopharmacology 67:297–305, 1980
138. Randrup A, Braestrup C: Uptake inhibition of biogenic amines by newer antidepressant drugs; Relevance to the dopamine hypothesis and depression. Psychopharmacology 53:309–314, 1977
139. Pert A, Rosenblatt J, Sivit C, et al: Long-term treatment-lithium prevents the development of dopamine receptor supersensitivity. Science 201:171–173, 1978
140. Chiodo LA, Antelman SM: Repeated tricyclics induce a progressive dopamine autoreceptor subsensitivity independent of daily drug treatment. Nature 287: 451–454, 1980
141. Mendels J, Stinnett JL, Burns D, et al: Amine precursors and depression. Arch Gen Psychiatry 32:22–30, 1975
142. Pare CMB, Sandler M: A clinical and biochemical study of a trial of iproniazid in the treatment of depression. J Neurol Neurosurg Psychiat 22:247–251, 1959
143. Van Praag HM: A critical investigation of the significance of MAO inhibition as a therapeutic principle in the treatment of depression. Thesis, University of Utrecht, 1962
144. Ashcroft GW, Crawford TBB, Eccleston D, et al: 5-hydroxyindole compounds in the cerebrospinal fluid of patients with psychiatric or neurological diseases. Lancet 2:1049–1052, 1966

145. Coppen A: The biochemistry of affective disorders. Brit J Psychiat 113:1237-1264, 1967
146. Lapin IP, Oxenkrug GF: Intensification of the central serotonergic processes as a possible determinant of the thymoleptic effect. Lancet 1:132–136, 1969
147. Kalin NH, Risch SC, Murphy DL: Involvement of the central serotonergic system in affective illness. J Clin Psychopharmacology 1:232–237, 1981
148. Van Praag HM: Management of depression with serotonin precursors. Biol Psychiatry 16:291–310, 1981
149. Murphy DL, Campbell I, Costa JL: Current status of the indoleamine hypothesis of affective disorders. In Lipton MA, DiMascio A, Killam KF (eds): Psychopharmacology: A Generation of Progress. New York, Raven Press, 1978
150. Traskman L, Tybring G, Asberg M, et al: Cortisol in the CSF of depressed and suicidal patients. Arch Gen Psychiatry 37:761–767, 1980
151. Carroll BJ, Greden JF, Feinberg M: Suicide, neuroendocrine dysfunction and CSF 5-HIAA concentrations in depression. In Angrist B, Burrows GD, Lader M, et al (eds): Recent Advances in Neuropsychopharmacology. Oxford, Pergamon Press, 1981
152. Rodnight R: Body fluid indoles in mental illness. Internat Rev Neurobiol 3: 251–292, 1961
153. Coppen A, Shaw DM, Malleson A: Changes in 5-hydroxytryptophan metabolism in depression. Brit J Psychiat 111:105–107, 1965
154. Coppen A, Shaw DM, Malleson A, et al: Tryptamine metabolism in depression: Brit J Psychiat 111:993–998, 1965
155. Dewhurst WG: New theory of cerebral amine function and its clinical application. Nature 218:1130–1133, 1968
156. Wirz-Justice A: Theoretical and therapeutic potential of indoleamine precursors in affective disorders. Neuropsychobiology 3:199–233, 1977
157. Zarcone VP, Berger PA, Brodie HKH, et al: The indoleamine hypothesis of depression: An overview and pilot study. J Clin Psychiatry 38:646–653, 1977
158. Murphy DL, Baker M, Goodwin FK, et al: Tryptophan in affective disorders: Indoleamine changes and differential clinical effects. Psychopharmacologia 34:11–20, 1974
159. Prange AJ, Wilson IC, Lynn CW, et al: L-tryptophan in mania: Contribution to a permissive hypothesis of affective disorders. Arch Gen Psychiatry 30: 56–62, 1974
160. Farkas T, Dunner DL, Fieve RR: L-tryptophan in depression. Biol Psychiatry 11:295–302, 1976
161. Louvenberg W, Engelman K: Assay of serotonin, related metabolites and enzymes. Meth Biochem Anal 19:1–34, 1971
162. Bueno JR, Himwich HE: A dualistic approach to some biochemical problems in endogenous depression. Psychosomatics 8:82–94, 1967
163. Asberg M, Bertillson L, Tuck D, et al: Indoleamine metabolites in the cerebrospinal fluid of depressed patients before and during treatment with nortriptyline. Clin Pharmacol Ther 14:277–286, 1973
164. Asberg M, Thoren P, Traskman L, et al: "Serotonin depression"–A biochemical subgroup within the affective disorders? Science 191:478–480, 1976
165. Goodwin FK, Cowdry RW, Webster MH: Predictors of drug response in the affective disorders: Toward an integrated approach. In Lipton MA, DiMascio A, Killam KF (eds): Psychopharmacology: A Generation of Progress. New York, Raven Press, 1978

166. Kripke DF: Serotonin depression. Science 194:214, 1976
167. Koe BK, Weissman A: p-Chlorophenylalanine: A specific depletor of brain serotonin. J Pharmacol Exp Ther 154:499–516, 1966
168. Shopsin B, Gershon S, Goldstein M, et al: Use of synthesis inhibitors in defining a role for biogenic amines during imipramine treatment in depressive patients. Commun Psychopharmacol 1:239–249, 1975
169. Shopsin B, Friedman E, Gershon S: Parachlorophenylalanine reversal of tranylcypramine effects in depressed patients. Arch Gen Psychiatry 33:811–819, 1976
170. Ross SB, Renyi AL: Tricyclic antidepressant agents–I. Acta Pharmacol Toxicol (Copenh) 36:382–394, 1975
171. Randrup A, Braestrup C: Uptake inhibition of biogenic amines by newer antidepressant drugs: Relevance to the dopamine hypothesis of depression. Psychopharmacology 53:309–314, 1977
172. Van Praag HM: New evidence of serotonin-deficient depressions. Neuropsychobiology 3:56–63, 1977
173. Post RM, Goodwin FK: Effects of amitriptyline and imipramine on amine metabolites in the cerebrospinal fluid of depressed patients. Arch Gen Psychiatry 30:234–239, 1974
174. Bowers MB: Amitriptyline in man: Decreased formation of central 5-hydroxyindoleacetic acid. Clin Pharmacol Ther 15:167–170, 1974
175. Bertillson L, Asberg M, Thoren P: Differential effect of chlorimipramine and nortriptyline on cerebrospinal fluid metabolites of serotonin and noradrenalin in depression. Eur J Clin Pharmacol 7:365–368, 1974
176. Traskman L, Asberg M, Bertillson L, et al: Plasma levels of chlorimipramine and its desmethyl metabolite during treatment of depression. Clin Pharmacol Ther 26:600–610, 1979
177. Coppen AJ: Abnormalities of indoleamines in affective disorders. Arch Gen Psychiatry 26:474–478, 1972
178. Shaw DM, Camps FE, Eccleston EG: 5-hydroxytryptamine in the hindbrain of depressive suicides. Brit J Psychiat 113:1407–1411, 1967
179. Bourne HR, Bunney WE, Colburn RW, et al: Noradrenalin, 5-hydroxytryptamine, and 5-hydroxyindoleacetic acid in hindbrains of suicidal patients. Lancet 2:805–808, 1968
180. Pare CMB, Yeung DPH, Price K, et al: 5-hydroxytryptamine, noradrenalin, and dopamine in brainstem, hypothalamus and caudate nucleus of controls and of patients committing suicide by coal gas poisoning. Lancet 2:133–135, 1969
181. Lloyd KG, Farley IJ, Deck JHN, et al: Serotonin and 5-hydroxyindoleacetic acid in discrete areas of the brainstem of suicide victims and control patients. Adv Biochem Psychopharmacol 11:387–398, 1974
182. Gottfried CG, Oreland L, Wibert A, et al: Lowered monoamine oxidase activity in brains from alcoholic suicides. J Neurochem 25:667–673, 1975
183. Cochrane E, Robins E, Grote S: Regional serotonin levels in brain: A comparison of depressive suicides and alcoholic suicides with controls. Biol Psychiatry 11:283–294, 1976
184. Beskow J, Gottfries CG, Roos B-E, et al: Determination on monoamine and monoamine metabolites in the human brain: Post mortem studies in a group of suicides and in a control group. Acta Psychiatr Scand 53:7–20, 1976
185. Birkmayer W, Riederer P: Biochemical post-mortem findings in depressed patients. J Neural Transm 37:95–109, 1975

186. Moses SG, Robins E: Regional distribution of norepinephrine and dopamine in brains of depressive suicides and alcoholic suicides. Commun Psychopharmacol 1:327–337, 1975
187. Asberg M, Traskman L, Thoren P: 5-HIAA in the cerebrospinal fluid: A biochemical suicide predictor? Arch Gen Psychiatry 33:1193–1197, 1976
188. Traskman L, Asberg M, Bertillson L, et al: Monoamine metabolites in CSF and suicidal behavior. Arch Gen Psychiatry 38:642–646, 1981
189. Nakajima T, Kakimoto Y, Sano I: Formation of B-phenylethylamine in mammalian tissues and its effects on motor activity in the mouse. J Pharmacol Exp Ther 143:319–325, 1964
190. Borison RL, Mosnaim AD, Sabelli HC: Biosynthesis of brain 2-phenylethylamine: Influence of decarboxylase inhibition and D-amphetamine. Life Sci 14:1837–1848, 1974
191. Borison RL, Sabelli HC, Ho B: Influence of a peripheral monoamine oxidase inhibitor (MAOI) upon the central nervous system levels and pharmacological effects of 2-phenylethylamine (PEA). Pharmacologist 17:258, 1975
192. Yang HYT, Neff NH: B-phenylethylamine: A specific substrate for type B monoamine oxidase of brain. J Pharmacol Exp Ther 187:365–371, 1973
193. Squires RF: Multiple forms of monoamine oxidase in intact mitochondria as characterized by selective inhibitors and thermal stability: A comparison of eight mammalian species. Adv Biochem Psychopharmacol 5:355–370, 1972
194. Fuxe K, Grobecker H, Jonsson J: The effect of B-phenylethylamine on central and peripheral monoamine-containing neurons. Eur J Pharmacol 2:202–207, 1967
195. Sabelli HC, Borison RL: Non-catecholamine adrenergic modulators. Adv Biochem Psychopharmacol 15:69–74, 1976
196. Borison RL, Mosnaim AD, Sabelli HC: Brain 2-phenylethylamine as a mediator for the central actions of amphetamine and methylphenidate. Life Sci 17:1331–1344, 1975
197. Sabelli HC, Mosnaim AD, Borison RL, et al: Use of pharmacological agents in elucidation of central synaptic transmission. In Dhawan BN, Bradley PB (eds): Drugs and Central Synaptic Transmission. New York, Macmillan and Company, 1976
198. Sabelli HC, Borison RL, Diamond BI, et al: Phenylethylamine and brain function. Biochem Pharmacol 27:1707–1711, 1978
199. Mosnaim AD, Inwang EE, Sabelli HC: The influence of psychotropic drugs on the levels of 2-phenylethylamine in rabbit brain. Biol Psychiatry 8:227–234, 1974
200. Sabelli HC, Vasquez AJ, Mosnaim AD, et al: 2-phenylethylamine as a possible mediator for $D^9$-tetrahydrocannabinol-induced stimulation. Nature 248:144-145, 1974
201. Sabelli HC, Mosnaim AD: Phenylethylamine hypothesis of affective behavior. Am J Psychiatry 131:695–699, 1974
202. Sabelli HC, Giardina WJ, Mosnaim AD, et al: A comparison of the functional roles of norepinephrine, dopamine and phenylethylamine in the central nervous system. Acta Physiologia Polonica 24:33–40, 1973
203. Fischer E, Heller B, Miro AH: B-phenylethylamine in human urine. Arzneim-Forsch 18:1486, 1968
204. Mosnaim AD, Inwang EE, Sugerman JH: Ultraviolet spectrometric determina-

tion of 2-phenylethylamine in biological samples and it possible correlation with depression. Biol Psychiatry 6:235–257, 1973
205. Javaid JI, Davis JM: GLC analysis of phenylalkyl primary amines using nitrogen detector. J Pharm Sci 70:813–815, 1981
206. Fawcett J, Sabelli HC, Javaid JI, et al: Urinary phenylethylamine in affective disorders. Presented at the World Psychiatric Association Regional Meeting, New York, Oct. 30–Nov. 3, 1981
207. Diagnostic and Statistical Manual of Mental Disorders (DSM-III) (Third Edition). Washington, DC, The American Psychiatric Association, 1980
208. Potkin SG, Wyatt, RJ, Karoum F: Phenylethylamine (PEA) and phenylacetic acid (PAA) in the urine of chronic schizophrenic patients and controls. Psychopharm Bull 16:52–54, 1980
209. Sandler M, Ruthven CRJ, Goodwin BL, et al: Decreased cerebrospinal fluid concentration of free phenylacetic acid in depressive illness. Clin Chem Acta 93:169–171, 1979
210. Davis BA, Durden DA, Boulton AA: Plasma concentrations of p- and m-hydroxyphenylacetic acid and phenylacetic acid in humans: Gas chromatographic-high resolution mass spectrometric analysis. J Chromatography 230: 219–230, 1982
211. Boulton AA, Dyck LE, Durden DA: Hydroxylation of B-phenylethylamine in the rat. Life Sci 15:1673–1683, 1974
212. Tallman JF, Saavedra JM, Axelrod J: Biosynthesis and metabolism of endogenous tyramine and its normal presence in sympathetic nerves. J Pharmacol Exp Ther 199:216–221, 1976
213. Sandler M, Ruthven CRJ, Goodwin BL, et al: Phenylethylamine overproduction in aggressive psychopaths. Lancet 2:1269–1270, 1978
214. Sandler M, Ruthven CRJ, Goodwin BL, et al: Raised cerebrospinal fluid phenylacetic acid concentration: Preliminary support for the phenylethylamine hypothesis of schizophrenia? Commun Psychopharmacol 2:199–202, 1978
215. Karoum F, Linnoila M, Potter WZ, et al: Fluctuating high urinary phenylethylamine excretion rates in some bipolar affective disorder patients. Psychiatry Res 6:215–222, 1982
216. Liebowitz MR, Klein DF: Hysteroid dysphoria. Psychiatric Clinics of North America 2:555–575, 1979
217. Spitzer RL, Williams JBW: Hysteroid dysphoria: An unsuccessful attempt to demonstrate its syndromal validity. Am J Psychiatry 139:1286–1291, 1982
218. Kupfer DJ, Pickar D, Himmelhoch JM, et al: Are there two types of unipolar depression. Arch Gen Psychiatry 32:866–871, 1975
219. Wold PN, Dwight K: Subtypes of depression identified by the KDS-3A: A pilot study. Am J Psychiatry 136:1415–1419, 1979
220. Janowsky DS, El-Yousef MK, Davis JM, et al: A cholinergic-adrenergic hypothesis of mania and depression. Lancet 2:632–635, 1972
221. Sitaram N, Gillin JC: Development and use of pharmacological probes of the CNS in man: Evidence of cholinergic abnormality in primary affective illness. Biol Psychiatry 15:925–955, 1980
222. Risch SC, Kalin NG, Janowsky DS: Cholinergic challenges in affective illness: Behavioral and neuroendocrine correlates. J Clin Psychopharmacol 1:186–192, 1981
223. Jarvik ME: Drugs used in the treatment of psychiatric disorders. In Goodman

LS, Gilman A (eds): The Pharmacological Basis of Therapeutics. Fourth Edition. New York, The Macmillan Company, 1970
224. Janowsky DS, El-Yousef MK, Davis JM, et al: A cholinergic-adrenergic hypothesis of mania and depression. Lancet 2:632–635, 1972
225. Vasquez AJ, Sabelli HC, Ludmer RI, et al: Pharmacological analysis of evoked potentials in rabbit cortex. In Wortis J (ed): Recent Advances in Biological Psychiatry, Vol. 8. New York, Plenum Press, 1966
226. Detre T, Himmelhoch J, Swartzburg M, et al: Hypersomnia and manic-depressive disease. Am J Psychiatry 128:1303–1305, 1972
227. Kupfer DJ, Himmelhoch JM, Swartzburg M, et al: Hypersomnia in manic-depressive disease (A preliminary report). Dis Nerv Syst 33:720–724, 1972
228. Wender P' Minimal Brain Dysfunction in Children. New York, John Wiley and Sons, 1971
229. Wender PH: Diagnosis and treatment of adult minimal brain dysfunction: A replication. Presented at the American College of Neuropsychopharmacology, Maui, Hawaii, December, 1978
230. Schildkraut JJ, Orsulak PJ, Schatzberg AF, et al: Possible pathophysiological mechanisms in subtypes of unipolar depressive disorders based on differences in urinary MHPG levels. Psychopharm Bull 17:90–91, 1981
231. Edwards DJ, Spiker DG, Neil JF, et al: MHPG excretion in depression. Psychiatry Res 2:295–305, 1980
232. Klein DF, Gittelman R, Quitkin F, et al: Clinical management of Affective Disorders. In Klein DF, Gittelman R, Quitkin F, et al: Diagnosis and Drug Treatment of Psychiatric Disorders: Adults and Children. Second Edition. Baltimore, Williams and Wilkins Company, 1980
233. Schildkraut JJ: Norepinephrine metabolites and biochemical criteria for classifying depressive disorders and predicting response to treatment. Am J Psychiatry 130:695–699, 1973
234. Modai I, Apter A, Gulomb M, et al: Response to amitriptyline and urinary MHPG in bipolar depressive patients. Neuropsychobiology 5:181–184, 1979
235. Sacchetti E, Allaria E, Negri F, et al: 3-methoxy-4-hydroxyphenylglycol and primary depression: Clinical and pharmacological considerations. Biol Psychiatry 14:473–484, 1979
236. Feighner JP, Robins E, Guze SB, et al: Diagnostic criteria for use in psychiatric research. Arch Gen Psychiatry 26:57–63, 1972
237. Beckmann H, St. Laurent J, Goodwin FK: The effect of lithium on urinary MHPG in unipolar and bipolar depressed patients. Psychopharmacologia 42: 277–282, 1975
238. Greenspan K, Schildkraut JJ, Gordon EK, et al: Catecholamine metabolism in affective disorders—III. MHPG and other catecholamine metabolites in patients treated with lithium carbonate. J Psychiat Res 7:171–183, 1970
239. Pickar D, Sweeney DR, Maas JW, et al: Primary affective disorder, clinical state change, and MHPG excretion: A longitudinal study. Arch Gen Psychiatry 35:1378–1383, 1978
240. Cobbin D, Requin-Blow B, Williams LR, et al: Urinary MHPG levels and tricyclic antidepressant selection. Arch Gen Psychiatry 36:1111–1115, 1979
241. Hollister LE, Davis KL, Berger PA: Subtypes of depression based on excretion of MHPG and response to nortriptyline. Arch Gen Psychiatry 37:1107–1110, 1980
242. Gaertner HJ, Krueter F, Scharek G, et al: Do urinary MHPG and plasma drug

levels correlate with response to amitriptyline therapy. Psychopharmacology 76:236–239, 1982
243. Shopsin B, Wilk S, Sathananthan G, et al: Catecholamines and affective disorders revisited: A critical assessment. J Nerv Ment Dis 158:369-383, 1974
244. Prange AJ, Wilson IC, Knox AE, et al: Thyroid–imipramine clinical and chemical interaction: Evidence for a receptor deficit in depression. J Psychiat Res 9:187–205, 1972
245. Shopsin B, Wilk S, Gershon S: Collaborative psychopharmacologic studies exploring catecholamine metabolism in psychiatric disorders. In Usdin E, Snyder S (eds): Frontiers in Catecholamine Metabolism–Third International Catecholamine Symposium New York, Pergamon Press, 1973
246. Sacchetti E, Smeraldi E, Cagnasso P, et al: MHPG, amitriptyline and affective disorders: A longitudinal study. Int Pharmacopsychiatry 11:157–162, 1976
247. Coppen A, Rama Rao VA, Ruthven CRJ, et al: Urinary 4-hydroxy-3-methoxyphenylglycol is not a predictor for clinical response to amitriptyline in depressive illness. Psychopharmacology 64:94–97, 1979
248. Steiner M, Radwan M, Elizur A, et al: Urinary 3-methoxy-4-hydroxyphenylglycol (MHPG) excretion in depression. Japan J Exp Med 49:95–99, 1979
249. Spiker DG, Edwards D, Hanin I, et al: Urinary MHPG and clinical response to amitriptyline in depressed patients. Am J Psychiatry 137:1183–1187, 1980
250. Veith RC, Bielski RJ, Bloom V, et al: Urinary MHPG excretion and treatment with desipramine or amitriptyline: Prediction of response, effect of treatment, and methodological hazards. J Clin Psychopharmacology 3:18–27, 1983
251. Beckmann H, Murphy DI: Phenylzine in depressed patients: Effects on urinary MHPG excretion in relation to clinical response. Neuropsychobiology 3:49–55, 1977
252. Blackwell B: Current psychiatric research: MHPG in Depression. Psychiat Opinion 16:2,47,1979
253. Beckmann H, Goodwin FK: Urinary MHPG in subgroups of depressed patients and normal controls. Neuropsychobiology 6:91–100, 1980
254. Rosenbaum AH, Schatzberg AF, Maruta T, et al: MHPG as a predictor of antidepressant response to imipramine and maprotiline. Am J Psychiatry 137: 1090–1092, 1980
255. Schatzberg AF, Orsulak PJ, Rosenbaum AH, et al: Toward a biochemical classification of depressive disorders: IV. Pretreatment urinary MHPG levels as predictors of antidepressant response to imipramine. Commun Psychopharmacol 4:441–445, 1980
256. Maitre L, Waldmeier PC, Greengrass PM, et al: Maprotiline–its position as an antidepressant in the light of recent neuropharmacological and neurobiochemical findings. J Int Med Res 3(suppl2):2–15, 1975
257. Waldmeier PC, Baumann P, Greengrass PM, et al: Effects of chlomipramine and other tricyclic antidepressants on biogenic amine uptake and turnover. Postgrad Med J 52(suppl 3):33–39, 1976
258. Maas JW: Neurotransmitters and depression: Too much, too little, or too unstable? Trends in Neurosci 2:306–308, 1979
259. Schatzberg AF, Orsulak PJ, Rosenbaum AH, et al: Toward a biochemical classification of depressive disorders, V: Heterogeneity of unipolar depressions. Am J Psychiatry 139:471–475, 1982
260. Kety SS: Brain amines and affective disorders. In Ho BT, McIsaac WM (eds): Brain Chemistry and Mental Disease. New York, Plenum Press, 1971

261. Mendels J, Frazer A: Reduced central serotonergic activity in mania: Implications for the relationship between depression and mania. Brit J Psychiat 126:241–248, 1975
262. Ridges AP, Bishop FM, Goldberg IJL, et al: Urine amine metabolites in depression: A combined biochemical and general practice study: II. Biochemical aspects. J Int Med Res 8(suppl 3):37–44, 1980
263. Pearce JB: Fenfluramine in mania. Lancet 1:427, 1973
264. Murphy DL, Salter S, De La Vega CE, et al: The serotonergic neurotransmitter system in the affective disorders—A preliminary evaluation of the antidepressant and antimanic effects of fenfluramine. In Deniker P, Radouco-Thomas C, Villeneuve A (eds): Neuro-Psychopharmacology, Vol 1. Proceedings of the Tenth Congress of the Collegium Internationale Neuro-Psychopharmacologium. Oxford, Pergamon Press, 1978
265. Cole JO: Fenfluramine. In Cole JO (ed): Psychopharmacology Update. Lexington, Mass, The Collamore Press, 1980
266. Tissot R: The common pathophysiology of monoaminergic psychoses: A new hypothesis. Neuropsychobiology 1:243–260, 1975
267. Potter WZ, Calil HM, Extein I, et al: Specific norepinephrine and serotonin uptake inhibitors in man: A crossover study with pharmacokinetic, biochemical, neuroendocrine and behavioral parameters. Acta Psychiatr Scand 63 (suppl 290):152–170, 1981
268. Potter WZ, Calil HM, Extein I, et al: Crossover study of zimelidine and desipramine in depression: Evidence for amine specificity. Psychopharm Bull 17: 26–29, 1981
269. Siwers B, Ringberger VA, Tuck JR, et al: Initial clinical trial based on biochemical methodology of zimelidine (a serotonin uptake inhibitor) in depressed patients. Clin Pharmacol Ther 21:194–200, 1977
270. Coppen A: Indoleamines and affective disorders. J Psychiat Res 9:163–171, 1972
271. Kragh-Sorensen P, Hansen CE, Baastrup PC: Relationship between antidepressant effect and plasma level of nortriptyline: Clinical studies. Pharmakopsychiatr Neuropsychopharmakol 9:27–32, 1976
272. Glassman AH, Perel JM, Shostak M, et al: Clinical implications of imipramine plasma levels for depressive illness. Arch Gen Psychiatry 34:197–204, 1977
273. Carroll BJ, Greden JF, Haskett R, et al: Neurotransmitter studies of neuroendocrine pathology in depression. Acta Psychiatr Scand 61(suppl 280): 183–199, 1980
274. Davis KL, Hollister LE, Mathe AA. et al: Neuroendocrine and neurochemical measurements in depression. Am J Psychiatry 138:1555–1562, 1981
275. Zis AP, Goodwin FK: Novel antidepressants and the biogenic amine hypothesis of depression: The case for iprindole and mianserin. Arch Gen Psychiatry 36:1097–1107, 1979
276. Sabelli HC: A pharmacological strategy for the study of central modulator linkages. In Wortis J (ed): Recent Advances in Biological Psychiatry, Vol. 6. New York, Plenum Press, 1964
277. Fischer E, Ludmer RI, Sabelli HC: The antagonism of phenylethylamine to catecholamines on mouse motor activity. Presented at the Proceedings of the Third International Pharmacological Congress, Sao Paulo, July 24–30, 1966
278. Fischer E, Ludmer RI, Sabelli HC: The antagonism of phenylethylamine to catecholamines on mouse motor activity. Acta Physiol Latinoam 17:15–21, 1967

279. Maas JW: Clinical implications of pharmacological differences among antidepressants. In Lipton MA, DiMascio A, Killam KF (eds): Psychopharmacology: A Generation of Progress. New York, Raven Press, 1978
280. Maas JW, Dekirmenjian H, Fawcett JA: Catecholamine metabolism and stress. Nature 230:330–331, 1971
281. Redmond DE: New and old evidence for the involvement of a brain norepinephrine system in anxiety. In Fann WE, Karacan I, Pokorny AD, et al (eds): Phenomenology and Treatment of Anxiety. New York, Spectrum Publications, Inc., 1979
282. Cannon WB: Bodily Changes in Pain, Fear and Rage. New York, Appleton, 1915
283. Cannon WB: The James-Lange theory of emotions: A critical examination and an alternative theory. Am J Psychol 39:106–124, 1927
284. Everett GM, Tomas JEP: Mode of action of Rauwolfia alkaloids and motor activity. In Masserman J (ed): Biological Psychiatry. New York, Grune and Stratton, 1959
285. Berger PA, Barchas JD: Biochemical hyoptheses of affective disorders. In Barchas JD, Berger PA, Ciarenello RD, et al (eds): Psychopharmacology: From Theory to Practice. New York, Oxford University Press, 1977
286. Sweeney DR, Maas JW, Heninger GR: State anxiety and urinary MHPG. Psychosom Med 38:57, 1977
287. Sweeney DR, Maas JW, Heninger GR: State anxiety, physical activity, and urinary 3-methoxy-4-hydroxyphenylglycol excretion. Arch Gen Psychiatry 35:1418–1423, 1978
288. Post RM, Lake CR, Jimerson DC, et al: CSF norepinephrine in affective illness. In New Research Abstracts No. 24, American Psychiatric Association, 1977
289. Wheatley D: Comparative effects of propranolol and chlordiazepoxide in anxiety states. Brit J Psychiat 115:1411–1412, 1969
290. Stone WN, Glesar GC, Gottschalk LA: Anxiety and beta adrenergic blockade. Arch Gen Psychiatry 29:620–622, 1973
291. Tyrer PJ, Lader MH: Response to propranolol and diazepam in somatic and psychic anxiety. Brit Med J 2:14–16, 1974
292. Kellner R, Collins C, Shulman RS, et al: The short-term antianxiety effects of propranolol HCl. J Clin Pharmacol 14:301–304, 1974
293. Gottschalk LA, Stone WN, Glesar GC: Peripheral versus central mechanisms accounting for antianxiety effects of propranolol. Psychosom Med 36:47–51, 1974
294. Suzman MM: Propranolol in the treatment of anxiety. Postgrad Med J 52 (suppl 4):168–174, 1976
295. Gosling RH: Clinical experience with oxprenolol in treatment of anxiety in the United Kingdom. In Kielholtz P (ed): Beta-Blockers and the Central Nervous System. Baltimore, University Park Press, 1977
296. Lader MH, Tyrer PJ: Central and peripheral effects of propranolol and sotolol in normal human subjects. Brit J Pharmacol 45:557–560, 1972
297. Bonn JA, Turner P, Hicks DC: Beta-adrenergic-receptor blockade with practolol in treatment of anxiety. Lancet 1:814–815, 1972
298. Greenblatt DJ, Shader RI: Pharmacology of anxiety with benzodiazepines and beta-adrenergic blockers. In Lipton MA, DiMascio A, Killam KF (eds): Psychopharmacology: A Generation of Progress, New York, Raven Press, 1978
299. Robinson DS, Nies A, Ravaris CL, et al: The monoamine oxidase inhibitor

phenelzine in the treatment of depressive-anxiety states. Arch Gen Psychiatry 29:407–413, 1973
300. Ravaris CL, Nies A, Robinson DS, et al: A multiple dose, controlled study of phenelzine in depressive-anxiety states. Arch Gen Psychiatry 33:347–350, 1976.
301. Klein DF, Zitrin CM, Woerner MG: Antidepressants, anxiety, panic, and phobia. In Lipton MA, DiMascio A, Killam KF (eds): Psychopharmacology: A Generation of Progress. New York, Raven Press, 1978
302. Zitrin CM, Klein DF, Woerner MG: Behavior therapy, supportive psychotherapy, imipramine, and phobias. Arch Gen Psychiatry 35:307–316, 1978
303. Vetulani J, Sulser F: Action of various antidepressant treatments reduces reactivity of noradrenergic cyclic AMP-generating system in limbic forebrain. Nature 257:495–496, 1975
304. Sulser F, Vetulani J, Mobley PL: Mode of action of antidepressant drugs. Biochem Pharmacol 27:257–261, 1978
305. Sulser F: Pharmacology: Current antidepressants. Psychiatr Ann 10(suppl): 381–386, 1980
306. Nyback, H, Walters JR, Aghajanian GK, et al: Tricyclic antidepressants: Effects on the firing rate of brain noradrenergic neurons. Eur J Pharmacol 32: 302–312, 1975
307. Schultz J: Psychoactive drug effects on a system which generates cyclic AMP in brain. Nature 216:417–418, 1976
308. Osmond H, Smythies J: Schizophrenia: A new approach. J Ment Sci 98:309–315, 1952
309. Friedhoff AJ, Van Winkel E: The characteristics of an amine found in the urine of schizophrenic patients. J Nerv Ment Dis 135:550–555, 1962
310. Oon MCH, Murray RM, Rodnight R, et al: Factors affecting urinary excretion of endogenously formed dimethyltryptamine in normal human subjects. Psychopharmacology 54:171–175, 1977
311. Wyatt RJ, Termini BA, Davis J: Biochemical and sleep studies of schizophrenia: A review of the literature–1960–1970. Schizophrenia Bull 4:10–66, 1971
312. Pollin W, Cardon PV, Kety SS: Effects of amino acid feeding in schizophrenic patients treated with iproniazid. Science 133:104–105, 1961
313. Kety SS: Biochemical hypotheses and studies. In Bellak L, Loeb L (eds): Schizophrenic Syndromes. New York, Grune and Stratton, Inc., 1969
314. Cohen SM, Nichols A, Wyatt R, et al: The administration of methionine to chronic schizophrenic patients: A review of 10 studies. Biol Psychiatry 8: 209–225, 1974
315. Gillin JC, Stoff DM, Wyatt RJ: Transmethylation hypothesis: A review of progress. In Lipton MA, DiMascio A, Killam KF (eds): Psychopharmacology: A Generation of Progress. New York, Raven Press, 1978
316. Kety SS: Summary. The hypothetical relationships between amines and mental illness: A critical synthesis. In Himwich HE, Kety SS, Smythies JR (eds): Amines and Schizophrenia. Oxford, Pergamon Press, 1967
317. Bumpus FM, Page IH: Serotonin and its methylated derivatives in human urine. J Biological Chemistry 212:111–116, 1955
318. Axelrod J: Enzymatic formation of psychotomimetic metabolites from normally occurring compounds. Science 134:343, 1961
319. Axelrod J: The enzymatic N-methylation of serotonin and other amines. J Pharmacol Exp Ther 138:28–33, 1962

320. Fischer E, Fernandez Lagravere TA, Vasquez AJ, et al: A bufotenin-like substance in the urine of schizophrenics. J Nerv Ment Dis 133:441–444, 1961
321. Fischer E, Spatz H: Determination of bufotenin in the urine of schizophrenics. Int J Neuropsychiatry 3:226–228, 1967
322. Fischer E, Spatz H: Quantitative determination of an increased excretion of bufotenin in urine of schizophrenics. Archiv fur Psychiatric and Zeitschrift f.d. ges. Neurologie 211:241–249, 1968
323. Fischer E, Spatz H: Studies on urinary elimination of bufotenin-like substances in schizophrenia. Biol Psychiatry 2:235–241, 1970
324. Fischer E, Vasquez FA, Fernandez TA, et al: Bufotenin in human urine. Lancet 1:890–891, 1961
325. Brune GG, Hohl HH, Himwich HE: Urinary excretion of bufotenin-like substance in psychotic patients. J Neuropsychiatry 5:14–17, 1963
326. Himwich HE, Brune GG: Relationship between indole metabolism and schizophrenic behavior. In Rinkel M (ed): Biological Treatment of Mental Illness. New York, L.C. Page and Company, 1966
327. Tanimukai H, Ginther R, Spaide J, et al: Detection of psychotomimetic N, N-dimethylated indoleamines in the urine of four schizophrenic patients. Brit J Psychiat 117;421–430, 1970
328. Greenberg R: N,N-diemthylated and N,N-diethylated indoleamines in schizophrenia. In Sabelli HC (ed): Chemical Modulation of Brain Function. New York, Raven Press, 1973
329. Corbett L, Christian ST, Morin ED, et al: Hallucinogenic N-methylated and indolealkylamines in the cerebrospinal fluid of psychiatric and control populations. Brit J Psychiat 132, 139–144, 1978
330. Kopin IJ: Tryptophan loading and excretion of 5-hydroxyindoleacetic acid in normal and schizophrenic subjects. Science 129:835–836, 1959
331. Pollin W, Cardon PV, Kety SS: Effects of amino acid feedings in schizophrenic patients treated with iproniazid. Science 133:104–105, 1961
332. Brune CG, Pscheidt GR: Correlations between behavior and urinary excretion of indole amines and catecholamines in schizophrenic patients as affected by drugs. Fed Proc 20:889–893, 1961
333. Brune GG: Tryptophan metabolism in psychoses. In Himwich HE, Kety SS, Smythies JRP (eds): Amines and Schizophrenia. Elmsford, NY, Pergamon Press, 1967
334. Mandell AJ, Spooner CE: Psychochemical research studies in man. Science 162:1442–1453, 1968
335. Matthysse S, Kety SS (eds): Symposium on catecholamines and their enzymes in the neuropathology of schizophrenia, May 18–21, 1973, Strasbourg, France. J Psychiat Res. 11:1–364, 1974
336. Seeman P, Lee T: Brain dopamine receptors in schizophrenia. In the Abstracts of the Proceedings of the 12th CINP Congress, Goteborg, 1980
337. Carlsson A, Lindqvist M: Effect of chlorpromazine or haloperidol on the formation of 3-methoxytryptamine and normetanephrine in mouse brain. Acta Pharmacol Toxicol (Kobenhavn) 20:140–144, 1963
338. Randrup A, Munkvad I: Evidence indicating an association between schizophrenia and dopaminergic hyperactivity in the brain. Orthomol Psychiat 1:2–27, 1972
339. Stevens JR: An anatomy of schizophrenia? Arch Gen Psychiatry 29:177–189, 1973

340. Carlsson A: Antipsychotic drugs, neurotransmitters, and schizophrenia. Am J Psychiatry 135:164–173, 1978
341. Connell PH: Amphetamine Psychosis. London, Oxford University Press, 1958
342. Snyder S: Amphetamine psychosis: A "model" schizophrenia mediated by catecholamines. Am J Psychiatry 130:61–67, 1973
343. Snyder S, Banerjee SP, Yamamura HI, et al: Drugs, neurotransmitters and schizophrenia. Science 184:1243–1253, 1974
344. Snyder SH: The dopamine hypothesis of schizophrenia: Focus on the dopamine receptor. Am J Psychiatry 133:197–202, 1976
345. Janowsky DS, El-Yousef MK, Davis JM, et al: Provocation of schizophrenic symptoms by intravenous administration of methylphenidate. Arch Gen Psychiatry 28:185–191, 1973
346. Janowsky DS, Davis JM: Methylphenidate, dextroamphetamine and levamphetamine. Effects on schizophrenia symptoms. Arch Gen Psychiatry 33:304–308, 1976
347. Segal DS, Janowsky D: Psychostimulant-induced behavior effects: Possible models of schizophrenia. In Lipton MA, DiMascio A, Killam KF (eds): Psychopharmacology: A Generation of Progress, New York, Raven Press, 1978
348. Post RM: Cocaine psychoses: A continuum model. Am J Psychiatry 132: 225–231, 1975
349. Post RM, Kopanda RT: Cocaine, kindling, and psychosis. Am J Psychiatry 133:627–634, 1976
350. Yaryura-Tobias JA, Diamond D, Merlis S: The action of L-dopa in schizophrenic patients. Curr Ther Res. 12:528–581, 1970
351. Angrist BM, Sathananthan G, Gershon S: Behavioral effects of L-dopa in schizophrenia patients. Psychopharmacology 31:1–12, 1973
352. Rifkin A, Quitkin F, Kane J, et al: Are prophylactic antiparkinson drugs necessary? A controlled study of procyclidine withdrawal. Arch Gen Psychiatry 35:483–489, 1978
353. Bowers MB: 5-hydroxyindoleacetic acid (5-HIAA) and homovanillic acid (HVA) following probenecid in acute psychotic patients treated with phenothiazines. Psychopharmacologia 28:309–318, 1973
354. Bowers MB: Central dopamine turnover in schizophrenic syndromes. Arch Gen Psychiatry 31:50–57, 1974
355. Bowers MB: CSF acid monoamine metabolites as a possible reflection of central MAO activity in chronic schizophrenia. Biol Psychiatry 11:245–249, 1976
356. Post RM, Goodwin FK: Time-dependent effects of phenothiazines on dopamine turnover in psychiatric patients. Science 190:488–489, 1975
357. Post RM, Fink E, Carpenter WT, et al: Cerebrospinal fluid amine metabolites in acute schizophrenia. Arch Gen Psychiatry 32:1063–1069, 1975
358. Stein L, Wise CD: Possible etiology of schizophrenia: Progressive damage to the noradrenergic reward system by 6-hydroxydopamine. Science 171:1032–1036, 1971
359. Jimerson D, Gordon EK, Post RM, et al: Central norepinephrine function in man: VMA in the CSF. In The Scientific Proceedings of the American Psychiatric Association, 1975
360. Lake CR, Sternberg D, Van Kammen D, et al: Schizophrenia: Elevated cerebrospinal fluid norepinephrine. Science 207:331–333, 1980

361. Kemali D, Del Vecchio M, Maj M: Increased noradrenaline levels in CSF and plasma of schizophrenic patients. Biol Psychiatry 17:711–717, 1982
362. Berger PA: Biochemistry and the schizophrenias: Old concepts and new hypotheses. J Nerv Ment Dis 169:90–99, 1981
363. Wyatt RJ, Potkin SG, Kleinman JE, et al: The schizophrenia syndrome: Examples of biological tools for subclassification. J Nerv Ment Dis 169:100–112, 1981
364. Aghajanian GK: LSD and CNS transmission. Ann Rev Pharmacol 12:157–168, 1962
365. Freedman DX, Halaris AE: Monoamines and the biological mode of action of LSD at synapses. In Lipton M, DiMascio A, Killam KF (eds): Psychopharmacology: A Generation of Progress. New York, Raven Press, 1978
366. MacKay AVP, Yates CM, Wright A, et al: Regional distribution of monoamines and their metabolites in the human brain. Neurochem Res 30:841–848, 1978
367. Bowers MB: LSD-related states as models of psychosis. In Cole JO, Freedman AM, Friedhoff AJ (eds): Psychopathology and Psychopharmacology. Baltimore, Johns Hopkins Press, 1973
368. Sedvall G, Wade-Helgodt B: A relationship between abnormal 5-HIAA concentrations in the cerebrospinal fluid and family disposition for the disorder in schizophrenic patients. Presented at the 34th Annual Meeting of the Society of Biological Psychiatry, Chicago, Illinois, May 10–13, 1979
369. Potkin SG, Weinberger DR, Linnoila M, et al: Low CSF 5-hydroxyindoleacetic acid in schizophrenic patients with enlarged cerebral ventricles. Am J Psychiatry 140:21–25, 1983
370. Wise, CD, Stein L: Dopamine-beta-hydroxylase deficits in the brains of schizophrenic patients. Science 181:344–347, 1973
371. Farley IJ, Price KS, McCullough E, et al: Norepinephrine in chronic paranoid schizophrenia: Above-normal levels in limbic forebrain. Science 200:456–458, 1978
372. Lee T, Seeman P, Tourtellotte WW, et al: Binding of $^3$H-neuroleptics and $^3$H-apomorphine in schizophrenic brains. Nature 247:897–900, 1978
373. Owen F, Cross AJ, Crow TJ, et al: Decreased dopamine receptor sensitivity in schizophrenia. Lancet 2:223–226, 1978
374. Bird ED, Spokes EGS, Iversen LL: Increased dopamine concentration in limbic areas of brain from patients dying with schizophrenia. Brain 102:347–360, 1979
375. Bird ED, Spokes EG, Barnes J, et al: Increased brain dopamine and reduced glutamic acid decarboxylase activity in schizophrenia and related psychoses. Lancet 2:1157–1159, 1977
376. Kleinman J, Bridge P, Karoum R, et al: Catecholamines and metabolites in the brains of psychotics and normals: Postmortem studies. In Usdin E, Kopin IJ, Barchas J (eds): Catecholamines: Basic and Clinical Frontiers, Vol 2. Proceedings of the Fourth International Catecholamine Symposium. New York, Pergamon Press, 1979
377. Crow TJ, Baker HF, Cross AJ, et al: Monoamine mechanisms in chronic schizophrenia: Postmortem neurochemical findings. Brit J Psychiat 134: 249–256, 1979
378. MacKay AVP, Bird ED, Spokes EG, et al: Dopamine receptors and schizophrenia: Drug effect or illness; Lancet 2:915–916, 1980

379. Carlsson A: The impact of catecholamine research on medical science and practice. In Usdin E, Kopin IJ, Barchas J (eds): Catecholamines: Basic and Clinical Frontiers, Vol 1. Proceedings of the Fourth International Catecholamine Symposium. New York, Pergamon Press, 1979
380. Bird ED, Spokes EG, Iversen LL: Brain norepinephrine and dopamine in schizophrenia. Science 204:93–94, 1979
381. Fischer E, Spatz H, Saavedra JM, et al: Urinary elimination of phenylethylamine. Biol Psychiatry 5:139–147, 1972
382. Wyatt RJ, Gillin JC, Stoff DM, et al: B-phenylethylamine and the neuropsychiatric disturbances. In Usdin E, Hamburg DA, Barchas JD (eds): Neuroregulators and Psychiatric Disorders. New York, Oxford University Press, 1977
383. Sandler M, Reynolds GP: Does phenylethylamine cause schizophrenia? Lancet 1:70–71, 1976
384. Wyatt RJ, Potkin SG, Cannon HE, et al: Phenylethylamine (PEA) and chronic schizophrenia. In Usdin E, Kopin IJ, Barchas J (eds): Catecholamines: Basic and Clinical Frontiers, Vol 2. Proceedings of the Fourth International Catecholamine Symposium. New York, Pergamon Press, 1979
385. Potkin SG, Karoum F, Chuang L-W, et al: Phenylethylamine in chronic paranoid schizophrenia. Science 206:470–471, 1979
386. Jeste DV, Doongaji DR, Panjwani MD, et al: Cross-cultural study of a biochemical abnormality in paranoid schizophrenia. Psychiatry Res 5:341–352, 1981
387. Murphy D, Wyatt RJ: Reduced monoamine oxidase activity in blood platelets from schizophrenic patients. Nature 238:225–226, 1972
388. Borison RL, Havdala HS, Diamond BL: Chronic phenylethylamine stereotypy in rats: A new animal model for schizophrenia? Life Sci 21:117–122, 1977
389. Vasquez AJ, Tomas JEP: Some interactions of nicotine with other drugs upon central nervous function. Ann NY Acad Sci 142:201–215, 1967
390. Sabelli HC, Giardina WJ: The influence of inhibitors of amine metabolism on the effects of serotonin and its metabolites on the photic evoked potential in rabbits. Experientia 27:64–65, 1971
391. Jouvet M: Biogenic amines and the states of sleep. Science 163:32–41, 1969
392. Rothballer AB: The effects of catecholamines on the central nervous system. Pharmacological Reviews 11:494–547, 1959
393. Domino EF: Electroencephalographic and behavioral arousal affects of small doses of nicotine: A neuropsychopharmacological study. Ann NY Acad Sci 142:216–244, 1967
394. Stein L: Neurochemistry of reward and punishment: Some implications for the etiology of schizophrenia. J Psychiat Res 8:345–361, 1968

# Toxicology Evaluation

CHAPTER 4

# Laboratory Procedures Related to the Metals

NEIL B. EDWARDS

## INTRODUCTION

Most physicians can recall from their medical student days a learned professor standing at the lectern and saying, "if you just listen, your patient will tell you what is wrong." Some patients, however, cannot tell their story well. There simply are certain things in a patient's history which no patient no matter how intelligent or well versed would put into his/her "own story." For precisely this reason the review of systems is universally included as part of the medical history to pick up things that are wrong, which the patient has left out of his story. It is then up to the physician to find out how these symptoms are related to the presenting illness. It is our responsibility as physicians to elicit this data and to make sense of it. This is even more starkly the case when one considers the vast array of symptoms produced by disorders of metal metabolism or by metal poisoning. Consequently, any information which is obtained about these elements, in almost all cases, is the responsibility of the physician to elicit from specially designed historical questions and from the laboratory.

Laboratory analysis as an aid to diagnosis in psychiatry is not one of our richer traditions. In most instances, our use of such tests is on a pro forma basis. Consequently, when we admit a patient to the hospital, many psychiatrists do certain laboratory tests because they are required for admission to hospital. Or we order a white blood cell count to make sure that our patient who has now devel-

*Handbook of Psychiatric Diagnostic Procedures,* vol. 1, edited by R. C. W. Hall and T. P. Beresford. 

oped a sore throat is not developing agranulocytosis from the medication we are giving. On the clinical level, our consultation/liaison and biologically oriented colleagues remind us that certain body chemicals when elevated or deficient can cause approximations of some of the syndromes which we are fond of diagnosing. These reminders usually provoke the more observant of us to say somewhat uncomfortably to ourselves something such as "I'll look out for that more closely." Very few of us, however, actually change our diagnostic habits. Such a nonchalant attitude toward laboratory analysis can no longer hold sway in our specialty. This is especially true in the area of metal deficiencies and intoxications where the laboratory is absolutely indispensable. Disorders of metal metabolism (essential and nonessential) often produce syndromes which are either totally or partially psychiatric in their presentation [1].

This chapter deals with the laboratory procedures related to metal disorders. The essential metals are described first, followed by the nonessential metals.

## ESSENTIAL METALS

### Calcium (Ca)

Calcium has long been known to be an important element for man's internal homeostasis. It is essential in bone metabolism and for conduction of nerve impulses. In 1968 Peterson [2] demonstrated that elevated serum Ca is related to a variety of psychiatric disorders ranging from subtle personality changes to psychoses. Gatewood, et al [3] in 1978 noted a similar range of disorders in five cases. Carman and his associates have published a series of articles [4–7] relating both serum Ca and cerebrospinal fluid (CSF) Ca to cyclical affective disorders. These authors have demonstrated transient increases in serum Ca at the onset of agitated psychotic and manic states. Further, they have noted more enduring decreases in cerebrospinal fluid Ca of (1) depressed patients ad they improve and (2) manic and other agitated psychotic patients. Jimerson et al [8] demonstrated similar CSF findings in depressed patients as they improved and significant increases in CSF Ca in schizophrenics recovering from acute psychotic episodes. Weizman et al [9] reported on a series of twelve patients with hypercalcemia secondary to malignancy, seven of whom demonstrated psychiatric symptomatology ranging from mild anxiety and depression to severe depression and organic psychosis. Groat and Mackenzie [10] in 1980 reported a case of mania following intravenous Ca replacement. Decreases in serum Ca have been noted, in 1976, by Paterson [11] to be associated with a variety of psychiatric symptoms ranging from mild anxiety and irritability to severe depression and toxic psychosis. Prolonged decreases of serum Ca have been associated with irreversible dementia [11].

At the present the most useful and practical Ca measurement for the psychiatrist is the screen Ca. This is obtained in most medical centers as part of the routine SMA-12/60. It should be obtained fasting as an additional screening test to the SMA6-60 (glucose, BUN, Na, K, Cl and $CO^2$ profile. Normal serum Ca is 9.0-10.6 mg/dl or 4.5–5.3 mEq/L.[12]

Serum Ca is influenced by many factors. Hypomagnesemia through mechanisms not clearly understood, but probably involving parathyroid hormone, results in hypocalcemia [13–16]. Hypomagnesemia further renders many organisms refractory to parathyroid hormone [13], and hypercalcemia due to hyperparathyroidism results in hypomagnesemia [3]. Hence, paradoxically, low magnesium (Mg) can be associated with either high or low Ca. Of course, hypomagnesemia has its own associated psychiatric symptoms, as we shall see later, and care must be taken to define those related to Ca aberration from those related to hypomagnesemia. Part of this detective process should always include obtaining a serum Mg level in the face of any aberration of serum Ca. Patients on chronic lithium (Li) therapy can develop hypercalcemia presumably due to an ability of this element to produce hyperparathyroidism [17–22]. Although it would be unlikely that a patient's receiving Li would go unnoticed for very long, anything is possible: hence, any patient with hypercalcemia must be asked (hopefully re-asked) about Li therapy. Conversely, since hypercalcemia can produce psychiatric symptomatology resembling both depression and mania it is incumbent upon the physician to obtain a serum Ca in the face of the resurgence of any affective symptoms. Given a hypercalcemic state in such a patient, one is then faced with a vexing clinical question: Is the hyperclacemia producing the affective state a la Peterson [2] and Gatewood [3], or is the hypercalcemia a presage or early accompaniment of a true manic episode as has been observed by more recent authors?[4–7] Two clues can be helpful here: (1) Laboratory values sufficient to cause mania tend to be much higher than those merely accompanying it, and (2) the patient with true mania often has a previous history of affective swings. An important feature of Peterson's study [2] was the finding that the severity of psychiatric symptoms tended to roughly parallel the degree of hypercalcemia. Serum Ca levels between 10.5 and 14.5 mg/dl tended to be associated with subtle personality changes, moderate anxiety, or depression; levels between 12.6 and 16.5 mg/dl were accompanied by more severe affective disturbances; psychoses occurred between 14.6 and 18.0 mg/dl. Parathyroid adenomas often are slowly progressive and thereby increase serum Ca levels over the years. Hence one can easily envisage a patient, over a period of years, going from mild personality changes through neurotic-like symptoms to affective disturbances and/or toxic psychosis. In this light it is important to remember that this progression is extremely rare in functional psychiatric disorders; given such a picture, a serum Ca determination is essential. As Gatewood [3] has pointed out, decreased serum Ca can lead to a similar variety of psychiatric symptom-complexes. These patients tend to have confusion and neuromuscular irritability as part of their presenting picture. It is important to measure serum Ca in demented patients since chronically depressed serum Ca can lead to dementia, sometimes reversible, sometimes not. Finally, serum Ca is elevated in hereditary idiopathic hypercalcemia, presumably a disorder of increased sensitivity to vitamin D: It occurs in infancy and is characterized by mental retardation, elvin facies, and failure to thrive [23].

### Magnesium (Mg)

Magnesium, like Ca, has been known to be an essential element for decades. It is a potent inhibitor of nerve transmission and has been used for many years as an anticonvulsant and antihypertensive agent, especially in toxemia of pregnancy. Hypomagnesemia has been observed as a cause of anxiety, restlessness, depression, and psychotic episodes as early as 1954 [24]. These observations have been replicated by several other authors since then [25,26]. Magnesium deficiency has been demonstrated to occur frequently in chronic alcoholics, especially when delirium tremens is a complicating feature, as noted by Stendig-Lindberg [27], who also observed that the presence of hypomagnesemia in these patients may be a predictor of the later development of various alcoholic encephalopathies. Magnesium deficiency has also been demonstrated to interfere with the growth response produced by thiamine [28]. These separate observations add up to a fairly persuasive argument for a role of Mg in alcoholic encephalopathies, especially Wernicke-Korsakoff syndrome, where the role of thiamine is well known.

The laboratory test for Mg which is of practical interest to psychiatrists is the serum Mg level. No special instructions to the patient are required. Normal values are 1.8-3.0 mg/dl or 1.5-2.5 mEq/L [12].

The complex interrelationships of hypomagnesemia to hypo- and hypercalcemia have already been described. Again, whenever a serum Mg determination is requested from the laboratory, a serum Ca should be done also, and vice versa. Hypomagnesemia may be found in a variety of psychiatric states, notable anxiety, irritability, depression, and toxic psychoses. Usually varying degrees of neuromuscular irritability will be present also, e.g., hyperreflexia, muscle twitches, myoclonic jerks, and even convulsions. The common occurrence of anxiety and hyperreflexia together usually has no specific organic concomitant; however, on occasion, this symptom pair indicates the presence of hypomagnesemia. Serum Mg should be determined in all alcoholics and in all patients with a confusional psychosis even without a clear-cut history of alcoholism, since the tendency for alcohol abusers to minimize their problems is well-known. The presence of hypomagnesemia may be a predictor of future alcoholic encephalopathy [27]. Furthermore Stendig-Lindberg[27] demonstrated that the treatment of these hypomagnesemic patients with Mg replacement may prevent their encephalopathy. Hypermagnesemia does occur, almost always in the presence of compromised renal function and as a result of overzealous treatment of toxemia or constipation. To date, research on a role of hypermagnesemia in psychiatric disorders is highly conflicting [29].

### Copper (Cu)

Hepatolenticular Degeneration (HLD) (Wilson's disease) was first described by Wilson in 1912 [30]. Scheinberg and Sternlieb [30] characterized the disorder as due to a deficiency in ceruloplasmin (the plasma Cu transport protein) and an impairment of liver lysozymal excretion of Cu into the bile. This results in decreased serum Cu. Psychiatric symptomatology early in the disorder was recognized by Wilson in his original description [30] and has been described by many writers since [32-35]. Psychiatric manifestations of the disease are protean, leading Scheinberg [33] to state that HLD can mimic practically any psychiatric disorder. Serum Cu has been reported to be elevated in schizophrenia [36-38] and in autistic children [39]. CSF Cu has been reported to be lower in a group of schizophrenic patients compared with six normal controls [40]. Very low serum Cu levels have been demonstrated in Menkes' kinky-hair disease first described by Menkes and his colleagues in 1962 [41]. This disease is found in infants, usually in the first month of life, and is characterized by weak Moro reflexes, poor head control, seizures, severe mental retardation, and white stubby hair. The laboratory assay of most interest to the psychiatrist is the serum Cu level, normal being 70-140 mg/dl for males and 85-155 mg/dl for females [12]. Finally, 24-hour urinary amino acid nitrogen may be elevated in patients with Wilson's disease: The normal level for amino acid nitrogen is 50-200 mg/24 hr [12].

The tetrad of decreased serum Cu, decreased serum ceruloplasmin, increased 24-hour urinary Cu, and increased urinary 24-hour amino acid nitrogen excretion is diagnostic of Wilson's disease (HLD). This set of laboratory assays is extremely important to keep in mind since the psychiatric symptomatology is so varied and often precedes any physical symptomatology [1,31,32]. Adding to the importance of using these laboratory assays when indicated is the fact that unrelated HLD is invariably fatal, whereas treatment with potassium sulfide and pencillamine results in amelioration of symptoms and significant prolongation of life.

Serum Cu should be measured in any infant who is failing to meet developmental landmarks, particularly if the hair is white and kinky. Although indispensable for diagnosing Menkes' kinky-hair disease, knowledge of the serum Cu cannot materially affect prognosis. Treatment with Cu replacement has been very discouraging to date [42,43], and the outcome of the disorder is invariably fatal.

The findings of elevated serum Cu and depressed CSF Cu in some schizophrenic patients are of considerable academic interest. Cu is essential for the action of dopamine-β-hydroxylase (DBH): Further studies on CSF Cu in schizophrenia may prove exciting, since reduced DBH activity is postulated by some as being instrumental in the development of schizophrenia [35].

### Zinc (Zn)

The evidence for the importance of Zn in human homeostasis has been increasing over the past ten years. This element is essential for the function of more than 50 enzymes [45,46]. Zinc deficiency has been demonstrated to produce a large number of behavioral symptoms in humans, including apathy, mental retardation, psychosis, and paranoia [47]. Acrodermatitis enteropathica was demonstrated by Moynihan in 1976 [48] to be due to Zn deficiency. Psychiatric symptoms in this disorder include tearfulness, irritability, lack of smiling and laughing, and gaze aversion in infancy [48], and cyclical depressions if the patient survives into adulthood [49]. Decreased serum Zn has been associated with growth retardation, hypogonadism, hypogeusia (impaired taste), and hyposmia (impaired smell) [1]. Decreased learning ability has been demonstrated in Zn deficient rats and their offspring [50], and lowered Zn levels have been demonstrated in children with learning disability [39]. Zn deficiency has been implicated in impotence in male patients on renal dialysis [51,52]. Although Zn seems to have no CNS toxicity [47], excess CNS zinc has been found in the brains of patients with Pick's disease, especially in the hippocampus [53]. Zn antagonizes the absorption of Cu from the gut and has been suggested as a useful treatment in Wilson's disease [54]. Casper and his colleagues [46] have recently (1978) found significantly decreased serum Zn in 24 female patients with anorexia nervosa. This is by no means a reliable finding in this disorder. Finally, zinc deficiency has been demonstrated in cirrhotic alcoholic patients [55,56]. All of the discoveries cited above regarding zinc's role in various pathological states have been made in the past decade.

The laboratory assay of interest to psychiatrists is the serum Zn level. The normal level is 50–150 m/dl [12]: No special instructions to the patient are necessary. Hair Zn levels can also be obtained, the normal being 125 per mg/g of hair. A low serum Zn level in an infant who displays gaze aversion, lack of smiling and laughing, excessive tearfulness, plus an exfoliative bullous rash over the extremities, perianally and periorally, and chronic severe diarrhea is diagnostic of acrodermatitis enteropathica. Adult patients who have cyclical affective disorder and a history of any of the symptoms and signs of acrodermatitis enteropathica during infancy should have a serum Zn level drawn. In the infant Zn supplementation is usually lifesaving [48] and, in the adult, it relieves the affective disorder [49]. Zinc supplementation in male dialysis patients experiencing impotence has been reported to reverse their sexual dysfunction [51]. Hypozincemia in any of the other disorders noted (schizophrenia, Laennec's cirrhosis, and anorexia nervosa) is at present of considerable academic but little practical interest.

### Iron (Fe)

The importance of iron for the formation and function of hemoglobin is well known. Symptoms resulting from Fe deficiency, whether from inadequate dietary intake or blood loss, are entirely referable to the decreased ability of the blood to carry oxygen, in other words, to the anemia thereby produced. Inherited disorders resulting in low usable Fe, i.e., the hemoglobinopathies, also result in anemia with similar consequences. The easy fatigability, weakness, tingling of the extremities, faintness, and spots before the eyes seen with anemias are often also seen in depressions and hysteria [57]. Idiopathic hemochromatosis and exogneous Fe overload (e.g., due to Bantusiderosis and hemochromatosis secondary to chronic, heavy ingestion of iron-rich wines in alcoholics) result in deposition of large amounts of Fe in various tissues, notably liver, pancreas, and gonads [23]. Psychiatric symptoms are referable to the disorders produced by failure of these organs. Weakness, lassitude, loss of libido, and depression can be early symptoms associated with anemia. Jacobs, in 1977 [58], Leibel, in 1977 [59], and Oski and Honig, in 1978 [60], found lowered work and intellectual performance in mildly anemic subjects.

Anemia will be quickly revealed by a lowered hemoglobin or hematocrit. Normal values for hemoglobin are 1.35–18.0 g/dl for males and 12.0-16.0 g/dl for females [12]. In practice, the hemoglobin and hematocrit are usually obtained as part of the complete blood count (CBC). Other lab values which may be of interest in anemia are mean cell volume (MCV), mean cell hemoglobin (MCH), and mean cell hemoglobin concentration (MCHC). All of these (MCV, MCH, and MCHC) are decreased in Fe deficiency anemia, a microcytic, hypochromic anemia. Serum Fe is decreased and Fe-binding capacity increased in Fe deficiency anemia: Normal values are 50–150 mg/dl for the former and 250–370 mg/dl for the latter [23]. In hemochromatosis a number of laboratory values are askew, notably serum Fe and serum ferritin, both of which are elevated. Normal values for serum Fe are cited above: The normal range for serum ferritin is 10–200 mg/dl.

A screening hemoglobin and hematocrit should be obtained on all patients complaining of fatigue, lassitude, and depression. Similar symptoms can be early signs of hemochromatosis: usually other stigmata of the disease will be present, e.g., brown skin pigmentation or symptoms referable to pancretic, hepatic, or gonadal function. If in doubt, a serum Fe and serum ferritin should be obtained: The former often is 2X normal; the latter may be increased *thirty-fold* [23].

### Manganese (Mn)

During the past decade Mn has been found to be essential for the function of several human enzymes [45,61,62]. These enzymes subserve such important metabolic functions as oxidative phosphorylation, fatty acid metabolism, and the synthesis of proteins, mucopolysaccharides, and cholesterol [23]. Despite all of this, no deficiency state, either hereditary or acquired, has been established. Neither has an hereditary excess state been reported. However, an acquired toxic condition has been described and is known aptly as manganic madness. The psychiatric picture resembles disorganized schizophrenia complete with hallucinations, delusions, explosive and inappropriate laughing and crying, and compulsive acts [63]. Some patients display a milder psychiatric picture with gradual onset of fatigue and trouble concentrating [64], and some atypical organic psychosis [65,66]. Freqently the psychiatric picture is followed by a disorder indistinguishable from Parkinson's disease, with masked facies, bradykinesia, rigidity, and dystonia [63].

The serum Mn level is the laboratory value of interest, normal being less than 1 PPM. In manganic madness the serum level is dramatically increased. Hair levels may also be elevated. Normally there is no Mn in the hair.

## NONESSENTIAL METALS

### Lithium (Li)

Our use of Li in psychiatry forms the basis for perhaps the one exception to the general rule stated in the introduction to this chapter, viz., that our interest in laboratory studies has been, at best, peripheral to the mainstream of our thinking. From the very onset of the therapeutic use of this metal in the treatment of the cyclical affective disorders, laboratory measurement has been an integral part of its use because (1) the element is quite toxic, and (2) its therapeutic margin is narrow.

In 1949 Cade in Australia [67] successfully treated ten manic patients with Li. In the same year several deaths were reported in the United States in cardiac patients using lithium chloride as a salt substitute. These deaths putatively were due to the ingestion of toxic amounts of the substance by these patients. Despite Cade's findings, and despite many positive reports from other countries as to its efficacy over the ensuing years, Li was eschewed in this country for 20 years because of the deaths attributed to it in 1949. In 1970 Li was finally approved in this country for the treatment of acute mania and in 1974 for the prophylaxis of recurrent manic episodes. There is little, if any, doubt as to the effectiveness of Li in the treatment of mania and the prevention of future manic episodes, but its value in unipolar affective illness and in preventing depression in bipolar patients remains a matter of significant controversy [68]. It has also been purported to be effective in schizoaffective disorders [69], chronic alcoholism with depression [70,71], impulsive aggression [72], cluster headaches [70,73], hyperthyroidism [74,75], neutropenia secondary to chemotherapy [76], and the neutropenia of Felty's syndrome [77].

The laboratory assay of interest to psychiatrists is the serum Li level. The normal serum Li level is zero [12]. The therapeutic range is 0.6–1.4 mEq/L [22]. Jefferson and Greist [78] suggest 1.0–1.4 mEq/L for maintenance. Some patients may be effectively maintained on lower levels (0.4–0.8 mEq/L [78], especially if they experience mental dulling or organic brain syndrome secondary to the medication. The serum Li must be drawn at least 12 hours after the last dose and care must be taken to insure against red blood cell hydrolysis [12].

The serum Li level must be monitored in patients in Li therapy for two important reasons, (1) to gauge therapeutic effectiveness, and (2) to guard against toxicity. I shall discuss these in turn and in regard to only the treatment of those disorders in which Li has proven effectiveness both as a therapeutic and prophylactic agent, viz., the bipolar affective disorders.

Different formulae have been proposed for initiation of Li therapy. Cooper and his colleagues, in 1973 [79], proposed a means for determining the daily dosage after giving a single priming dose of 600 mg of lithium carbonate ($Li_2Co_3$). If in 24 hours the serum Li level was less than 0.05 mEq/L the required dosage was 1200 mg t.i.d.; a serum level of 0.05–0.09 mEq/l predicted a dose of 900 mg t.i.d.; 0.10–0.14 mEq/L, 600 mg t.i.d.; 0.15–0.19, 300 mg q.i.d.; 0.20–0.23 mEq/L, 300 mg t.i.d.; 0.24–0.30, 300 mg b.i.d.; and more than 0.30, 300 mg b.i.d. Jefferson and Greist [78] recommended 1200–1800 mg per day as the starting dose in acute mania but caution that this must be individualized. Of course, one can be considerably more aggressive in starting Li therapy on an inpatient basis because (1) serum levels can be more closely monitored, and (2) the clinical situation is usually more urgent. For inpatients, I usually obtain serum Li levels three times weekly until a therapeutic level is established. Once the patient reaches a therapeutic level, some adjustment of the dosage downward is often needed to avoid "over-shooting." After stabilization of the therapeutic level, I then obtain levels weekly until the patient has been clinically stable for at least a month. After that, levels can be obtained every one to three months depending on the state of the affective disorder and the presence of any other medical problems which might complicate treatment such as thyroid, cardiac, or renal disease, diuretic therapy, salt restriction, etc. On an outpatient basis, one can proceed somewhat more leisurely. Hence, most patients can be started on 900–1200 mg of $Li_2CO_3$ a day with weekly checks of the serum level. After a therapeutic level is obtained the level can be checked monthly for a few months, and then every one to three months as outlined above.

Acute toxicity due to Li is rarely encountered below serum levels of 1.5, but has been reported [80]. Mild toxicity occurs at levels of 1.5–2.5 mEq/L, serious intoxication between 2.5–3.5 mEq/L and life-threatening toxicity at levels greater than 3.5 mEq/L [22]. Toxic symptoms are referable to the nervous sytem, the GI tract, and the cardiovascular system. From the neuromuscular standpoint, patients may proceed from a fine tremor of the hands through hyperreflexia and myoclonic jerks to grand mal seizures and finally coma and death; a confusional state may be present at any stage in this progression; also dysarthria, nystagmus, and ataxia are frequently seen. Nausea, vomiting, and diarrhea are the usual toxic GI symptoms. Cardiovascular symptoms include hypotension and various arrhythmias, probably secondary to sinus node dysfunction [81,82]. Lithium is reabsorbed in the kidney by the proximal tubule as is Na; when Na is less available for reabsorption at the proximal tubule, as in the cases of low salt diets, excessive salt loss due to hot temperatures and/or heavy exercise, and the use of salt-losing diuretics, Li is preferentially reabsorbed thus enhancing the possibility of toxicity. When a patient must be put on a low salt diet or a salt-losing diuretic, or is likely to lose large amounts of salt through heavy daily sweating, the Li dosage may need to be adjusted downward and more frequent serum Li levels drawn.

Whether or not chronic Li therapy can lead to renal insufficiency through interstitial fibrosis is a controversial issue [83–85]. Nonetheless, few authors recommend more caution than a serum creatinine every few months. Certainly a serum creatinine should be obtained before initiation of lithium therapy and periodically thereafter since any compromise in renal function, whatever the cause, can result in enhanced probability of Li toxicity. Lithium also causes diabetes insipidus, with resultant inability of the kidney to concentrate the urine [83–85]. This is an innocent disorder and usually disappears with discontinuation of Li, but it has been noted to persist for months or even years [83]. Lithium also causes hypothyroidism in some patients and goiter in others; elevation of TSH is a frequent finding in Li-treated patients. Vestergaard and his associates [85] recommend that TSH be determined every six months in patients on Li therapy. It is also a good idea to determine TSH, $T_3$, and $T_4$ before beginning Li therapy and every six months to a year thereafter. If a patient becomes clinically hypothyroid during Li therapy this may present as a depressive disorder thus confusing the picture; thyroid replacement would be recognized here rather than any change in the patient's psychotropic drugs. As mentioned previously, Li can produce hyperparathyroidism with consequent hypercalcemia [17-22]. The many psychiatric pictures which can be produced by hypercalcemia, including depressed and manic-like states, can mimic recrudescences in the affective illness and hence confuse the picture. Therefore in the face of an apparent return of the affective illness one must obtain a serum Ca (and Mg).

### Aluminum (Al)

Elevated levels of this element in the dialysate of patients on renal dialysis have been implicated repeatedly in dialysis dementia over the past six years [86–90]. Also, aluminum hydroxide and aluminum carbonate preparations are given orally to patients with chronic renal failure to maintain normal serum phosphate levels [89].

Increased brain Al has been posited as having an etiological significance in Alzheimer's disease by Crapper et al., in 1975 [91], and Duckett, in 1976 [92]. However, McDermott, in 1977 [93], could find no difference in brain Al levels between normal and Alzheimer patients.

The laboratory value of interest for this element is serum Al. The normal level for serum Al is 19 mg/dl [94].

Serum levels of Al in dialysis dementia may reach 230–550 mg/dl [94]. The disorder is always fatal with no treatment, and frequently so even after withdrawal from the Al source(s) [89].

## Lead (Pb)

Lead intoxication typically produces encephalopathy in children and peripheral neuropathy in adults. In 1972 Bryce-Smith [95] asserted that 25% of children with one episode of lead intoxication will display mental retardation later, 100% if there is more than one episode. Numerous studies have shown deficits in children with blood levels not classically thought to be toxic (40–70 mg/dl) [1]: Learning disability, mental retardation, hyperkinesis, and deficits in fine and gross motor movements have all been observed.

Whole blood Pb level is the important measurement, although coproporphyrin III is frequently present in the urine of Pb-intoxicated patients. "Normal" whole blood levels range from 0–50 mg/dl, with 60–70 mg/dl being the area above which intoxication is generally accepted to be present.

It is important to keep in mind that recent evidence suggests that levels above 40 mg/dl may be quite dangerous, especially to children. It is important also to recall that Pb is excreted *very* slowly (three times more slowly than it is absorbed): prior to excretion it is stored in bone from which it can be re-released in large quantities, especially in the face of acute infection or alcoholic sprees. Therefore a patient previously "effectively treated" who has normal blood levels one day may be toxic the next. This can occur months or even years after blood levels have returned to normal.

From the above it is clear that Pb levels should be checked in children who display mental retardation, learning disability, or hyperkinesis or who have difficulty with fine and/or gross motor development. Any patient with a previous history of intoxication should have levels redrawn if acute illness or alcoholism ensues, especially if any sings of toxicity are present. Removal of the patient from the source of ingestion will result in a rapid shift of most of the Pb into bone with alleviation of symptoms.

## Mercury (Hg)

This metal is toxic in any form in which it exists, elemental inorganic salts and organomercurials. Elemental and organomercurial poisoning tend to result in syndromes of psychiatric importance. Commonly seen is a classical depression complete with loss of energy, loss of interests, social withdrawal and interpersonal irritability [1]. A peculiar oversensitivity and proclivity to embarrassment are often seen as well as a tendency for sweating and blushing (erethism). Hallucinations and delusions may occur. The phrase "mad as a hatter" stems from the frequent occurrences of psychosis in people working in the felting industry where organomercurials are used.

The critical laboratory assay for Hg intoxication is 24-hour urine excretion with toxicity appearing in the range of 30–100 mg/24 hr and above [12]. Identification of the disorder is critical since it is frequently fatal and treatment is often effective. Penicillamine is useful in treatment of elemental mercury poisoning and BAL in intoxication by inorganic salts. Organomercurials are stored in the brain and are not removed by chelating agents. Hence the treatment in this case is removal from the source and "wait and see": The latter can take a long time and be quite discouraging, chronic morbidity and death being frequent.

### Thallium (Tl)

Thallium does not normally appear in human tissues in any appreciable quantities, but when it does it is highly toxic. Before 1934, when Munch reported 778 cases of poisoning with a 6% death rate [96], it was commonly used as a depilatory agent, especially for treatment of ringworm of the scalp. In the United States the use of Tl has been restricted to industrial pesticides, but in many other countries there are no such restrictions so intoxication still occurs with fair frequency. Psychiatric symptoms are frequent and include poor concentration, irritability, somnolence, fatigue, anorexia, psychosis, and organic brain syndrome. Neurological symptoms can be protean and severe leading to convulsions, coma, and death. Tl is accumulated in all tissues and causes direct damage to all. Hence, death can occur from renal, hepatic, cardiovascular, or CNS failure. Alopecia occurs 1-2 weeks after exposure and hence is not a useful diagnostic or prognostic sign as the disorder progresses quite rapidly.

Diagnosis depends on demonstration of Tl in blood, urine, or stool. The disorder is so protean as to be almost totally nonspecific (and therefore nondiagnostic) from a clinical point of view. Even the alopecia which *is* more specific occurs in patients already on the road to recovery. Hence the laboratory and a careful environmental history are absolutely essential.

### Bismuth (Bi)

Bismuth intoxication has been reported as a result of treatment with various medications: bismuth subgallate used orally in the regulation of colostomies [97], bismuth subnitrate used in some constipation preparations [98], and Bi-containing skin-lightening creams [99]. All of these reports have been published in the last eight years and all in Europe [100]. Organic hallucinosis is a frequent feature as are various other neurologic signs ranging from intention tremor to seizures.

The finding of Bi in blood or urine is diagnostic: Normally human tissues contain none or only trace quantities of the element. In cases of intoxication, blood levels have ranged from 100-2900 mg/L, mean levels being 600-700 mg/L [100].

A careful medication history plus blood Bi level are essential for diagnosing this rare but often lethal disorder. Removal from the source often results in recovery. Death, when it occurs, is secondary to the encephalopathy.

## CONCLUSIONS

Most of the laboratory studies I have outlined in this chapter are not, and should not be, carried out on most psychiatric patients. In most instances the diagnosis will depend on maintaining a high index of suspicion and obtaining a very careful and thorough history: Thus we are led to appropriate laboratory procedures. However, there are some laboratory procedures which should be carried out on most patients. These would include: CBC; SMA6-60 and 12-60; and serum Mg. Of course, when organic brain disease is present, further screening for various metal disorders should be done. However, this finding can by no means be a limiting factor; the physician must use his best diagnostic skills, the full range of literature available to him, and the laboratory to rule in or out these uncommon but important disorders.

## REFERENCES

1. Edwards NB: Mental disturbances related to metals. In Hall RCW: Psychiatric Presentations of Medical Illness: Somatopsychic Disorders. New York, Spectrum Publications, pp. 283–308, 1980
2. Peterson P: Psychiatric disorders in primary hyperparathyroidism. J Clin Endocrinol 28:1491–1495, 1968
3. Gatewood JW, Organ CH, Jr, Mead BT: Mental changes associated with hyperparathyroidism. Am J Psychiatry 132:129–132, 1975
4. Carman JS, Wyatt JR: Calcium: Bivalent cation in the bivalent psychoses. Biol Psychiatry 14:195–235, 1979
5. Carman JS, Post RM, Runkle DC, et al: Increased serum calcium and phosphorous with the "switch" into manic or excited psychotic states. Br J Psychiatry 135:55–61, 1979
6. Carman JS, Wyatt RJ: Calcium: pacesetting the periodic psychoses. Am J Psychiatry 136:1035–1039, 1979
7. Carman JS, Wyatt RJ: Use of calcitonin in psychotic agitation or mania. Arch Gen Psychiatry 36:72–75, 1979
8. Jimerson DC, Post RM, Carman JS, et al: CSF Calcium: Clinical correlates in affective illness and schizophrenia. Biol Psychiatry 14:37–51, 1979
9. Weizman A, Eldar M, Shoenfeld Y, et al: Hypercalcaemia-induced psychopathology in malignant diseases. Br J Psychiatry 135:363–366, 1979
10. Groat D, Mackenzie T: The appearance of mania following intravenous calcium replacement. J Nerv Ment Dis 168:562–563, 1980
11. Paterson CR: Hypocalcemia: Differential diagnosis and investigation. Ann Clin Biochem 13:578–584, 1976
12. Todd-Stanford's Clinical Diagnosis by Laboratory Methods. Davidson I, Henry JB (eds) 15th Edition. Philadelphia, WB Saunders, 1974
13. Shils ME: Magnesium deficiency and calcium and parathyroid hormone interrelations. In Prasad AS, Oberleas D (eds): Trace Elements in Human Health and Disease, II. New York, Academic Press, 1976
14. Nordio S, Donath A, Macagno F, Gattis R: Chronic hypomagnesemia with

magnesium dependent hypocalcemia, I: A New Syndrome with Intestinal Magnesium Malabsorption. ACTA Paediat Scand 60:441–448, 1971
15. Lombeck I, Ritzl R, Schnippering HG, et al: Primary hypomagnesemia. Z. Kinderheilk 118:249–258, 1975
16. Madelle R, Waterhouse C, Hahan TJ: Vitamin D resistance in magnesium deficiency. Am J Clin Nutrition 29:854–858, 1976
17. Herman SP: Lithium, hypercalcemia, and hyperparathyroidism. Biol Psychiatry 16:593–595, 1981
18. Davis BM, Pfefferbaum A, Krutzik S, et al: Lithium's effect on parathyroid hormone. Am J Psychiatry 138:489–492, 1981
19. Fu-Hsiung S, Sheppard JF: Lithium-induced hyperparathyroidism: An alteration of the "set-point." Anns Int Med 96:63–65, 1982
20. Rothman M: Acute hyperparathyroidism in a patient after initiation of lithium therapy. Am J Psychiatry 139:362–363, 1982
21. Franks RD, Dubovsky SL, Lifshitz M, et al: Long-term lithium carbonate therapy causes hyperparathyroidism. Arch Gen Psychiatry 39:1074–1077, 1982
22. Lewis DA: Lithium in internal medicine and psychiatry: An outline. J Clin Psychiatry 43:314–320, 1982
23. Harrison's Principles of Internal Medicine, Ninth Edition. Isselbacher KJ, Adams RD, Braunwald E, et al (eds). New York, McGraw-Hill, 1980
24. Flink EB, Stutzman Fl, Anderson AR, et al: Magnesium deficiency after prolonged parenteral fluid administration and after chronic alcoholism complicated by delerium tremens. J Lab Clin Med 43:167–183, 1954
25. Fishman RA: Neurological aspects of magnesium metabolism. Arch Neurol 12:562–569, 1965
26. Hall RCW, Joffe JR: Hypomagnesemia: Physical and psychiatric symptoms. JAMA 224:1749–1751, 1973
27. Stendig-Lindberg G: Hypomagnesemia and local encephalopathies. ACTA Psychiatry Scand 50:465–480, 1974
28. Zieve L, Doizaki WM, Stenroos LE: Effect of magnesium deficiency on growth response to thiamine in thiamine-deficient rats. J Lab Clin Med 72: 261–267, 1968
29. Ananth, Y, Yassa J: Magnesium in mental illness. Comp Psychiatry 20:475–482, 1979
30. Wilson SAK: Progressive lenticular degeneration: A familial nervous disease associated with cirrhosis of the liver. Brain 34:295, 1911–1912
31. Scheinberg IH, Sternlieb I: Copper toxicity and Wilson's Disease. In Prasad IAS, Oberleas D (eds): Trace Elements in Human Health and Disease. New York, Academic Press, 1976
32. Walker S, III: The psychiatric presentation of Wilson's Disease (Hypatholenticular Degeneration) with an etiologic explanation. Behav Neuropsychiatry 1:38–43, 1968
33. Scheinberg IH: A psychogenetic anecdote. Psychosom Med 37:368–371, 1975
34. Walshe JM: Missed Wilson's Disease (Letter). Lancet 2:405, 1975
35. Dobyns WB, Goldstein NP, Gordon H: Clinical spectrum of Wilson's Disease (hepatolenticular degeneration). Mayo Clin Proc 54:35–42, 1979
36. Baron M, Perlman R, Levitt M, et al: Plasma, copper and dopamine-B-Hydroxylase in schizophrenia. Bull Psychiatry 17:115–120, 1982
37. Pfeiffer CC, Iliev VA: A study of zinc deficiency and copper excess in the schizophrenias. Int Rev Neurobiol (Supp) 1, 1972

38. Rahman B, Rahman MA, Hassan Z: Copper and ceruloplasmin in schizophrenia. Biochem Soc Trans 4:1138–1139, 1976
39. Kirscher KN: Copper and zinc in childhood behavior. Psychopharm Bull 14: 58–59, 1978
40. Tyrer SP, Delves HT, Weller MPI: CSF copper in schizophrenia. Am J Psychiatry 136:937–939, 1979
41. Menkes JH, Alter M, Steigleder GK, et al: A sex-linked recessive disorder with retardation of growth, peculiar hair, and focal cerebral and cerebellar degeneration. Pediat 29:764–779, 1962
42. Bauer JD, Ackermann PG, Toro G: Clinical Laboratory Methods, 8th Edition. St. Louis, Mosby, 1974
43. Danks DN, Campbell PE, Walker-Smith J, et al: Menkes' kinky-hair syndrome. Lancet 1:1100–1102, 1972
44. Dekaban AS, Steussing JK: Menkes' kinky-hair disease treated with subcutanceous copper sulfate (Letter). Lancet 1:1236, 1975
45. Tuman RW, Doisy RJ: The role of trace elements in human nutrition and metabolism. In Jeanes A, Hodge J (eds): Physiological Effects of Food Carbohydrates. Washington, D.C., Amer Chem Soc, 1975
46. Casper RC, Kirscher B, Jacob RA: Zinc and copper status in anorexia nervosa. Psycholpharm Bull 14:53–55, 1978
47. Pfeiffer CC, Braverman ER: Zinc, the brain and behavior. Biol Psychiatry 17: 513–532, 1982
48. Moynihan EJ: Zinc deficiency and disturbances of mood and visual behavior (Letter). Lancet 1:91, 1976
49. Olholm-Larsen P' Untreated acrodermatitis enteropathica in adults. Dermatologica 156:155–166, 1978
50. Caldwell DF, Oberleas D, Prasad AS: Psychobiological changes in zinc deficiency In Prasad AS, Oberleas D (eds): Trace Elements in Human Health and Disease, vol 1. New York, Academic Press, 1976
51. Antoniou LD, Shalhoeb RJ, Sudhakter T, et al: Reversal of uraemic impotence by zinc. Lancet 2:895–898, 1977
52. Antonion LD, Shalhoe RJ: Zinc and sexual dysfunction (Letter). Lancet 80: 1034–1035, 1980
53. Constantinidis J, Tissot R: Role of glutamate and zinc in the hippocampal lesions of Pick's disease. Adv Biochem Psychopharmacol 7:413–422, 1981
54. Hoogenraad TU, Vanden Hamer CJA, Koevoet R, et al: Oral zinc in Wilson's Disease. Lancet 2:1 262, 1978
55. Smith JC, Jr., Brown ED, White SC, et al: Plasma vitamin A and zinc concentrations in patients with alcoholic cirrhosis (Letter). Lancet 1:1251–1252, 1975
56. Hartoma TR, Sotaniemi EA, Pelkonen O, et al: Serum zinc and serum copper and indices of drug metabolism in alcoholics. Eur J Phar 12:147–151, 1977
57. Popkin MK: Psychiatric presentations of hematological disorders. In Hall RCW (ed): Psychiatric Presentations of Medical Illness: Somatopsychic Disorders. New York, Spectrum, 1980
58. Jacobs A: The non-hematological effects of iron deficiency. Clin Sci Mol Med 53:105–109, 1977
59. Leible RL: Behavioral and biochemical correlates of iron deficiency. J Am Diet Assn 71:398–404, 1977
60. Oski FA, Hoenig AS: The effects of therapy on the developmental scores of iron-deficient infants. J Pediat 92:21–25, 1978

61. Davies IJT: The clinical significance of the essential biological metals. London, William Hunemen Medical Books Ltd, 1972
62. Sanstead HH: Some trace elements which are essential to human nutrition: Zinc, copper, manganese, and chromium. Prog Food Nutr Sci 1:371–391, 1975
63. Mena I: The role of manganese in human disease. Ann Clin Lab Sci 4:487–491, 1974
64. Abd El Naby S, Hassanein M: Neuropsychiatric manifestations of chronic manganese poisoning. J Neurol Neurosurg Psychiatry 28:282–288, 1965
65. Cook DG, Fahn S, Bratt KA: Chronic manganese intoxication. Arch Neurol 30:52–58, 1974
66. Banteta RG, Markesberry WR: Elevated manganese levels associated with dementia and extrapyramidal signs. Neurol 27:213–216, 1977
67. Cade J: Lithium salts in the treatment of manic excitement. Med J Australia 36:349–352, 1949
68. Peselow ED, Dunner DL, Fieve RR, et al: Lithium prophylaxis of depression in unipolar, bipolar II, and cyclothymic patients. Am J Psychiatry 139:747–752, 1982
69. Prien RJ: Lithium in the treatment of schizophrenia and schizoaffective disorders. Arch Gen Psychiatry 36:852–853, 1979
70. Schou M: Lithium in the treatment of other psychiatric and non-psychiatric disorders. Arch Gen Psychiatry 36:856–859, 1979
71. Merry J, Reynolds CM, Bailey J, et al: Prophylactic treatment of alcoholism by lithium carbonate: A controlled study. Lancet 2:481–482, 1976
72. Sheard MH, Marini JL, Bridges CI, et al: The effect of lithium on impulsive-aggressive behavior in man. Am J Psychiatry 133:1409–1413, 1976
73. Bussone G, Boiaroi A, Merati B, et al: Chronic cluster headache: Response to lithium treatment. J Neurol 221:181–185, 1979
74. McKenzie JM, Zakarija M: Hyperthyroidism. In DeGroot LJ, Cahill GF, Martini L, et al (eds): Endocrinology, vol 1. New York, Grune & Stratton, 1979
75. Hedley JM, Turner JG, Brownlie BEW, et al: Low dose lithium-carbimazole in the treatment of thyrotoxicosis. Aust NZ J Med 8:628–630, 1978
76. Lyman GH, Williams CC, Preston D: The use of lithium carbonate to reduce infection in leukopenia during systemic chemcotherapy. N Engl J Med 302: 257–260, 1980
77. Gupta RC, Robinson WA, Kurnick JE: Felty's syndrome: Effect of lithium on granulopoiesis. Am J Med 61:29–32, 1976
78. Jefferson JW, Greist JM: Primer of lithium Therapy. Baltimore, University Park Press, 1978
79. Cooper TB, Bergner PE, Simpson GM: The 24-hour serum lithium level as a prognosticator of dosage requirements. Am J Psychiatry 130:601–603, 1973
80. Fetzer J, Kader G, Danahy S: Lithium encephalopathy: A clinical, psychiatric, and EEG evaluation. Am J Psychiatry 138:1622–1623, 1981
81. Roose SP, Nurnberg JI, Dunner DL, et al: Cardiac sinus node dysfunction during lithium treatment. Am J Psychiatry 136:804–806, 1979
82. Hagman A, Arnman K, Ryden L: Syncope caused by lithium treatment. Acta Med Scand 205:467–471, 1979
83. Ramsey TA, Cox M: Lithium and the kidney: A review. Am J Psychiatry 139: 443–449, 1982
84. Lippmann S: Is lithium bad for the kidneys? J Clin Psychiatry 43:220–224, 1982

85. Vestergaard P, Schou M, Thomsen K: Monitoring of patients in prophylactic lithium treatment: An assessment based on recent kidney studies. Br J Psychiatry 140:185–187, 1982
86. Scheiber SC, Zeistat HJR: Dementia dialytica: A new psychotic organic brain syndrome. Comp Psychiatry 17:781–785, 1976
87. Dunea G, Mahurkas SD, Mamdoni B, et al: Role of aluminum in dialysis dementia. Ann Intern Med 88:502–504, 1978
88. Elliott HL, Drybergh F, Fell GS, et al: Aluminum toxicity during regular haemodialysis. Br Med J 1:101–103, 1978
89. Sideman S, Manor D: The dialysis dementia syndrome and aluminum intoxication. Nephron 31:1–10, 1982
90. Dialysis Dementia in Europe: Report from the Registration Committee of the European Dialysis and Transplant Association. Lancet 8:190–192, 1980
91. Crapper DR, Krishnan SS, DeBoni U, et al: Aluminum: a possible agent in Alzheimer's disease. Trans Am Neurol Assn 100:154–156, 1975
92. Duckett S: Aluminum and Alzheimer's disease (Letter). Arch Neurol 33: 730–731, 1976
93. McDermott JR, Smith AL, Igbal K, et al: Aluminum and Alzheimer's Disease (letter). Lancet 2:710–711, 1977
94. Masselot JP, Adhemar JP, Jaudon MC, et al: Reversible dialysis encephalopathy: Role for aluminum containing gels. Lancet 2:1386–1387, 1978
95. Bryce-Smith D: Behavioral effects of lead and other heavy metal pollutants. Chem Br 8:240–243, 1972
96. Munch JC: Human thallotoxicosis. JAMA 102:1929–1934, 1934
97. Burns R, Thomas DW, Barron VJ: Reversible encephalopathy possibly associated with bismuth subgallate ingestion. Br Med J 1:220–223, 1974
98. Loiseau P, Henry P, Jallon P, et al: Iatrogenic myoclonic encephalopathies caused by bismuth salts. J Neurol Sci 27:133–143, 1976
99. Kruger G, Thomas DJ: Disturbed oxidative metabolism in organic brain syndrome caused by bismuth in skin creams. Lancet 1:485–487, 1976
100. LeQuesne PM: Toxic substances and the nervous system: The role of clinical observation. J Neurol Neurosurg Psychiatry 44:1–8, 1981

# Laboratory Evaluation of Treatment

CHAPTER 5

# Plasma Concentration Monitoring of Antipsychotic and Tricyclic Antidepressant Treatment

JOHN M. DAVIS, JAVAID I. JAVAID, and WILLIAM MATUZAS

## INTRODUCTION

### History

The history of plasma levels in psychiatry goes back to World War II, when the pharmacologist Shannon (later head of NIH) was trying to develop synthetic antimalarial drugs as substitutes for quinine. Until more was known in this field, differing rates of metabolism obscured important clinical findings. B.B. Brodie, a student of Shannon's, developed fundamental knowledge about the clinical pharmacology of many drugs used in internal medicine. His student, Julius Axelrode (later to win the Nobel Prize), became interested in the metabolism of amphetamine and, as a consequence, discovered the liver microsomal enzymes that metabolize amphetamine. Subsequent work indicated that these liver microsomal enzymes metabolize

*Handbook of Psychiatric Diagnostic Procedures,* vol. 1, edited by R. C. W. Hall and T. P. Beresford. 

a great variety of drugs including antipsychotics and tricyclic antidepressants. A student of Axelrode's, Snyder, developed an assay for antipsychotic drugs which involved measuring the dopamine-receptor properties of drug and/or metabolites in plasma, rather than a chemical measure of the drug itself. Another student of Brodie's, Stephen Curry, developed a method for measuring chlorpromazine [1]. Davis, Janowsky, and Marshall (students of Curry's) determined correlations between antipsychotic drug plasma levels and clinical effects in man [2–5]. Yet another student of Brodie's, Sjoqvist [6], developed a method for monitoring plasma tricyclic levels. Subsequently, students of his in Sweden and Denmark related tricyclic plasma levels to clinical response.

### Conceptual Basis of Plasma Level/Clinical Effects Relationship

The assumption which underlies plasma level studies is that the rate of absorption, metabolism, distribution, plasma binding, and other factors, vary the quantity of drug that reaches the receptor site in different individuals. The classic plasma-level/clinical-response curve is the sigmoid dose-response curve (see top panel of Figure 1) [7]. With a constant dose, clinical pharmacologic factors determine how much drug reaches the brain or other site of action. The left part of the curve shows the relative lack of clinical response with low plasma levels. Plasma levels are linearly related to clinical effects in the middle (linear) part of the curve. Beyond the linear part of the curve, as larger quantities of drug reach the brain, the curve flattens–indicating a level of diminishing return. Once enough drug has reached the receptor to provide all the benefits it is capable of producing, the curve flattens out, approaching an asymptotic limit. A plasma-level/toxicity relationship is demonstrated for the various side effects (middle panel). If total clinical benefit to the patient is plotted against plasma level, the curve is an inverted U (bottom panel). Improved clinical response is seen as plasma level rises; as this curve begins to level off, the patient is in the segment of optimal benefit. When plasma levels are further elevated, the resulting detrimental side effects may outweigh the beneficial therapeutic effects. Adding the therapeutic and side effect curves yields an inverted U-shape curve.

For most drugs, the upper end of the therapeutic window is defined by toxicity. In addition, however, certain drugs lose their clinical effectiveness above a critical plasma level. We would speculate that a different pharmacological property of the drug counteracts or supercedes the drug's therapeutic property. For example, a drug may stimulate one receptor at a certain concentration but inhibit a second receptor at higher concentrations. Consequently, there are two meanings to the upper end of the therapeutic window: one refers to dose-related side effects; the second refers to the loss of therapeutic benefits above a critical plasma level. As with all definitional issues, it would have been better, perhaps, if the upper end of the therapeutic window could be given a different name for each of the two

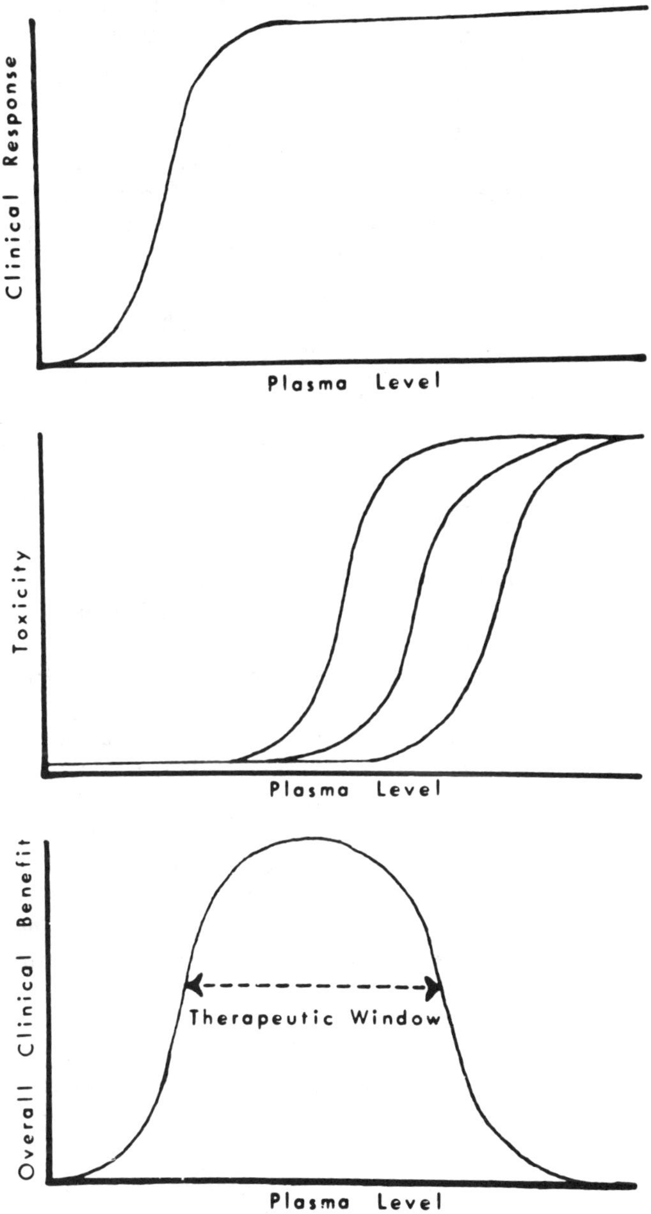


Figure 1. Theoretical concept of therapeutic window.

different types of upper limits. A drug which has neither of these effects, i.e., neither paradoxical loss of clinical effector nor serious toxicity, would not display a descending limb of the inverted U-shaped curve since the upper portion of the therapeutic window is absent. The ability to measure drug in plasma allows us to work with these individual differences to determine empirically the nature of the relationship between plasma level and clinical response or a given side effect.

Factors other than the plasma concentrations can also affect the quantity of drug that reaches the receptor site. Plasma-protein binding, which alters the amount of free drug, is one such factor and volume of distribution is another. In valid plasma-level studies, a constant dose is often used, and the clinical pharmacologist assesses how such factors as distribution, binding, and plasma concentration affect the quantity of drug reaching the receptor site.

## INDICATIONS

### When Are Plasma Levels Useful?

What are the circumstances under which plasma levels are potentially of greatest clinical use? Plasma levels are useful when there is wide interindividual variation in plasma levels. If individual differences did not exist, plasma levels would correlate perfectly with dose and provide no special new information. Plasma levels can be useful when there is a long interval between drug administration and clinical response. Dosage cannot be adjusted by clinical response as a number of weeks may need to pass before the clinical response occurs. If a drug produces an immediate effect, then the clinician can adjust the dosage to this clinical effect. Plasma levels of inhalation anesthetics, for example, may not be clinically useful because the anesthesiologist can directly monitor the clinical stages of anesthesia. Plasma levels are particularly useful when there is a narrow therapeutic index. When there is a wide therapeutic index, the clinician can administer an oral dose sufficient to produce adequate plasma levels for all patients. Plasma levels are also useful in the event of clinically silent toxicity or when there is a possibility of sudden toxicity. If minor side effects occur, the dose can be adjusted downward; however, if catastrophic toxicity occurs, it is too late for reducing the dose. In this case, plasma levels can be useful as an early warning. In contrast, plasma levels may be particularly useful when minor side effects occur at blood levels lower than those required for a therapeutic response or early in the course of treatment. Knowledge of low plasma levels in a patient experiencing early minor side effects at low doses can encourage both patient and physician to achieve and maintain a higher dose and perhaps obtain a more gratifying clinical response. The object of treatment is to obtain an adequate clinical response with a minimum of toxicity. Hence, the clinically pertinent variables to monitor are not plasma levels, but clinical response and toxicity. It may be useful, however, to document the plasma level at which a patient responds because this information may be relevant to the treatment of episodes in the future. Finally, when a drug is used for prophylaxis, it may take many months for a relapse to occur at less than optimal blood levels. You cannot monitor the absence of symptoms. When symptoms occur, it may be too late. Plasma levels may provide early indication of an increased risk of relapse.

It is pertinent to ask the question: Under what circumstances will a lab test lead to bad clinical practice? If a clinician makes the right judgment nine out of ten times but the lab test is only 50% accurate, then the clinician will lower the quality of his clinical practice if he follows the lab test. Generally speaking, if a patient has no clinical response and no side effects, the clinician will raise the dose. If the patient is having a good clinical response but several side effects, the clinician may lower the dose. The clinician who believes the lab test and disregards the clinical indications might indeed make the wrong decision. The correct question to answer about clinical utility of laboratory tests is whether they supplement or add to the clinical information.

## ANTIDEPRESSANTS

Although it has been 15 years since the 30–40 fold interindividual variability of steady-state tricyclic antidepressant plasma concentrations was first recognized, we still do not know the relationship between steady-state plasma concentrations and clinical response for most antidepressants.

### Literature Review

In this section, we summarize evidence on plasma levels from empirical studies. We make an effort to combine the data from multiple studies to see if the results are consistent. For authors who did not publish a table of data but did present graphs, we read the data off the graph by visual inspection. If an investigator reported amitriptyline and nortriptyline data on two separate graphs, and a given data point matches up uniquely to a given improvement score, we can also recover the total amitriptyline plus nortriptyline level or the total imipramine plus desipramine level. (When two or more patients have an identical improvement score, we have, of course, no way to recover this data.) Some investigators do not present complete data but only the number of patients above or below a certain cut-off point. When this occurs, we present data summarizing results from many studies using these cut-off points. The empirical investigations on the relationships between antidepressant plasma level and therapeutic response have been summarized in Tables 1–2 and Figures 2–3. In one instance, an investigator reported a preliminary trial and then apparently extended the trial to a large number of patients.

**Table 1. Plasma Levels vs. Clinical Response in Patients Treated with Imipramine**

| | | Plasma levels (ng/ml) | | |
|---|---|---|---|---|
| | | 0-180 | 180-240 | +240 |
| Glassman et al, 1977 [9] | R | 8 | 22[a] | |
| Perel et al., 1978 [11] | NR | 21 | 8[a] | |
| Matuzas et al, 1982 [13] | R | 1 | 1 | 0 |
| | NR | 6 | 2 | 0 |
| Matuzas et al, 1983 [81] | R | 5 | 1 | 2 |
| | NR | 5 | 2 | 1 |
| Reisby et al, 1977[b] [12] | R | 11 | 4 | 18 |
| | NR | 23 | 5 | 5 |
| Oliver-Martin et al, 1975[b] [10] | R | 0 | 2 | 4 |
| | NR | 3 | 1 | 4 |
| Simpson et al, 1982 [14] | R | 8 | 3 | 7 |
| | NR | 6 | 1 | 2 |

Key: R = Responder; NR = nonresponder.
[a]Author gave plasma levels only as below or above 180
[b]Endogenous + Nonendogenous

If we identified identical values in the larger series on amitriptyline, nortriptyline, and the clinical response to those that occurred in the preliminary report, we assume that the preliminary data was included in the larger series, so we counted these cases only once. For investigators who reported plasma levels drawn on several different weeks, we averaged those plasma levels to obtain a mean plasma level and related this to the best measure of clinical response available.

Three tricyclic antidepressants (imipramine, nortriptyline, and amitriptyline) have been studied in four or more independent investigations. The results for

**Table 2. Desipramine Plasma Level and Clinical Response**

| | | Plasma level ng/ml | | |
|---|---|---|---|---|
| | | 0-92 | 82-115 | 115+ |
| Amin et al, 1978 [17] | R | 0 | 0 | 2 |
| | NR | 1 | 0 | 2 |
| Hrdina et al, 1981 [16] | R | 0 | 0 | 3 |
| | MR | 3 | 0 | 1 |
| Nelson et al, 1982 [15] | R | 2 | 1 | 8 |
| | NR | 13 | 5 | 1 |

R = Responder; NR = nonresponder.

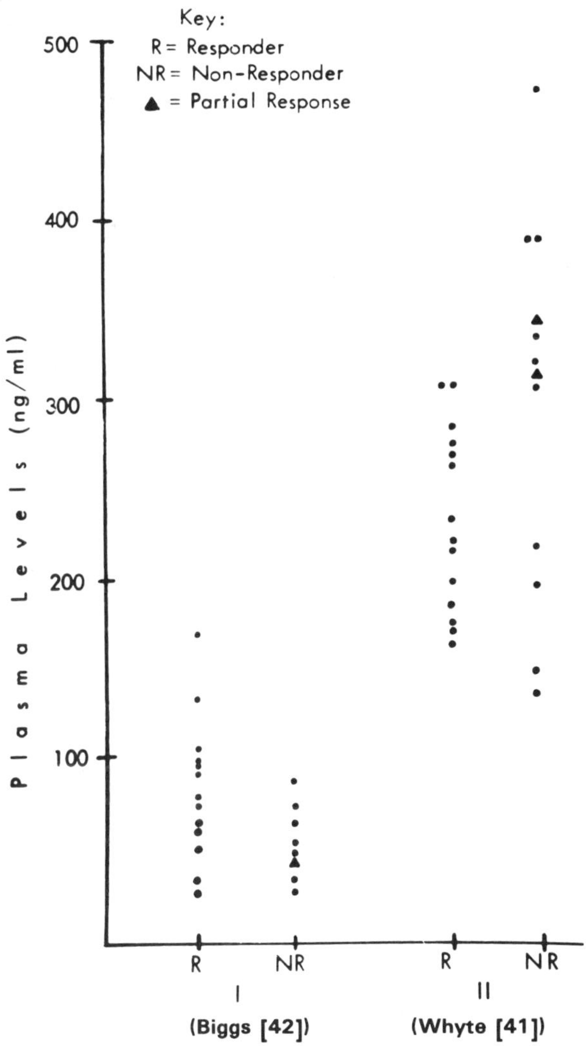


**Figure 2.** Protriptyline plasma levels and clinical response.

imipramine are probably the most consistent and are presented in Table 1. When plasma levels of imipramine plus its metabolite, desipramine, were higher than 240 ng/ml, most patients were considered responders. In contrast, for levels lower than 180 ng/ml, most patients were considered nonresponders. Response in the range of 180–240 ng/ml was mixed. Imipramine did not appear to lose its efficacy at high plasma levels, but toxicity did occur [8–14].

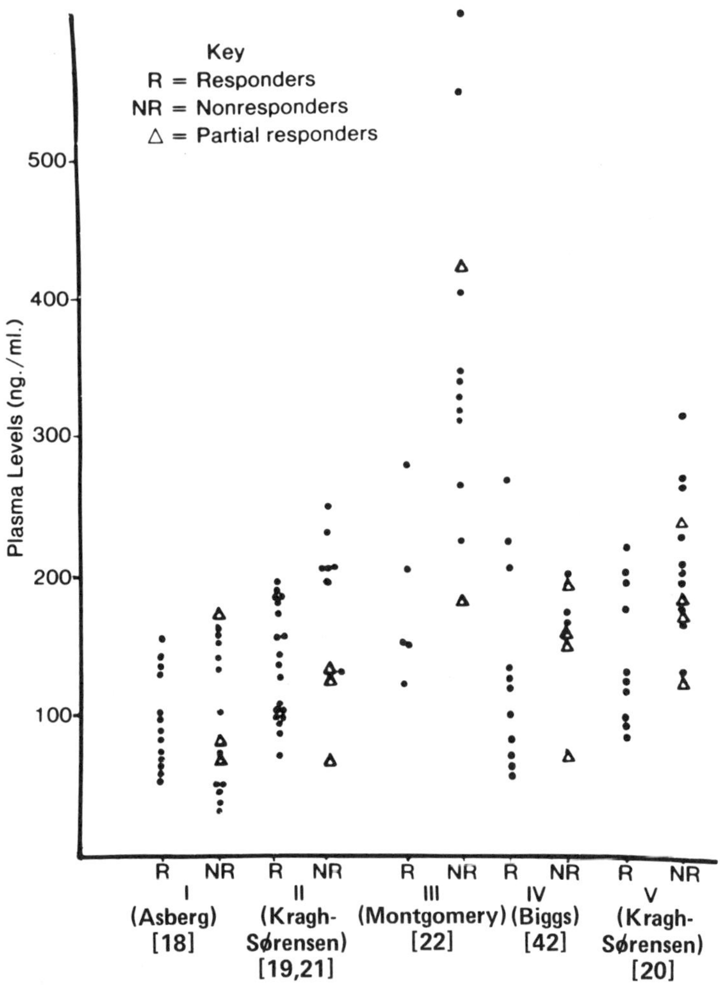


**Figure 3.** Nortriptyline plasma levels and clinical response (Hamilton scores). Cubic regression model.

Nelson et al [15] found that 89 percent of patients with desipramine plasma levels above 115 ng/ml had a good clinical response; in contrast, only 14 percent of patients with plasma levels below 115 ng/ml were responders. A study by Hrdina et al. [16] found a good response in three out of four patients with plasma levels above 115 ng/ml and no responders among three patients with desimipramine plasma levels below that concentration. However, Amin et al [17] found two out of four patients to be responders at plasma levels above 115 ng/ml and one nonresponder with a plasma level below 115 ng/ml (Table 2).

Figure 3 demonstrates the inverted U-shaped relationship observed between plasma nortriptyline levels and clinical response. Asberg et al found that if plasma levels were very low (less than 50 ng/ml), all patients failed to respond [18]. Asberg et al also found that patients who had plasma levels above 140 ng/ml tended to show a poor clinical response. That did not appear to be due to toxicity, but rather to a loss of therapeutic effectiveness. Most of these studies were directed only to high dosage. Many studies agree that there is an upper end to dose effectiveness, but disagree about exactly where it is. Kragh-Sorenson et al [19–21] and Montgomery et al [22] found poor response with plasma nortriptyline levels above 175 ng/ml and 209 ng/ml, respectively. Montgomery et al [22] noted that of 16 patients with high plasma levels who had their dosages reduced, 12 improved within a week or so. Kragh-Sorenson et al [20], using a valid and innovative design, studied patients whose doses had been adjusted to either above 180 ng/ml or below 150 ng/ml and found that more patients in the first group showed a poor clinical response than in the second group. That study continued to a second phase, where a randomly chosen subgroup of five patients in the high plasma-level group (greater than 180 ng/ml) had their doses lowered so plasma levels fell to the therapeutic range. All five patients improved. In contrast, all six patients who continued on their previous dosage and continued to have high plasma levels did poorly. The upper end of the therapeutic window varies substantially from study to study; hence, on examination of the pooled data, it cannot be precisely defined. Note that the 150 ng/ml upper limit, so widely quoted in secondary sources, is actually well within the range of the therapeutic window reported by most of the studies.

Two fixed-dose studies have failed to find a significant relationship between plasma levels of nortriptyline and clinical response. In the first study by Burrows and his associates [23], patients were treated for 4 weeks with a fixed dose of nortriptyline. In examining the data and taking as a definition of response a 50% decrease on the Hamilton at 4 weeks, we noted that there were 16 responders and 16 nonresponders. There were 6 patients who had plasma levels below 50 ng/ml at either 2 or 4 weeks. Of these 6 patients with low plasma levels, 5 were nonresponders. Of the 26 patients with plasma levels above 50 ng/ml at both 2 and 4 weeks, 11 were nonresponders. This indicated a tendency to have poorer response when plasma levels were low for at least one of the two blood drawings. This trend did not reach the 5% confidence level. The p value was 0.09 on the Fishers Exact Test (one-tailed).

In the second fixed-dose study of plasma concentration and clinical response, Davies, Burrows, and Scoggins [24] nevertheless made an interesting clinical observation in 12 patients who had a history of good response to tricyclics with relapses when dose was reduced. Each of these patients underwent a dosage reduction regime and all patients deteriorated when plasma levels were decreased and then improved when levels were raised again. The doctor who did the ratings of depression was unaware of the dose change. Although the plasma levels differed widely, it seemed that there was a critical plasma level for these patients in that when dose was reduced and plasma level dropped below this critical level, the patient became worse. This suggests that the plasma-level/response relationship may not be a constant and may be influenced by an as yet undetermined factor (i.e., RBC concentration [8], hydroxy metabolites, binding, etc.). This would provide some rationalization for the difficulty encountered in establishing reliable plasma level correlates of clinical response in some studies.

Burrows et al [25] did a subsequent study where patients were treated with a moderate dose of nortriptyline for 2 weeks and then randomly assigned to receive either a low dose or a high dose, either in the third week or the fourth week, using a crossover design. That is, half the patients at week 3 had a dose of 50 mg a day and half the patients had a dose of 200 mg a day. At week 4, the patients were crossed over so that those patients who received 50 mg a day at week 3 now received 200 mg and vice-versa. In analyzing this data, we classified as temporarily worsening a patient who had an increase of three or more points on the Hamilton during the week the patient received the low dose. Of the 6 patients who showed a worsening by this definition, 3 showed plasma levels at or below 50 ng/ml. Of the patients whose plasma levels were above 50 ng/ml during the trial of 50 mg a week, 3 out of 16 showed a worsening by this definition. This trend had a p value on Fishers Exact Test of 0.18 (one-tailed) which did not reach the conventional 5% level. In none of Burrows' studies was there evidence for an upper end of the therapeutic window.

Finally, Burrows et al [26] reported an interesting sequential design where patients were randomly assigned to receive low dose or high dose treatment. In the low-dose protocol, patients had plasma levels monitored, and the plasma level was kept under 49 ng/ml. There was no statistically significant difference between the degree of improvement on either dose regime. The rating physician was blind to whether the patient was in the high or low dose group. The design of this study can be criticized as follows: The upper end of the therapeutic window has been stated

**Table 3. Result of Rickel's Study Compared with Other Studies**

| Clinical Results | Low (less than 100 ng/ml) | High (greater than 100 ng/ml) |
|---|---|---|
| | Rickel's Study | |
| Good | 0 | 4 (20%) |
| Moderate | 8 (67%) | 15 (75%) |
| Poor | 4 (33%) | 1 (5%) |
| | Combined Data from Other Studies | |
| Good | 12 (34%) | 106 (50%) |
| Moderate | 11 (32%) | 38 (18%) |
| Poor | 12 (34%) | 66 (32%) |

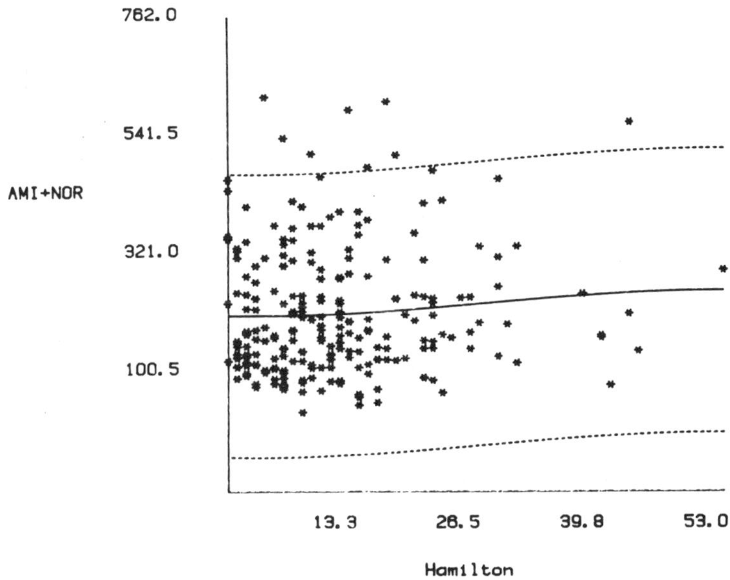


**Figure 4.** Amitriptyline plus nortriptyline plasma levels and clinical response.

by some to be 150 ng/ml, by others to be 175 ng/ml, etc., so it seems clear that some patients in the high-dose group likely would have had plasma levels above the assumed upper end of the therapeutic window, although undoubtedly some patients in the high plasma level group clearly would be within the usual therapeutic window. While it would have been preferable to have a design comparing the patients under 49 ng/ml with patients whose plasma levels were adjusted between 100 and 150 ng/ml, the fact that the "low" plasma level group did no worse than the "high" plasma level group does not provide evidence supporting the 50 ng/ml limit for the lower end of the therapeutic window.

With amitriptyline, there is similar disagreement as to where the upper and lower limits of the therapeutic window are located. Furthermore, it is not clear that there is an upper end of the therapeutic window. Rickels and his co-workers found that four out of five nonresponders had plasma levels below 100 ng/ml [27]. Overall findings from ten amitritpyline studies [17,28–38] showed that at low plasma levels patients divided equally between responders, partial responders, and nonresponders (Table 3).

Total amitriptyline plus nortriptyline plasma levels and final Hamilton scores for the ten studies were entered into a cubic regression model and plotted (Figure 4). No systematic relationship between plasma levels and clinical response was found ($r^2 = 0.006$). In addition, we classified patients as responders or nonresponders

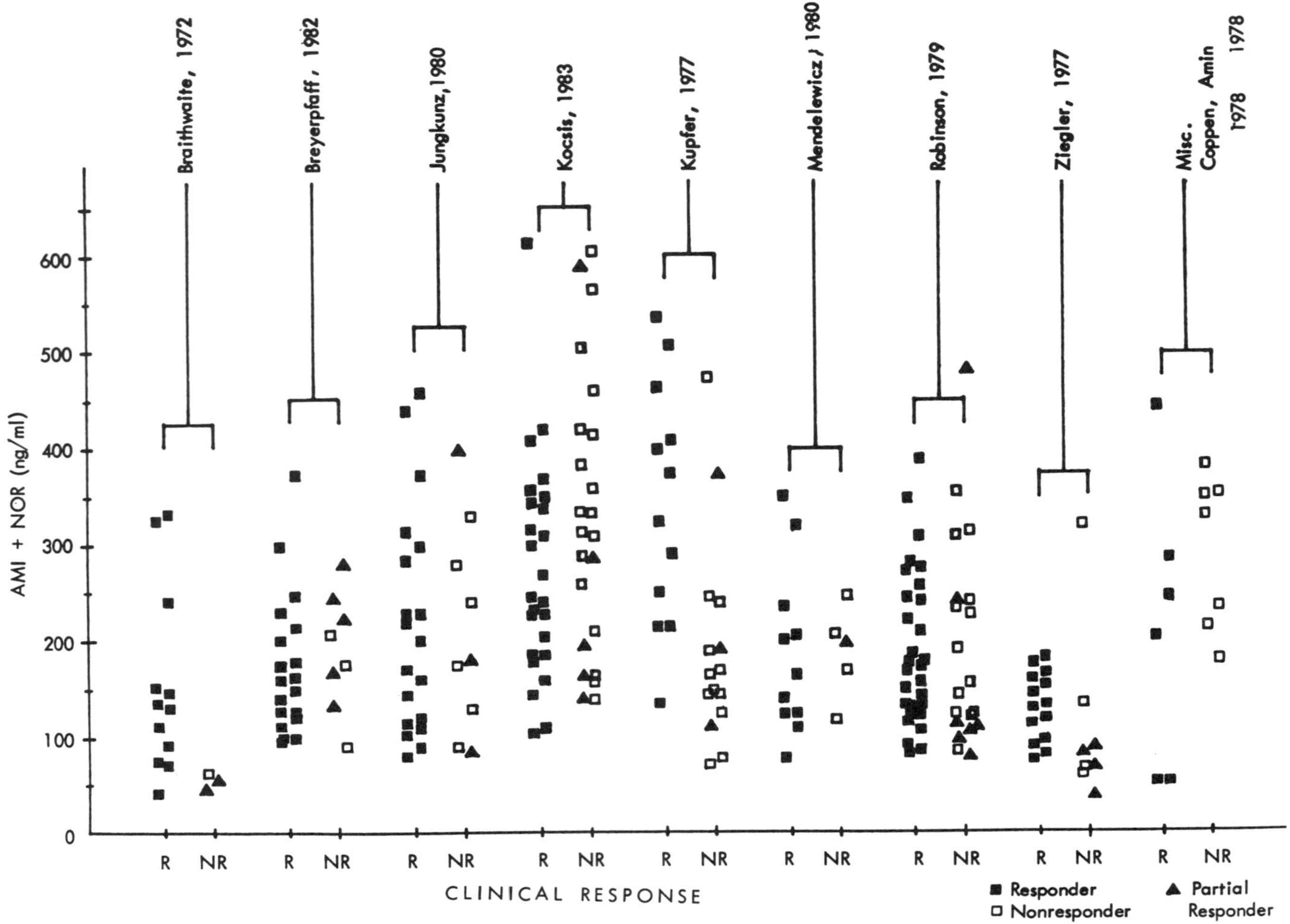


**Figure 5.** Amitriptyline vs. clinical response (Hamilton scores).

**Table 4a. Results of Corona Study**

| | | Amitriptyline | | Nortriptyline | |
|---|---|---|---|---|---|
| | | Low (less than 110[a]) | High (110 plus) | Low (less than 110) | High (110 plus) |
| Bipolar Depressed | R[b] | 8 (53%) | 17 (81%) | 16 (62%) | 9 (90%) |
| | NR | 7 (47%) | 4 (19%) | 10 (38%) | 1 (10%) |
| | | (less than 110) | (110 plus) | (less than 70) | (70 plus) |
| Unipolar Depressed | R | 24 (71%) | 9 (45%) | 26 (68%) | 5 (36%) |
| (Involutional and Neurotic) | NR | 10 (29%) | 11 (55%) | 12 (32%) | 9 (64%) |

**Table 4b. Results of Other Studies Combined**

| | | Amitriptyline | | Nortriptyline | |
|---|---|---|---|---|---|
| | | Low (less than 110[a]) | High (110 plus) | Low (less than 110) | High (110 plus) |
| | R[b] | 79 (72%) | 52 (70%) | 95 (71%) | 36 (67%) |
| | NR | 31 (28%) | 22 (30%) | 38 (29%) | 18 (33%) |
| | | | | less than 70 | 70 plus |
| | R | – | – | 61 (72%) | 70 (69%) |
| | NR | – | – | 24 (28%) | 32 (31%) |

[a]ng/ml
[b]R = Responder, NR = nonresponder

in order to see if there was a quantitative relationship between degree of clinical response and plasma level. A scatter graph indicating amitriptyline plus nortriptyline plasma levels and clinical response is presented in Figure 5. Again, no relationship between plasma level and clinical response is noted.

Several authors have separately looked at amitriptyline plasma levels and nortriptyline plasma levels and also inspected data with several different cut-off points to see if amitriptyline itself or nortriptyline itself did correlate with clinical response. Johnstone et al [39] examined the relationship between amitriptyline plasma levels and Hamilton depression scores. Tabular data were not presented, but the authors indicated that no significant relationship between plasma level and Hamilton-D scores was found. Corona et al [40] examined plasma levels of amitriptyline and clinical response and nortriptyline and clinical response. Their findings are summarized in Table 4a. Corona's data suggests that unipolar and bipolar patients may have a different plasma level relationship of clinical response to amitriptyline. Corona found a trend for bipolar patients to respond if amitriptyline plasma levels are higher than 110 ng/ml, but for unipolar patients to respond if plasma levels are below 100 ng/ml. If plasma level results for bipolar and unipolar patients are combined, patients with low or high plasma levels do about equally well. Corona suggests a different therapeutic window for nortriptyline for bipolar vs. unipolar patients, 110 ng/ml or 70 ng/ml being the cut-off points, respectively.

Data from the ten studies of amitriptyline and nortriptyline plasma levels were organized using Corona and his co-workers's criteria for high and low plasma levels of amitriptyline and nortriptyline and are presented in Table 4b. Comparison of the data reveals that the percentage of responders and nonresponders is similar for patients with either low or high plasma levels. The percentage of clinical responders and nonresponders at nortriptyline plasma levels above or below 70 ng/ml for the ten studies was also calculated. We found an almost equal percentage of responders in the low as in the high plasma level group at either the 70 or 110 ng/ml cut-off point. Although we do not break down the data from the other ten studies into unipolar vs. bipolar classification, we could not confirm that either the 110 or the 70 ng/ml cutoff point is correlated with clinical response.

Data from two studies on protriptyline are presented in Figure 2. Secondary sources often report that an inverted U-shaped relationship exists here; Whyte et al [41] did indeed find several nonresponders with high plasma levels and two nonresponders who have low plasma levels. Biggs et al [42] found nonresponders generally to have low plasma levels. What is particularly striking is that Whyte's patients overall had higher plasma levels than Biggs'. The studies disagree with each other as to absolute plasma levels. If patients are at steady-state on a constant dose and if a specific method is used, plasma level should be comparable from study to study and, in that sense, would be an absolute value. The steady-state assumption is not met in practice; patients are not necessarily at steady-state. This is particularly true with protriptyline, which has an unusually long half-life. In addition, not all methods are completely specific. Sometimes fluorometric methods, for example, are less specific than mass spectroscopic methods. It is incorrect to state the therapeutic window limits for protriptyline as the studies disagree. Figure 2 illustrates why the upper and lower ends of the therapeutic window should not be considered to be written in stone.

Although commercial laboratories advertise the limits of the therapeutic windows, it is difficult to state that these are established for most tricyclics. For example, if limits are set from Biggs' protriptyline data, then it must be assumed Whyte's data is wrong or vice-versa. The reason this has been missed in previous reviews is that one study uses gram units and the other uses molar units. (We converted the latter to the former.) Similar considerations apply to amitriptyline.

Some reviews list whether or not a study shows a correlation between plasma level and clinical efficacy and, if so, whether the correlation is linear or inverted U. The protriptyline data indicate that such a manner of summarizing studies can be inaccurate. Two studies may agree that the correlation is an inverted U, but find a markedly different absolute level. We feel that some form of presentation of raw data is required in the reporting of laboratory studies for the following reasons:

1. The type of relationship may vary from study to study. One investigator may be fortunate in that most of his patients have plasma levels on the linear part of the traditional dose-response curve. Another investigator may have a much wider range of plasma levels, and he may have an appreciable number of patients below and/or above the linear portion of the typical sigmoid dose-response curve. A linear correlation may not provide a good fit to the latter investigator's data. The same considerations apply to the inverted U-shaped curve.

2. Two investigators may get the same shape of curve, but they may have markedly different data, as was seen in the protriptyline studies. In studies where simple linear relationships are found, the simple correlation may adequately summarize the data, but in plasma-level studies where a variety of relationships are possible, there is no substitute for the direct presentation of raw data, either in the form of a table or a graph.

3. An excellent relationship between plasma levels and clinical response may be obscured by a lot of noise in the data. Patients who respond with the passage of several weeks' time may constitute 20 to 40% of the population of depressed patients. Patients who will never respond to any dose of antidepressants can constitute a further 10 to 30%. In both of these cases, you would expect no relationship between plasma level and clinical efficacy because the former case always responds and the latter case never responds. Hence, large sample sizes are necessary to see a real relationship. Undoubtedly, methodological variables may explain contradictory results. One investigator may have a large number of treatment-resistant patients in a sample. Another may have a large number of placebo responders. Only by combining data from many studies will valid relationships be found or be ruled out.

4. Where many curves are expected, it is likely that by optimal choice of cut-off points, investigators can often find statistically significant results which may, to a large part, be a function of just choosing an optimal cut-off point. Only by inspection of raw data from many studies can we rule out artifacts of optimal choice of cut-off points capitalizing on chance variation.

### Methodologic Considerations

It should be noted that the time plasma levels were collected differs substantially among the studies. In some studies, peak plasma level is drawn 2–3 hours after the last oral dose; in others, trough level is drawn 12–24 hours after the last oral dose. Kragh-Sorensen made the measurements during the fourth week, at which point practically all patients would have achieved steady-state. Asberg et al [18] measured tricyclics during the first 2 weeks, when some patients would not yet have reached steady-state. If the clinician markedly increased the dose based on incorrect interpretation, he would produce a potentially toxic plasma level. A dosage normogram to predict steady-state levels from plasma levels before steady-state has been achieved would be helpful.

Careful attention should also be given to blood collection methods prior to the measurement of plasma levels of tricyclic antidepressants. Methodological studies by Cochran et al [43] and Veith et al [44] have shown that prolonged contact of blood with the rubber stoppers of vacutainer tubes can result in markedly low plasma levels of tricyclic antidepressants. Under these conditions, increasing the dose based on artifactually lower plasma levels, will be completely unwarranted.

## Interpretation

Interpretation of tricyclic plasma levels is clouded by the fact that some 20–40% of patients improve on placebo with the passage of 3–4 weeks' time. Other patients are unresponsive to drug irrespective of dose. Thus improvement at a given plasma level does not automatically identify the drug as the cause of such improvement, nor does failure to improve necessarily implicate the plasma level seen in that patient. It is clear that factors other than plasma levels determine response. Thus the observed plasma-level/clinical-effect correlations have been statistically significant, but of only modest magnitude because of the presence of other factors. Generally, the cause of the low correlation is a good clinical response at low concentrations. Much less often there is poor response at high concentrations.

However, plasma concentrations of tricyclic antidepressants can be useful in some circumstances. One example is the patient who has failed to respond to apparently adequate doses. Plasma concentrations can indicate whether levels are too low, thereby suggesting further increases in dose, or whether levels are relatively high, thereby indicating treatment resistance and suggesting the need to try a different medication. A second example is the patient who experiences intolerable side effects at relatively low doses. Again, plasma concentrations will indicate whether levels are low, suggesting the clinician switch medication, or whether they are relatively high, suggesting the patient is a slow metabolizer who may do well with low doses. There should always be a lower end of the therapeutic window. The ultimate lower end is a zero plasma level. If a valid plasma level study cannot define a lower end, then all patients must be receiving doses substantially above the lower end. This suggests that excessively high doses are being administered, unnecessarily placing patients at risk of toxicity.

The adjustment of doses to achieve particular plasma levels is generally straightforward. Plasma levels after a single dose of tricyclics are highly correlated with the multiple-dose steady-state plasma levels as found by Alexanderson [45] and replicated by many other studies. It is possible to predict steady-state levels from single-dose plasma levels. Roughly speaking, plasma levels should be proportional to dosage; therefore, a knowledge of steady-state plasma levels for given dosages should allow the prediction of dose necessary to produce a wanted plasma level by adjusting dose as a simple proportion. For example, it is quite likely that a patient might not respond to nortriptyline with a plasma level at 51 ng/ml, but will respond if the dose is doubled to yield a plasma level of 100 ng/ml. On the other hand, a patient who is responding at an imipramine plasma level of 900 ng/ml, but is experiencing many side effects could have the dose reduced. In the context of dosage, therapeutic effects, and side effects, plasma levels provide additional information from which inferences can be made as to appropriate treatment. This underscores the fact that results generally have been limited to the total plasma concentrations of the antidepressants. Other pharmacokinetic variables which may affect clinical outcome, such as free fraction, red-blood cell concentrations or the hydroxylated metabolites, have not been studied in relation to clinical response.

It should be pointed out that in adjusting the dose on the basis of total (instead of free) plasma levels, one may inadvertently take a patient out of the therapeutic range if that individual has highly increased protein binding. This might occur in infections or inflammatory conditions which increase the concentrations of $alpha_1$-acid glycoprotein, the main binding protein for tricyclic antidepressants [46].

### Future Directions

The further elaboration of our understanding of blood-level/clinical-response relationships will depend upon the accumulation of data from studies that have benefitted from the methodological insights gained from earlier studies. The standardization of clinical ratings, duration of treatment, time of blood sampling, the use of fixed-dose design, and so on will add substantially to the clinical value of future studies. However, it seems unlikely that plasma level studies alone will be sufficient to create a substantially greater degree of predictability than already achieved. This is so because a number of factors in addition to plasma concentrations may play a role in determining drug concentrations at relevant receptor sites. Thus, further studies might focus on such factors as plasma protein binding and red blood cell (RBC) concentrations in addition to total plasma concentrations.

A recent pilot study has presented an encouraging suggestion that studies of both plasma and red blood cell concentrations will enhance our understanding of "blood level"/response relationships [8]. In this study, both plasma and red blood cell concentrations were determined in 16 patients after 4 weeks of treatment with a fixed 150 mg/day dose of imipramine. It appeared that red blood cell concentrations were more significantly correlated with clinical response than were plasma concentrations. Surprisingly, however, it was the RBC/plasma ratio of total drug concentrations that seemed to be the best discriminator of responders from nonresponders. This measure separated these groups with no overlap whatsoever. This observation suggests that the distribution of imipramine may be one factor shaping clinical response at given plasma concentrations.

## ANTIPSYCHOTICS

There have been relatively few controlled investigations of plasma levels of antipsychotic drugs and clinical efficacy. Most studies find that there is an inverted U-shaped relationship between plasma levels of antipsychotic drugs and therapeutic efficacy, so it is quite possible there may be a better relationship between plasma levels and antipsychotic efficacy than there is between plasma levels and antidepressant efficacy. Nevertheless, there are only a relatively limited number of studies. The same methodological considerations for the use of a fixed dose apply to neuroleptics as apply to tricyclic antidepressants. Flexible dose studies are methodologically flawed and are worthless in deriving conclusions about the relationship of plasma levels to efficacy. In addition, it is necessary to study patients who are having an acute episode. This is an important methodologic requirement, and so we will discuss it at some lenght here.

There are some patients who do not improve with neuroleptics because they are not floridly ill. Their degree of psychosis during hospitalization is about the same as before hospitalization. They may be admitted to the hospital because of some deterioration in their social situation. Patients admitted without a relapse in their disease, i.e., with only their residual psychopathology, do not constitute an adequate population for therapeutic trials. In a therapeutic trial, it is necessary to study patients who have florid illness and, therefore, have the capacity to show a substantial degree of therapeutic improvement. Valid plasma-level studies should exclude schizophrenics who have only residual symptoms and include only floridly ill patients. In suitable floridly-ill patients, improvement with antipsychotics should be measured over a time course of two or three weeks.

Placebo responders will recover regardless of plasma level, and some patients will not respond to neuroleptics at all, no matter what the dose. In such cases, one would anticipate no correlation between plasma levels and therapeutic response.

It is important to distinguish rate of improvement from the maximal improvement possible. Some schizophrenics will improve to a point of complete remission of symptoms. Many patients, however, after adequate drug treatment and substantial improvement, will still have residual symptoms. The degree of residual symptoms indicates the patient's maximal capacity to improve, and there may be no correlation between plasma levels and the maximal improvement possible. This probably reflects the underlying psychopathology.

In assessing the relationship between clinical response and plasma level in chronic patients, it is important to measure rate of drug-induced improvement, as distinct from capacity to improve. Taking patients off drugs for several weeks is not necessarily an adequate clinical procedure. There is a substantial body of data to show that patients relapse very slowly after the discontinuance of antipsychotic drugs. A drug-free interval of one year perhaps would be necessary to ensure that 80% or so of the patient population would have relapsed in that period of time.

### Literature Review

The first investigations were the studies by Curry, Marshall, Janowsky, and Davis [2–5] which noted that there were marked individual differences in plasma levels among patients on comparable doses of drug. A wide range of almost 20-fold (approximately 25 to 500 ng/ml) in plasma levels was seen in patients on reasonable clinical doses. A few patients who had a very low level of chlorpromazine failed to show side effects or clinical response. Another patient with a high chlorpromazine plasma level showed excessive sedation. When the dose was lowered, plasma levels fell, and this patient showed a clinical response. It is necessary that these exploratory open studies be verified by properly controlled studies.

### Controlled Studies of Chlorpromazine

There have been very few methodologically-appropriate investigations of the relationship between antipsychotic drug-plasma levels and clinical efficacy. The first study by Curry, Lader, and their co-workers [47–48] treated a small number of schizophrenics and manics with 300 mg of chlorpromazine daily. Complicating the study is the fact that the original sample deliberately included nonfloridly-ill patients (because investigators chose patients amenable to psychophysiological studies) who are inappropriate for the study of therapeutic effects. Lader extended the study to include a larger group of new patients, many of whom were floridly-ill. Three-hundred milligrams is probably lower than the ED 50 dose of chlorpromazine (the average dose necessary to produce 50% of maximal improvement). For this reason, it would be very unlikely that any patient would have plasma levels above the therapeutic window, although some may have plasma levels below the therapeutic window. The expected relationship between plasma level and clinical efficacy would, therefore, be a linear one at this dose. This dose would be useful to define the lower end of the therapeutic window. Patients with low plasma levels would be expected to have poor clinical response, whereas patients with slightly higher levels would be expected to have a good clinical response. In a recent report of results on the first 32 patients, the investigators found a correlation of –0.32 between clinical efficacy and plasma levels, which is of borderline significance ($p = 0.04$ level, one-tailed).

Wode-Helgodt, Sedvall, and co-workers [49–50] did a methodologically excellent study on patients who were treated with randomly-assigned fixed doses of 200, 400, or 600 mgs of chlorpromazine per day. A 200 mg or 400 mg fixed-dose schedule would be considered low, whereas 600 mg would be a moderate dose. In 15 male schizophrenics, there was a positive correlation ($r = 0.82$, p less than 0.01) between improvement and prolactin elevation at 4 weeks. There was a similar correlation between plasma levels and clinical response. Van Putten, May, Wilkins, and co-workers [51–52] studied schizophrenic patients generally treated with chlorpromazine (6.6 mg per kg per day) for 28 days. Plasma chlorpromazine and prolactin levels did not differentiate between the patients who did or did not do well or those who developed side effects and those who did not.

Chlorpromazine theoretically can be metabolized to 168 different metabolites. It is known that many metabolites of chlorpromazine may be active. If a chemical assay measures only the unchanged chlorpromazine, and if the clinical effects are produced to a fair extent by metabolites, and if the amount of metabolite is not well correlated with the amount of unchanged drug, then the presence of active metabolites may obscure the correlation between chlorpromazine-plasma levels and therapeutic efficacy. In other words, if what is producing improvement in the brain is active metabolites, then stable plasma chlorpromazine levels would not be expected to correlate well with clinical efficacy, since the clinical improvement is produced by something else. This may complicate the interpretation of the chlorpromazine studies.

### Other Antipsychotics

Cotes et al [53] treated patients with a fixed dose of flupenthixol and noted a correlation of 0.56 between prolactin levels and total symptom changes (p less than 0.05).

Davis (unpublished data) and Smith et al [54] have both found an inverted U-shaped relationship between haloperidol levels and clinical response. Brown and co-workers [55] found that for patients on maintenance antipsychotics, those who relapse tend to have low plasma levels.

Our group has studied plasma fluphenazine levels and finds an inverted U-shaped relationship between fluphenazine and clinical response [56]. Most nonresponders have either very low fluphenazine levels or very high fluphenazine levels. We also have unpublished data on patients treated with haloperidol showing an inverted U-shaped relationship. Nonresponders have either very low or very high plasma haloperidol levels.

### Use of Free or RBC Levels

It is the concentration of free drug which is in equilibrium with tissue-drug levels. Quantification of free drug is technically impossible at this time, yet potentially quite important. Drugs must cross the blood–brain barrier to reach central receptor sites. Various factors of distribution, in addition to rate of metabolism,

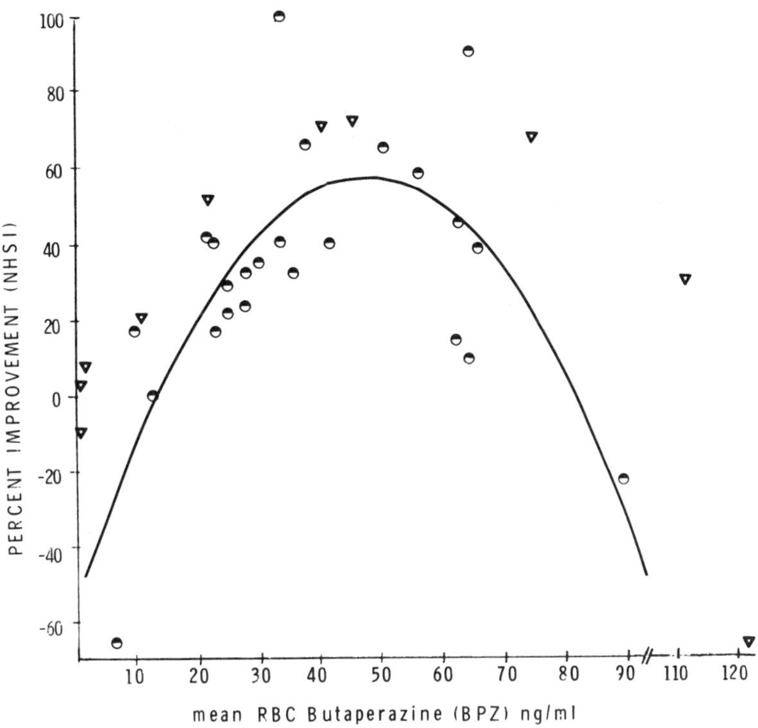


**Figure 6.** Butaperazine RBC level and clinical improvement.

will determine the amount of drug at receptor site. If some of the mechanisms involved in the drug's distribution across the red blood cell membrane mimic those governing the passage of drug through the blood-brain barrier, then drug levels within RBC (or RBC/plasma ratio) may give additional information that total plasma levels alone cannot. In fact, Manian et al. [57] have shown similarities between RBC and rat-brain synaptosomes-chlorpromazine levels. If the assumption is valid, then RBCs may be a preferred tissue for measurement.

Since chlorpromazine has a great many metabolites, certain active metabolites unmeasured by chemical methods may compllicate the interpretation of plasma-level efficacy studies [58–59]. For this reason, it may be desirable to use antipsychotic drugs without active metabolites to work out plasma level vs. therapeutic efficacy relationships. The metabolism of many antipsychotic drugs has not been worked out, so it is difficult to be sure which drugs do or do not have active metabolites. Simpson, Cooper, and co-workers [60–61] have suggested that butaperazine may be a particularly fruitful drug to investigate for this and other reasons.

Garver, Davis, and their co-workers [62-64] administered butaperazine on a constant dose schedule to acutely symptomatic schizophrenic patients while measuring plasma and RBC levels. Although both plasma and RBC levels vs. response were best characterized by an inverted U-shaped curve, the relationship using RBC levels was more striking (see Figure 6). These results support the hypothesis that RBC levels of antipsychotic drugs are a better correlate of clinical response and side effects than are plasma levels. Our group has replicated this study in a completely new sample of patients. An inverted-U relationship between both plasma and RBC levels and clinical response was again observed [65] (see Figure 6). Once again, the relationship of clinical response to RBC levels was more striking.

Most schizophrenics respond in some degree to neuroleptic drugs and then return home. However, there are occasional patients who show no response to drugs whatsoever and need to be hospitalized continuously on a lifetime basis in a chronic state hospital. Since some of these chronic patients are fast metabolizers, and therefore fail to respond to drugs, this might explain their chronicity. Our research group [66] studied such a chronic population and found that both their plasma and red cell levels were substantially below those seen in the acute population. In Figure 7, we have presented as a bar graph (in the right column) the plasma and red cell levels of our acute patients. This includes both relatively good and relatively poor responders. In the left bar graph is the mean response of the chronic, very unresponsive group. We also studied a similar group of very unresponsive patients in an acute setting. Many of these patients had absolutely no clinical response to antipsychotic drugs; many were, indeed, considered for transfer to a chronic facility. In essence, this was the same population as the chronic nonresponders, but identified in an acute setting. These patients also had extremely low plasma and red cell levels (see middle graph in Figure 7). A fair number of these nonresponders did respond when given higher than normal doses of fluphenazine enanthate or decanoate. Since chlorpromazine undergoes first-pass metabolism, an intramuscular formulation may bypass this first-pass effect to achieve an adequate plasma level.

### CSF-Plasma Level Correlation

Ideally, we should measure the concentration of the drug at the receptor site. Since CSF level may reflect free levels in plasma, it is relevant to note that Alfredsson et al [67] found that plasma-chlorpromazine levels are highly correlated to CSF chlorpromazine levels ($r = 0.91$).

### Bioavailability of Oral Antipsychotic

There was a marked difference in plasma levels following oral administration as compared to IV or IM administration [2-5, 68-73]. This is explained in part by

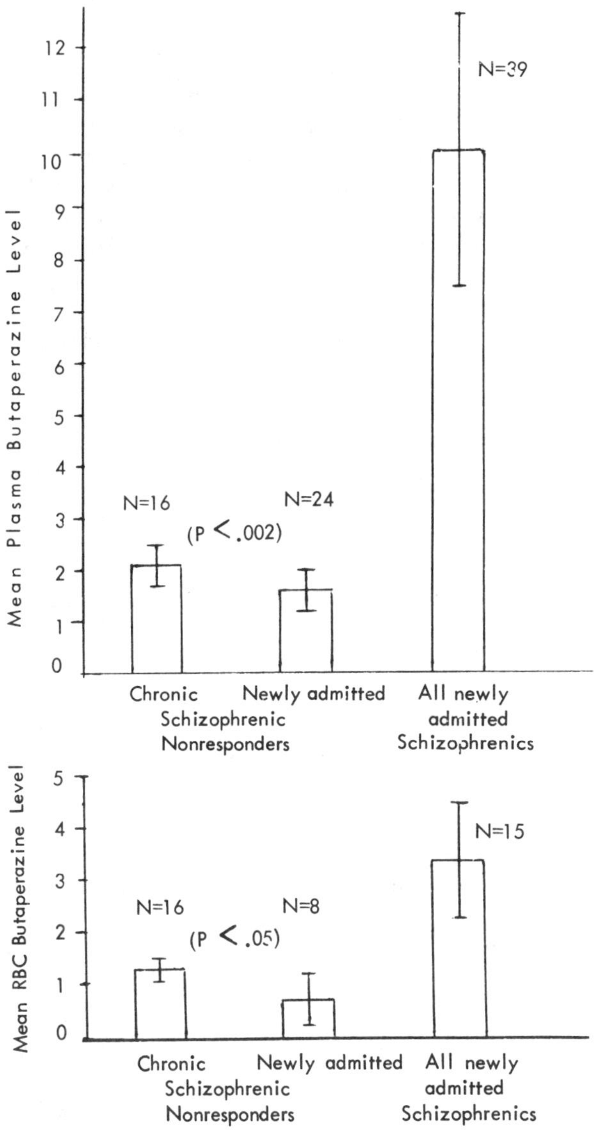


**Figure 7.** Mean plasma and RBC butaperizine levels in acute and chronic patients and responders and nonresponders.

"first-pass" metabolism in the liver. However, in the rat, plasma levels of chlorpromazine were roughly similar in IV vs. IP administration even though IP-administered drug also undergoes the "first-pass" metabolism [69-73]. In laboratory animals administered radioactive chlorpromazine, all modes of administration led to comparable plasma levels of radioactivity [72-74], indicating that the chlorpromazine is absorbed; i.e., chlorpromazine or its metabolites do reach the systemic circulation [55-57]. The urinary excretion of chlorpromazine and its metabolites was roughly similar in IM vs. oral doses in humans [74-75]. In our studies, chlorpromazine was not excreted as such in the feces [2-5]. In *in vitro* studies, where chlorpromazine was injected inside an isolated loop of rat intestine, large amounts of drug were metabolized to biologically inactive metabolites in the mucosal wall, suggesting that chlorpromazine is degraded to a large extent in the mucosal wall of the small intestine [73]. Clinically, there is a substantially greater degree of sedation and postural hypertension in patients given IV or IM chlorpromazine than is seen following oral administration. We suggest that drug nonresponders may have an excess of chlorpromazine-metabolizing enzyme in the gut that would metabolize orally administered chlorpromazine so fast that only a very small amount of unchanged chlorpromazine would reach the plasma and brain. These patients would be expected to have a larger proportion of the chlorpromazine reach the plasma as inactive metabolites. Conversely, the patient with a deficiency in chlorpromazine metabolism may have a larger amount of unchanged chlorpromazine and a smaller amount of metabolites in plasma.

## INTERPRETATION

### Laboratory Norms

Clinical laboratories sometimes publish norms for their laboratory. Such norms are not necessarily valid statements of a therapeutic window. Usually such norms are just the plasma levels determined by that particular laboratory. For example, if a given laboratory does a great deal of toxicologic work, its norms would be falsely high. If clinicians who send samples to that laboratory use high doses, that laboratory will have high norms. If another laboratory has clinicians who use low doses, it will have low levels. If many clinicians use the laboratory to check for compliance in patients who tend to be noncompliant, that laboratory will have low norms.

Similarly, if a commercial laboratory defines norms from the literature, it may use studies which are generally invalid for a variety of methodological reasons or may define norms from a valid study which uses different methodology, such as methods of differing specificity.

The advertising by commercial laboratories of upper and lower limits of a putative therapeutic window suggests that nonresponders surely fall either below or above these limits. Inspection of the data clearly establishes this not to be the case; most of the nonresponders have plasma levels within the therapeutic window.

We feel plasma levels can, indeed, be useful clinically, but that the advertisement of the limits of the therapeutic window by commercial vendors creates the false impression that there is a one-to-one relationship between therapeutic window limits and clinical response. This type of thinking suggests that the clinician makes dose adjustments to bring the plasma level within predefined limits. We feel this is not a precise or thoughtful way to use this information because the clinician goes from plasma level and therapeutic limits to dose adjustment without any intervening step—a one-to-one correlation. The clinician should integrate the observed plasma level, the dose and duration of treatment, side effects, clinical response, and other variables in order to figure out what is going on and then make the dosage adjustment based on an understanding of the total clinical picture.

Plasma levels sampled a few hours after the last dose would be higher than plasma levels drawn 12 hours after the last dose. The use of random plasma levels from a clinical laboratory to define a therapeutic window may yield invalid norms. If a given side effect appears at the same plasma level as is necessary to produce the therapeutic effect, then monitoring plasma levels will not avoid that particular side effect. Indeed, there is evidence that the dose-response relationship between certain side effects may even be shifted to the left of clinical efficacy. In other words, a slightly lower plasma level is necessary to produce certain side effects than it is to produce therapeutic effects. If a high plasma level is needed to produce a given side effect, then we might be able to avoid it by measuring plasma levels. Clearly, at high plasma levels, such as are observed after an overdose of drugs with suicidal intent, there is a good correlation between plasma levels and prolongation of the QRS complex on EKG.

## CONCLUSIONS

When does an assay go from experimental stage to routine clinical practice stage? This is somewhat analogous to a drug moving through the first three stages of early drug evaluation to win approval by the FDA and then passing into routine clinical practice. By analogy, phase 1 might consist of working out the assay in normal subjects or a small sample of patients and normal volunteers to be sure the laboratory can accurately measure plasma levels observed in humans on comparable doses. Phase 1 studies would also work out a rough estimate of the pharmacokinetic properties, bioavailability, etc. Phase 2, by analogy, would correspond to the first few exploratory studies of plasma levels vs. efficacy and related problems. Phase 2 studies would also provide much confirmatory information on pharmacokinetics and bioavailability in a large sample of patients. Phase 3 consists of replication studies that would verify that the assumed lower and upper limits of the therapeutic window are really true and show that studies agree about where these limits are. Since plasma levels are without risk, it is certainly reasonable to require fewer studies for an assay to pass from research to clinical use than for a drug to do the same. There is always the problem of equating many small sample studies against a few large sample studies. In addition, how much agreement between studies constitutes substantial agreement? We would feel that three large studies with consistent results, or four or five smaller studies with consistent results are necessary to establish that a finding is really true. We do not feel that one study is enough to demonstrate an empirical finding beyond a reasonable doubt. Consequently, we find that there are not enough studies of plasma levels of antipsychotics to establish their clinical utility. Clearly, there are a substantial number of studies which show that there are large differences in plasma levels between patients on constant doses of antipsychotics, and there is some evidence to suggest that these plasma or red cell differences do correlate with clinical response. This provides one rationale for why a clinican should adjust dose to clinical response. We feel that this data is fairly consistent. We do not feel that there are enough studies, however, to demonstrate just exactly what the therapeutic window is for different drugs. The therapeutic window must be worked out for each drug separately, so a substantial body of information is required before a rough approximation of the therapeutic window can be determined. We feel the use of antipsychotic plasma levels is experimental at this point.

More work is needed to precisely define therapeutic windows for plasma levels to be clinically useful. Not only must good data define a therapeutic window's existence, but it is also necessary for laboratories to agree on its exact location. Our graphs will give the reader a view of the data on plasma level. It is incorrect to think a drug plasma level is like a sodium plasma level–low, normal, or high. Since drug plasma levels differ widely among individuals due to differences in their rate of liver metabolism, the clinician must adjust the dose for each patient individually to achieve maximum benefit with minimal side effects. Accurately determined plasma levels can occasionally aid in dose adjustment when the literature provides enough data to make sense of the value obtained. We believe the best way to understand plasma levels is not through arbitrarily selected numbers defining the upper or lower end to the therapeutic window, but by placing a given plasma level in the context of the data which we have presented graphically.

## REFERENCES

1. Curry SH: Determination of nanogram quantities of chlorpromazine and some of its metabolites in plasma using gas-liquid chromatography with an electron-capture detector. Anal Chem 40:1251–1256, 1968
2. Curry SH, Davis JM, Janowsky D, et al: Intrapatient variation in physiological availability of chlorpromazine as a complicating factor in correlation studies of

drug metabolism and clinical effect. In A Carletti, FJ Bove (eds): The Present Status of Psychotropic Drugs Vol. 6. Amsterdam, Excerpta Medica Foundation, 1968
3. Curry SH, Marshall JHL: Plasma levels of chlorpromazine and some of its relatively non-polar metabolites in psychiatric patients. Life Sci 7:9–17, 1968
4. Curry, SH, Davis JM, Marshall JHL, et al: Factors affecting chlorpromazine plasma levels in psychiatric patients. Arch Gen Psychiatry 22:209–215, 1970a
5. Curry SH, Marshall JHL, Davis JM, et al: Chlorpromazine plasma level and effects. Arch Gen Psychiatry 22:289–296, 1970b
6. Hammer W, Sjoquist F: Plasma levels of monmethylated tricyclic antidepressants during treatment with imipramine-like compounds. Life Sci 6:1895–1903, 1967
7. Davis JM, Ericksen S, Dekirmenjian H: Plasma levels of antipsychotic drugs and clinical response," in MA Lipton, A DiMascio, KD Killam (eds): Psychopharmacology: A Generation of Progress, New York, Raven Press, 1978
8. Matuzas W, Javaid JI, Uhlenhuth EH, Davis JM, Glass RM: Plasma and red blood cell concentrations of imipramine and clinical response among depressed outpatients. Paper presented at Annual Meeting, American Psychiatric Association, New York, 1983
9. Glassman AH, Perel JM, Shostak M, et al: Clinical implications of imipramine plasma levels for depressive illness. Arch Gen Psychiatry 34:197–204, 1977
10. Olivier-Martin R, Marzin D, Buschenschutz E. et al: Concentrations plasmatiques de l'imipramine et de la desmethylimipramine et effect antidepresseur au cours d'un traitement controle. Psychopharmacol 41:187–195, 1975
11. Perel J, Stiller R, Glassman AH: Studies on plasma levels/effects relationships in imipramine therapy. Commun in Psychopharmacology 2:429–439, 1978
12. Reisby N, Gram LF, Bach P, et al: Imipramine: Clinical effects and pharmacokinetic variability. Psychopharmacology 54:263–272, 1977
13. Matuzas W, Javaid JI, Glass R, et al: Plasma concentrations of imipramine and clinical response among depressed outpatients. J Clin Psychopharmacology 2: 140–142, 1982
14. Simpson G, White KL, Boyd JL, et al: Relationship between plasma antidepressant levels and clinical outcome for inpatients receiving imipramine. Am J Psychiatry 139(3):358–360, 1982
15. Nelson JC, Jatlow P, Quinlan D, et al: Desipramine plasma concentration and antidepressant response. Arch Gen Psychiatry 39:1419–1422, 1982
16. Hrdina P, Lapierre Y: Clinical response, plasma levels and pharmacokinetics of desiprimine in depressed patients. Prog Neuro-Psychopharmacol 4:591–600, 1981
17. Amin M, Cooper R, Khalid R, et al: A comparison of desipramine and amitriptyline plasma levels and therapeutic response. Psychopharmacol Bull 14: 45–46, 1978
18. Asberg M, Cronholm B, Sjoqvist F. et al: Relationship between plasma levels and therapeutic effect of nortriptyline. Br Med J 3:331, 1971
19. Kragh-Sorensen, P, Hansen LE, Asperg M: Plasma levels of nortriptyline in the treatment of endogenous depression. Acta Psychiatr Scand 49:445–456, 1973
20. Kragh-Sorensen P, Eggert-Hansen C, Banstrup PC, et al: Self-inhibiting action of nortriptyline antidepressive effect at high plasma levels. Psychopharmacologia 45:305–312, 1976

21. Kragh-Sorenson P, Asberg M, Eggert-Hansen C: Plasma nortriptyline levels in endogenous depression. Lancet 1:113, 1973
22. Montgomery S, Braithwaite R, Dawling S, et al: High plasma nortriptyline levels in the treatment of depression. J Clin Pharmacol Ther 23:309–314, 1978
23. Burrows GD, Davies B, Scoggins BA: Plasma concentration of nortriptyline and clinical response in depressive illness. Lancet Sept. 23, 619–623, 1972
24. Davies B, Burrows GD, Scoggins B: Plasma nortriptyline and clinical response. Aust NZ J Psychiatry 9:249–253, 1975
25. Burrows GD, Maguire KP, Scoggins BA: Plasma nortriptyline and clinical response – a study using changing plasma levels. Psychiat Med7:87–91, 1977
26. Burrows GC, Turecek LR, Davies B, et al: A sequential trail comparing plasma levels of nortriptyline. Aust NZ J Psychiatry 8:21–23, 1974
27. Rickels K, Weise C, Case G, et al: Tricyclic plasma levels in depressed outpatients treated with amitriptyline. Psychopharmacology 80:14–18, 1983
28. Braithwaite RA, Goulding R, Theano G, et al: Plasma concentration of amitriptyline and clinical response. Lancet 1:1297–1300, 1972
29. Breyer-Pfaff U, Gaertner HJ, Kreuter F, et al: Antidepressive effect and pharmacokinetics of amitriptyline with consideration of unbound drug and 10-hydroxynortriptyline plasma levels. Psychopharmacology 76:240–244, 1982
30. Coppen A, Ghose K, Montgomery S, et al: Amitriptyline plasma-concentration and clinical effect: A World Health Organization collaborative study. Lancet 1:63–66, 1978
31. Jungkunz G, Kuss HJ: On the relationship of nortriptyline: Amitriptyline ratio to clinical improvement of amitriptyline-treated depressive patients. Pharmacopsychiatr Neuropsychopharmakol 13:111–116, 1980
32. Kocsis J, Bowden CL, Chang S, et al: Tricyclic plasma levels and clinical response. Syllabus and Scientific Proceedings 136:128, 1983
33. Kupfer, DJ, Hanin, I., Spiker, DG, et al: Amitriptyline plasma levels and clinical response: II. Commun Psychopharmacol 2:441–450, 1975
34. Kupfer DJ, Hanin I, Spiker DG, et al: Amitriptyline plasma levels and clinical response in primary depression. Clin Pharmacol Ther 22:904–911, 1977
35. Mendelewicz J, Linkowski P, Rees JA: A double-blind comparison of doxepin and amitriptylinc in patients with primary affective disorder: Serum levels and clinical response. Brit J Psychiatry 136:154–160, 1980
36. Robinson DS, Cooper TB, Ravaris CL, et al: Plasma tricyclic drug levels in amitriptyline-treated depressed patients. Psychopharmacology (Berlin) 63: 223–231, 1979
37. Ziegler VE, Co BT, Taylor JR, et al: Amitriptyline plasma levels and therapeutic response. Clin Pharmacol Ther 19:795–801, 1976
38. Ziegler VE, Clayton PJ, Biggs JT: A comparison study of amitriptyline and nortriptyline with plasma levels. Arch Gen Psychiatry 34:607–612, 1977
39. Johnstone EC, Bourne RC, Crow TJ, et al: The relationship between clinical response, psychological variables and plasma levels of amitriptyline and diazepam in neurotic outpatients. Psychopharmacol 72:233–240, 1981
40. Corona GL, Pinelli P, Zerbi F, et al: Amitriptyline, nortriptyline plasma levels and clinical response in women with affective disorders. Pharmacopsychiatry 13:102–110, 1980
41. Whyte SF, MacDonald AJ, Naylor GJ, et al: Plasma concentration of protriptyline and clinical effects in depressed women. Br J Psychiatry 128:384–390, 1976

42. Biggs JT, Zeigler VE: Protriptyline plasma levels and antidepressant response. Clin Pharmacol Ther 22:269–273, 1978
43. Cochran E, Carl J, Koslow S, et al: Effects of vacutainer stoppers on plasma tricyclic levels: A reevaluation. Commun Psychopharmacol 2:495-503, 1978
44. Veith RC, Raisys VA, Perera C: The clinical impact of blood collection methods on tricyclic antidepressants as measured by GC//MC-SIM. Commun Psychopharmacol 2:491–494, 1978
45. Alexanderson B: Predictions of steady state plasma levels of nortriptyline from single oral dose kinetics, studied in twins. Eur J Clin Pharmacol 6:44–53, 1973
46. Javaid JI, Hendricks K, Davis JM: Alpha$_1$-Acid glycoprotein involvement in high affinity binding of tricyclic antidepressants to human plasma. Biochem Pharmacol 32:1149–1153, 1983
47. Sakalis G, Curry SH, Mould GP, et al: Psychologic and clinical effects of chlorpromazine and their relationship to plasma level. Clin Pharmacol Ther 13:931–946, 1972
48. Lader M: Monitoring plasma concentrations of neuroleptics. Pharmacopsychiatry 9:170–177, 1976
49. Wode–Helgodt B, Borg S, Fyro B, et al: Clinical effects and drug concentrations in plasma and cerebrospinal fluid in psychotic patients tested with fixed doses of chlorpromazine. Acta Psychiatr Scand 58:149–173, 1978
50. Sedvall G, Grumm V: Cerebrospinal fluid and plasma as tools for obtaining biochemical and pharmacologic data in neuroleptic therapy. In GO Burrows, T Norman (eds): Psychotropic Drugs: Plasma Concentration and Clinical Research, Dekker, New York, 1981
51. May PRA, Van Putten T, Jenden D, et al: Chlorpromazine blood and saliva levels and the outcome of treatment in schizophrenic patients. Arch Gen Psychiatry 38:202–207, 1981
52. Van Putten T, May P, Jenden D: Does a plasma level of chlorpromazine help? Psychol Med 11:729–734, 1981
53. Cotes PJ, Crow TJ, Johnstone EC, et al: Neuroendocrine changes in acute schizophrenia as a function of clinical state and neuroleptic medication. Psychol Med 8:657–665, 1978
54. Smith RC, Vroulis G, Shvartsburd A, et al: RBC and plasma levels of haloperiodol and clinical response in schizophrenia. Amer J Psychiatry 139:1054–1056, 1982
55. Brown WA, Laughren T, Chisholm E, et al: Low serum neuroleptic levels predict relapse in schizophrenic patients. Arch Gen Psychiatry 39:998, 1982
56. Dysken MW, Javaid JI, Chang SS, et al: Fluphenazine pharmacokinetics and therapeutic response. Psychopharmacology 73:205–210, 1981
57. Manian AA, Piette LH, Holland D, et al: Red blood cell drug binding as a possible mechanism for tranquilization. In IS Forrest, CJ Carr, E Usdin (eds.): Advances in Biochemical Psychopharmacology. New York, Raven Press, 1974
58. Manian AA, Efron DH, Goldbert ME: A comparative pharmacological study of a series of monohydroxylated and methoxylated chlropromazine derivatives. Life Sci 4:2425–2438, 1965
59. Manian AA, Efron DH, Harris SR: Appearance of monohydroxylated chlorpromazine metabolites in the central nervous system. Life Sci 10:679–684, 1971
60. Simpson GM. Lament R, Cooper TB, et al: The relationship between blood levels of different forms of butaperazine and clinical response. J Clin Pharmacol 13:288–297, 1973

61. Cooper TB, Simpson GM, Haber EJ, et al: Butaperazine pharmacokinetics. Arch Gen Psychiatry 32:903–905, 1975
62. Davis JM, Janowsky DS, Dekerke I, et al: The pharmacokinetics of 6butaperazine in serum. In: I Forrest, C Carr, and E Usdin (eds.): The Phenothiazines and Structurally Related Drugs. New York, Raven Press, 1974
63. Garver DL, Dekirmenjian H, Davis JM, et al: Neuroleptic drug levels and therapeutic response: Preliminary observations with red blood cell bound butaperazine. Am J Psychiatry 134:304–307, 1977
64. Garver D, Davis JM, Dekirmenjian H, et al: Pharmacokinetics of red blood cell phenothiazine and clinical effects: Acute dystonic reactions. Arch Gen Psychiatry 33:862–866, 1976
65. Casper R, Garver DL, Dekirmenjian H, et al: Phenothiazine levels in plasma and red blood cells. Arch Gen Psychiatry 37:301–305, 1980
66. Smith RC, Crayton JW, Dekirmenjian H, et al: Blood levels of 6neuroleptic drugs in nonresponding chronic schizophrenic patients. Arch Gen Psychiatry 36:579–584, 1979
67. Alfredsson G, Wode-Helgodt B, Sedvall G: A mass fragmentographic method for the determination of chlorpromazine and two of its active metabolites in human plasma and CSF. Psychopharmacology 48:123–131, 1976
68. Curry SH: Theoretical changes in drug distribution resulting from changes in binding to plasma proteins and to tissues. J Pharm Pharmacol 22:753–757, 1970
69. Curry SH: Chlorpromazine: Concentrations in plasma, excretion in urine and duration of effect. Proc R Soc Med 64:285–289, 1971
70. Adamson L, Curry SH, Bridges P, et al: Fluphenazine decanoate trial in chronic inpatient schizophrenics failing to absorb oral chlorpromazine. Dis Nerv Syst 34:181–191, 1973
71. Curry SH, Adamson L: Double blind trial of fluphenazine decanoate. Lancet 2:543–544, 1971
72. Curry SH: Metabolism and kinetics of chlorpromazine in relation to effect. In G Sedval, U Uvnas, Y Zotterman (eds): Antipsychotic Drugs: Pharmacodynamics and Pharmacokinetics, Oxford, Pergamon Press, 1976
73. Curry SH, D'Mello A, Mould, GP: Destruction of chlorpromazine during absorption in the rat in vivo and in vitro. Br J Pharmacol 42:403–411, 1971
74. Curry SH, Derr JE, Maling HM: The physiological disposition of chlorpromazine in the rat and dog. Proc Soc Exp Biol Med, 132:314–318, 1970
75. Hollister LE, Curry SH: Urinary excretion of chlorpromazine metabolites following single doses and in steady-state conditions. Res Commun Chem Pathol Pharmacol 2:330–338, 1971

CHAPTER 6

# Lithium Monitoring


## JAMES W. JEFFERSON


### HISTORY

Prior to 1949 when lithium was introduced to modern psychiatry by Cade [1], the drug had a rather "checkered" medical history [2]. In the second half of the nineteenth century it was used extensively to treat "uric acid disorders" (which included headache, epilepsy, high blood pressure, angina, asthma, gout, rheumatism, and melancholia) and dosing was based on finding a balance between therapeutic and adverse effects. Of interest is the recommended daily dose of lithium carbonate given in the 1892 "Materia Medica in Therapeutics" of 0.7-2.0 grams per day which closely approximates the dosage range used today for the treatment of manic depressive disorder (see [3]).

When Cade first effectively treated mania with lithium, he stated "the original therapeutic dose decided on fortuitously proved to be the optimum." Once the patient responded, two months of further hospitalization were needed, in part, due to "the necessity of determining a satisfactory maintenance dose" [4]. This was achieved by clinical trial and error and it was not until many years later that blood level monitoring became a useful and essential part of lithium therapy.

While the toxicity of lithium had been recognized by the turn of the century, little heed was paid to appropriate monitoring when lithium chloride was used as a salt substitute in the late 1940's. Serious intoxications and deaths resulted [5].

Although lithium concentrations were measured in both serum and urine in the early 1950's, a well defined relationship between therapeutic effects, side effects, and toxicity could not be established [6]. Talbot [3] studied the use of


*Handbook of Psychiatric Diagnostic Procedures*, vol. 1, edited by R. C. W. Hall and T. P. Beresford.

lithium chloride as a salt substitute and concluded that adverse reactions occurred only in association with serum lithium levels greater than 1.0 mEq/l (mmol/l), although he also noted levels as high as 2.9 mEq/l in the absence of untoward effects. Noack and Trautner [7] concluded "So far it has not been possible to find a laboratory test which would indicate optimum dosage or impending intoxication, and which could replace the careful observation of the patient."

Schou et al [8] found variations in serum lithium level between 0.5 and 2.0 mEq/l during treatment but did not find a good correlation between level and outcome. They felt that "the serum level is not a reliable indicator of the lithium concentration in tissues" but did acknowledge that "the serum lithium concentration is of some value as a guide for therapy" and that they would be "hesitant to institute lithium therapy under conditions when the serum lithium level could not be checked regularly."

In 1959, Schou [9] advised that the serum lithium level be kept below 2.0 mEq/l to prevent intoxication but otherwise suggested that maintenance dose be established by achieving a clinical balance between therapeutic and side effects. This approach was not unique having its medical counterpart in digitalis, another drug with a narrow therapeutic margin, whose effective use was and still is governed largely by clinical judgment.

Amdisen, a leading force in establishing guidelines for lithium monitoring, notes that for 15-20 years following 1949, individual dosage was adjusted by clinical observation with insufficient knowledge of lithium pharmacokinetics to allow serum levels to be therapeutically useful [6,10–14]. He commented that not only historically but, unfortunately, currently it is common to find serum lithium values and ranges used without any reference to a standardized monitoring protocol. He states quite appropriately: "This lack most often makes the information incomprehensible, and may, when guidance is concerned, even be dangerous" [10]. The value of serum lithium levels for monitoring lithium therapy depends on standardization of the sampling procedure and elimination or control of variables that would otherwise render the results meaningless [12].

It is fortunate that the use of lithium in psychiatry has been paralleled by the development of inexpensive, commercially available, sensitive, reliable techniques for quantitatively measuring lithium in the body [15]. While qualitative spectroscopic techniques were available in the mid-1800s, the development and application of flame emission photometry and atomic absorption spectrophotometry in the last 30 years has truly made serum lithium determinations a routine clinical laboratory procedure.

## METHODS FOR LITHIUM MEASUREMENT

The methods commonly used today for measuring lithium concentration in the body are flame photometry (atomic emission) and atomic absorption spectrophotometry [13,15–17]. These procedures are widely available in modern clinical laboratories and for the routine monitoring of serum lithium levels both are sensitive and precise and neither is to be preferred.

The methods are based on measuring the intensity of light emitted or absorbed by free atoms of lithium [16,17]. As explained by Cooper [18], when a lithium solution is introduced into a flame, some of the lithium is converted to free atoms which then absorb additional energy and become transferred to a higher energy level (become excited). When the atoms return to their non-excited state "by collisional non-radiative deactivation and by spontaneous emission of light" an equal amount of energy is released [16]. The emission of energy in the form of light is the basis for flame photometry while the absorption of energy is the basis for atomic absorption spectrophotometry (AAS).

### Flame Emission (Flame Photometry, Flame Spectrometry)

In flame photometry, a sample is prepared in an appropriately diluted solution and introduced into the flame by nebulization, a process which creates a mist of droplets of appropriate size and uniformity. The solvent is vaporized by the flame leaving dry aerosol particles (desolvation) which, in turn, are volatized and dissociated to form free lithium atoms. A portion of these free atoms are then transformed to higher energy levels. When the excited lithium atoms return to their original energy level, radiation of a characteristic wavelength is emitted which is proportional to the amount of lithium present. A filter system is used to separate radiation characteristics of lithium from those of other elements. The signal is then amplified and recorded [16,17].

Problems which arise in the use of flame photometry can be caused by glasswork contamination; the presence of serum protein; the concentrations of other elements such as sodium, potassium, and calcium; the type of fuel gas used; and the type of photocell used [15].

### Atomic Absorption Spectrophotometry

The principles of atomic absorption spectrophotometry (AAS) were outlined by Coombs et al [15]:

> If an element is heated in a flame, as well as emitting light at particular wavelengths it will also absorb light at the same wavelengths. If the light of specific wavelengths produced by heating an element in a lamp is shone through a

flame, the amount of light of these wavelengths absorbed by the flame will vary directly with the amount of that element in the flame.

Thus, in AAS the purpose of the flame is only to atomize the lithium while in flame photometry the flame serves to both atomize and excite the element.

Possible problems with AAS can arise from improper dilution of serum and interference by other elements [15].

### Flame Photometry versus Atomic Absorption Spectrophotometry

While the two techniques are not identical with regard to factors such as sensitivity and interference, these differences are not of sufficient magnitude to be clinically important. Given the precision and accuracy of both techniques, either should be well suited for use in a clinical laboratory. The technique itself, however, succeeds or fails depending on the competence of the laboratory that employs it and high level quality control is essential. For example, the Clinical Toxicology Laboratory of the University of Wisconsin Hospital assesses quality control daily using a product with standardized, highly specific performance characteristics (Lab-Trol Chemistry Control from Dade Diagnostics, Inc.) to determine the accuracy and precision of their flame photometry lithium assay. The cumulative quality control data for a representative month (20 days) are as follow: mean concentration 0.649 mEq/l; standard deviation (SD) 0.015 mEq/l; coefficient of variation 2.0%; range (2 SD) 0.62-0.68 mEq/l.

### Other Techniques

Newer procedures are being investigated for measuring lithium in biological fluids but have not attained widespread clinical acceptance. These include flameless atomic absorption spectroscopy in which the sample is dried, ashed, and atomized in a graphite furnace [16,18,19], a process several times more sensitive than flame methods and suited for use with microliter samples; inductively coupled argon emission spectrometry [16]; and mass spectrometry, either field desorption [20] or thermal ionization [21], which promise a much greater sensitivity than currently used spectrometric techniques. When used therapeutically, however, lithium is present in serum in relatively high concentrations; consequently, detection methods which provide extreme sensitivity offer no clinical advantages over conventional techniques.

## BLOOD COLLECTION AND SAMPLE PREPARATION

Under routine clinical conditions, venous blood samples are collected in plain, anticoagulant-free tubes and the lithium concentrations measured in serum. Plasma can also be used for the analysis (plasma and serum lithium concentrations are the same) but caution must be taken to avoid using an anticoagulant that contains lithium (e.g., lithium-heparin).

The lithium concentration in plasma or serum remains quite stable over time with stability in serum at room temperature for at least eight days [22], and in frozen plasma for at least a year [23], having been demonstrated. A small amount of hemolysis will have no clinically important effect on the plasma lithium concentration [24].

Methods have been described for measuring lithium in microliter samples of blood, thus allowing the use of capillary samples from fingertip or ear lobe [18-25]. Cooper et al [26] found that simultaneous venous and capillary samples contained comparable concentrations of lithium (correlation coefficient 0.99). While microtechniques can be quite sensitive and precise, such procedures are not available in many clinical laboratories and for routine purposes, the use of a venous blood sample is preferred.

## LABORATORY MONITORING OF LITHIUM THERAPY

In his classic 1975 article, Amdisen described the pharmacokinetics of lithium and applied them to clinical practice [6]. In subsequent papers he revised and elaborated on these concepts and in doing so made major contributions that are critical to the safe and effective use of lithium [10–14].

Admisen makes the very important point that blood level monitoring lagged well behind the use of clinical observation to regulate lithium dosage. In retrospect, it seems obvious that blood levels obtained in a nonstandardized fashion would correlate poorly, if at all, with therapeutic outcome and side effects. In recent years, much has been done to minimize pharmacokinetic and other variables and standardize the monitoring of serum lithium levels so that the procedure is now a valuable and necessary tool for the effective treatment of patients. Unfortunately, even today many clinicians remain unaware of or disregard this information so that blood level monitoring of their patients may be meaningless or even harmful. Scientific papers continue to be published in which no mention is made of standardized blood level monitoring—a factor which greatly compromises or even invalidates the research.

### The Twelve-Hour Standardized Serum Lithium

Standardizing the timing of blood drawing in relation to the last dose of lithium is critical if serum levels are to be meaningful. Following a dose, the serum level peaks within a few hours and then as lithium is both distributed to the tissues and excreted, the level falls in a biphasic fashion with the second phase being more gradual than the first. The exact shape of this curve depends on factors which include dose, dosage interval, and bioavailability and dissolution characteristics of the lithium preparation used. Nonetheless, the generalization can be made that a blood sample obtained within hours after a dose will have a considerably higher lithium concentration than a sample taken many hours later. For example, two hours after a dose the level might be 2.0 mEq/l, twelve hours later a more therapeutic 1.0 mEq/l and 20 hours later only 0.6 mEq/l. Thus, with time as the only variable, a patient's dosage might be erroneously adjusted downward or upward or fortuitously left unchanged to achieve a "therapeutic" level of 1.0 mEq/l.

In order to eliminate this confusing and mischievous variable, the concept of the twelve hour standardized serum lithium (12h-stSLi) has been introduced and widely accepted. Amdisen specifies [12]:

(a) The blood sample should be drawn in the morning before the first dose of the day exactly 12 hours (± 30 minutes) after the evening dose.
(b) A multiple dose regimen should be used. The time of intake should always be the same in the individual patient, at least on the day before each control of 12h-stSLi.
(c) The patient should always be in steady state.
(d) Preference should be given to lithium preparations with the narrowest tolerance in terms of $Li^+$ content, bioavailability, and in vivo release course.
(e) The patient should be so thoroughly instructed and trained that complete compliance to the regimen is secured. In case of noncompliance, the 12h-stLIi may be of more danger than usefulness.

The use of 12 hours as a standard sampling interval is somewhat arbitrary and it is not known if this represents the optimal interval between last dose and blood sampling. It is conceivable that maximum, minimum, mean, or yet another level would be better, yet none of these could be easily and consistently determined. Twelve hours appears to be a reasonable compromise since it is convenient to patients and it is in a time range during which blood lithium levels are neither increasing nor falling rapidly. Insisting that patients closely adhere to this sampling interval would do much to reduce a major cause of inconsistent results.

### Therapeutic Serum Lithium Levels

The ranges of serum lithium most likely to be both effective and safe for acute and maintenance therapy were not developed in studies which strictly adhered to the 12h-stSLi [13,27]. Amdisen refers to only one prospective study in which this sampling interval was used [12]. Consequently, therapeutic ranges remain subject to further study and revision.

Currently recommended therapeutic ranges vary depending on the information source but are generally similar. The package inserts used in the United States currently give 1.0–1.5 mEq/l as an effective serum lithium level for acute mania and 0.6 to 1.2 mEq/l as a desirable serum level for long-term control.

Amdisen suggests that acute mania will respond to a 12h-stSLi of 1.2 mEq/l in "practically all potential lithium responders" [12]. There are, of course, exceptions and an occasional nonresponder at 1.2 mEq/l will respond at a higher level [28]. In such situations, extreme caution must be exercised since the risk of lithium intoxication is substantial. We suggest that for acute mania, the serum level be adjusted initially to between 0.8 and 1.2 mEq/l and only if the patient does not respond and if the drug is well tolerated should higher levels be used.

Some patients, especially the elderly, may be unusually sensitive to lithium so that clinical response and adverse reactions may occur at lower than expected serum levels. Blind adherence to the result of a laboratory test, especially in the face of clinical evidence to the contrary, can only be considered foolhardy.

For maintenance therapy, serum levels between 0.6–1.0 mEq/l (12 hour sample) are likely to be therapeutic in most lithium responders. On the other hand, the work of Hullin [29] and the experience of most clinicians indicate that a substantial number of persons will respond to maintenance levels between 0.4–0.6 mEq/l and some to even lower levels. Unfortunately, there is no way to determine the lowest effective maintenance level other than through the tedious and sometimes risky process of clinical trial and error.

Amdisen [11] cautions that patients who relapse despite a maintenance level of 0.8–1.0 mEq/l (12 hour sample) should not be considered nonresponders until they have an adequate trial at a level of about 1.2 mEq/l. Furthermore, it may take many months for a maximum prophylactic effect to develop so that one must not prematurely conclude that relapse early in the course of treatment is synonymous with lithium nonresponsiveness.

In brief, a 12h-stSLi for acute mania should be in the range of 0.8–1.2 mEq/l and for maintenance therapy in the range of 0.6–1.0 mEq/l. One must be aware, however, of the exceptions and caveats expressed elsewhere in this paper.

### Time of Day

Convenience to both patients and laboratory dictates that most blood samples be obtained in the morning with the last lithium dose taken the evening before (12 hours earlier). Occasionally, however, late afternoon or evening sampling may be more practical, yet the meaning of such results must be interpreted with caution. This is because there may be a marked variation in lithium elimination half-life between daytime and nighttime (possibly due to the effects of posture on lithium clearance) with nighttime half-life being as much as two times longer than daytime [30]. For example, one subject had a daytime elimination half-life of 13.5 hours and a nighttime elimination half-life of 33.5 hours [6].

### How Often to Do Blood Levels

When initiating treatment, a therapeutic, non-toxic blood level is the goal. According to first-order kinetics the maximal accumulation of a drug will occur after about 4 half-lives, after which the rate of administration will be balanced by the rate of elimination and the blood level will remain constant (assuming other variables are controlled). Since the elimination half-life of lithium is in the range of 15–30 hours (or longer in the presence of impaired renal function or in the elderly), steady state blood levels will not be reached for at least 2-1/2 to 5 days after starting treatment or changing dose. Thus, blood sampling more often than every 5–7 days is not necessary unless toxicity is a concern. Blood levels obtained prior to reaching steady state may actually be misleading and result in premature dosage adjustment. For example, Schou suggests that if treatment is initiated with large doses, a blood level be obtained after two days (since the risk of toxicity is high) but if treatment is started gradually with a low dose that weekly blood tests should be adequate until the desired level is attained. Then he suggests monthly levels for six months with even longer intervals permissible after that if the patient remains clinically stable [31]. In addition, blood levels should also be obtained whenever clinically indicated; for example, during relapse, suspected toxicity, possible drug interactions, intercurrent illness, and major change in diet.

### Dosage Schedule

Whether it is best to administer lithium in a single daily dose or in divided doses is not known. In this country, divided dosing is the rule and even the slow-release preparations are recommended at least twice daily. Amidsen has been quite emphatic in recommending divided dose [11,14]. He argues that existing knowledge correlating blood levels with therapeutic response is based on divided dose studies and would be invalid if a single daily dose schedule was used. For example, using computer-simulated concentration curves, he demonstrated that a 12h-stSLi based on a single daily dose would be considerably higher than if the same daily dose were administered in four parts (1.37 mEq/l versus 1.0 mEq/l) [11]. The differences in 12h-stSLi using two, three, or four doses daily are much less substantial. In addition, proponents of divided daily dosing suggest that the high peak concentration reached during single daily dosing might cause annoying side effects and be especially toxic to kidney and other tissues.

On the other hand, arguments favoring single daily dosing include ease of administration (improved compliance), the occurrence of peak-dependent side effects during sleep, and the possibility that the lower minimum lithium concentration reached between doses would be less noxious to body tissues and actually be less nephrotoxic [32].

Preliminary evidence appears to favor a single daily dose schedule. In a comparison of two major Danish lithium centers, one using single daily dose standard lithium and the other twice daily slow-release lithium, the single dose regimen was associated with significantly less polyuria [33]. Another study found both urine volume and changes in kidney morphology to be significantly less in patients receiving a single daily dose regimen [32]. Perry et al evaluated 8 patients who were switched from twice daily to once daily dosing for a period of 12 days [34]. They found no significant change in lithium half-life or renal lithium clearance but 24 hour urine volume did significantly decrease during the single daily dose phase.

Further work must be done to resolve the dosage schedule issue (and consider compromises such as single daily dosing of slow-release preparations or more extreme approaches such as every other day lithium). For example, while the mean 12 hour serum lithium concentrations were the same in the two studies that compared them [32,33], the mean 24 hour lithium dose was lower in the group receiving the single daily dose regimen. It would be premature to conclude that all patients should be treated with or could tolerate single daily dosing with a standard lithium preparation. It should be remembered that the meaning of the 12 hour serum lithium concentration has been reasonably well established only for a divided daily dose schedule. Nonetheless, therapeutic outcome seemed no worse nor toxicity more common in the Danish center using the single daily dose schedule [33].

## Lithium Preparations

The controlled release (Eskalith CR) and slow-release (Lithobid) preparations available in the United States differ from standard lithium preparations in having more gradual rates of absorption and lower peak serum levels following equivalent doses. On the other hand, the total amounts of lithium absorbed are similar and, assuming divided doses are used, the differences in the 12 hour serum levels are small enough to be of no clinical importance. Consequently, the same serum monitoring procedures can be applied to the standard and slower-release forms.

## Patient Instruction

A well informed, cooperative patient is essential if blood level determinations are to be effectively used for monitoring lithium therapy. Our booklet, *Lithium and Manic Depression: A Guide* [35] addresses questions such as "How should lithium be taken?," "Why are lithium blood tests necessary?," "How often is a lithium blood test needed?," and "What preparation is needed before a lithium blood test?" Schou offers similar advice in *Lithium Treatment of Manic-Depressive Illness: A Practical Guide* [31]. Patient compliance with those facets of treatment necessary to ensure the usefulness of blood level monitoring is certain to be enhanced if written instructions are available.

Before a blood test, we emphasize to patients: "(1) Be sure no doses of lithium have been forgotten in the last several days, and (2) be sure the blood test is done as closely as possible to 12 hours after the last dose of lithium" [35]. We also state that blood tests are usually done in the morning with the first dose of the day taken *after* the blood sample is obtained. Patients need not be fasting for the blood test since the lithium taken the night before is already absorbed. We further stress that while blood tests may be an inconvenience, they are necessary to ensure the safety and effectiveness of lithium therapy and that they should be done when requested by the doctor. Patients and relatives are also educated to recognize the early signs of affective relapse and lithium intoxication and encouraged to seek both clinical and laboratory evaluation when appropriate.

## Variables Affecting Serum Lithium Level

In general, once stabilized the 12 hour serum lithium level tends to be quite consistent over time. Should a particular level deviate substantially from the usual, an explanation should be sought. The most common causes are lapses in compliance (especially forgotten doses) and in sample timing (taking the morning dose prior to blood sampling). Other factors include laboratory error, variability in dissolution and bioavailability characteristics of different lithium preparations, changes in dietary sodium intake, drug interactions that either increase or decrease lithium clearance (thiazide diuretics and some of the nonsteroidal antiinflammatory agents cause substantial lithium retention), renal disease, dehydration, mood state, and more subtle factors such as position, temperature, and exercise.

If no apparent explanation is forthcoming and if the patient is clinically stable, the test should be repeated rather than readjusting dosage based on one aberrant result. More often than not, the second determination will be in the patient's usual range.

## LITHIUM INTOXICATION

Lithium poisoning is a serious matter since the ultimate outcome may be death or permanent neurological and/or renal damage. The subject has been reviewed elsewhere [36–38] so that this discussion will be limited to the use of blood level monitoring in the diagnosis and treatment of intoxication.

Guidelines offered by experts are admittedly based on clinical experience rather than experimental study so that they must be viewed with some flexibility. The severity of intoxication depends on the magnitude and duration of exposure as well as individual sensitivity. An acute overdose is more likely to be associated with a relatively high serum level in relationship to tissue saturation with lithium and, consequently, clinical symptoms may not be extreme. On the other hand, a long exposure to a high concentration of lithium results in higher tissue levels, a greater likelihood of serious consequences, and a longer recovery time.

Amdisen advises that a serum lithium level be obtained "urgently" at the slightest suggestion of intoxication and that this level and the time of last dosing be used to estimate the 12 hour value. Since the serum lithium concentration falls in an exponential fashion, the 12 hour level can be estimated even if the first samples are drawn many hours or even days later. Samples are obtained every three hours and the results plotted semilogrithmically with the resulting straight line extended back to a point 12 hours after the last dose [13,14,37].

According to Amdisen, a 12 hour value above 3.5 mEq/l should be considered life-threatening while a 12 hour value between 2.5-3.5 mEq/l should also be viewed as quite dangerous. In both instances he suggests that hemodialysis should be instituted without delay (peritoneal dialysis is less effective but preferable to no dialysis). He further recommends that if the 12 hour concentration is below 2.5 mE1/l, that serum levels be obtained every three hours and if the level falls less than 10% over each period that dialysis also be instituted [14].

Schou also considers hemodialysis "the treatment of choice in patients with clinically moderate to severe lithium poisoning" [37]. He comments that hemodialysis *may* also be indicted if serum concentrations have been high (above 3.0 mEq/l) even if clinical findings are mild or absent. Finally, he points out that if symptoms of intoxication are mild and the serum concentration has not exceeded 3.0 mEq/l, general supportive therapy may be adequate.

If hemodialysis is employed, treatment should be continued until serum levels *remain* below 1.0 mEq/l. Following dialysis, there is a redistribution of lithium from tissue to blood and a "rebound" rise in serum lithium level. Thus, a level below 1.0 mEq/l immediately after dialysis may rise substantially over the next several hours and necessitate further treatment. A serum lithium level done about six hours after dialysis will reflect the final redistribution of lithium and when this value falls below 1.0 mEq/l treatment can be stopped [10,14,38].

It should be stressed that these guidelines must be used flexibly and adapted to each clinical situation. Some patients may suffer irreparable harm at serum levels that the guidelines suggest are "safe" while others may tolerate dangerous levels and recover completely with only conservative treatment. Amdisen concludes "It should of course be noticed that only a certain number of patients with 12h-stSLi levels above 2.50 or 3.50 mmol/l would die or be permanently disabled, but since such patients cannot be identified in advance it is necessary to offer to all of them the most advanced treatment" [14].

## DOSAGE PREDICTION

Three methods have been employed to estimate dosage requirement and circumvent the conventional and sometimes time-consuming approach of gradually adjusting dosage based on previous serum lithium level.

1. Cooper et al developed and popularized the 24-hour serum lithium level as a prognosticator of dosage requirement [18,25,39,40]. They gave a single 600 mg dose of lithium carbonate and found that the serum level at 24 hours could be used to predict the daily dose of lithium necessary to attain a steady state serum level between 0.6–1.2 mEq/l. Others have confirmed the usefulness of this or similar approaches [18,41–45].

On the other hand, the accuracy and reproducibility of the test depend on certain prerequisites being met (such as correct sample timing, laboratory accuracy, physiological stability, patient compliance, and characteristics of the lithium preparation) [14,25]. Davis et al [46] were unable to confirm the predictive value of this test; Naiman et al [47] found that 30% of their patients (4/13) did not attain the desired steady-state serum level; and Gengo et al [43] described one patient whose daily dose was predicted to be twice as high as actually necessary. With regard to the 24 hour prognostication test, Amdisen concluded: "So many variabiles influence such a standardized serum concentration that the risk of calculating a wrong 24 hour dose is too great to be acceptable" [11]. This may be overstated but if the test is used, 24 hour values that are low must be interpreted with caution since they would predict high dosage requirements (for example, a 24 hour level of less than 0.5 mEq/l would predict a dosage requirement of 3600 mg/day—an amount with which only the ill-advised would initiate treatment).

2. Renal lithium clearance following a single dose of lithium has also been used to estimate lithium dosage requirement [14,42,44,48]. Since lithium is excreted almost entirely by the kidney, daily intake should be proportional to renal clearance. This technique has not been as widely used or standardized as the 24-hour serum level test and requires measurement of urine as well as serum lithium concentration. It cannot be recommended for general clinical use.

3. Amdisen described a safe but "admittedly laborious" method which involves giving a low lithium dose daily for a week, then checking the 12 hour lithium

level daily for three days and calculating by direct proportionality a maintenance dose [14,27]. This approach has not been widely used.

Overall, no dosage prediction test has gained widespread acceptance. While the 24-hour prognostication test has been reasonably well studied and does seem to have some practical utility, most clinicians continue to feel more comfortable adjusting dosage based on previous blood level, a knowledge of lithium pharmacokinetics, and the clinical status of the patient.

## THE LITHIUM RATIO (RED BLOOD CELL/PLASMA RATIO)

The red blood cell lithium concentration and the ratio between red blood cell and plasma lithium have been extensively investigated with regard to diagnosis, clinical state, response prediction, side effect and toxicity prediction, and as an indicator of compliance. Despite a considerable interest and expenditure of effort and resources, the area remains controversial in all regards and the lithium ratio cannot be recommended for routine clinical use [13,17,49-56].

The lithium ratio can be determined both in vivo [57] and in vitro [58] and the correlation between the two techniques is apparently quite good (Pearson correlation coefficient 0.99) [58]. Using the in vitro technique, Ostrow et al have shown that a number of drugs can alter the lithium ratio and suggest that this is one factor that has contributed to conflicting results found in other studies with regard to diagnosis and response prediction [58].

The lithium ratio has been suggested as a means of detecting that rare breed of noncomplier who takes lithium only immediately before blood tests in order to hoodwink the physician. In such patients, the red blood cell lithium concentration and lithium ratio would be lower than had sufficient time been allowed for steady state conditions to be established between red cell and plasma (summarized in [59]). For such a test to be useful, it would be necessary to establish stable baseline lithium ratios for patients and then prove that deviations from these baselines were due only to noncompliance. Whether a laboratory test designed to "trap" a patient would be of any value in improving compliance instead of eroding an already tenuous doctor-patient relationship is open to question. The use of the lithium ratio as an insurer of compliance has little future.

## LITHIUM MONITORING USING SAMPLES OTHER THAN BLOOD

### Saliva Lithium

At least 56 articles have been published on the subject of saliva lithium levels (source: Lithium Information Center, January 1983). It has been suggested that the use of saliva would eliminate the need for venipuncture, reduce patient inconvenience and discomfort, and even allow the patient to mail samples to the laboratory and avoid a clinic visit [46,60,61].

The actual measurement of lithium in saliva is said to be "a simple estimation, well within the compass of a district hospital biochemistry department" [60], yet collection and analysis techniques have varied considerably from study to study [61-66]. Guelen points out that wide intraindividual variations of saliva potassium concentration can artifactually alter the apparent saliva lithium concentration if measured by flame photometry and that failure to correct for this may account for the inconsistent results in many clinical studies [67].

Lithium is concentrated in saliva so that a saliva/plasma ratio of 2–3:1 is found. This ratio varies considerably among individuals but remains much more constant within a given individual. It has been suggested that once the ratio has been established for an individual, that further lithium monitoring might be done using only saliva samples [60–62,65,68]. Rosman et al [63] state that to use saliva to estimate serum lithium concentration, a linear regression equation derived from intrasubject data must be applied. In patients who were clinically unstable, they found that the saliva lithium concentration correlated poorly with serum levels.

Despite the work that has been done, the use of saliva for monitoring lithium therapy has no utility in routine clinical practice. It is doubtful if saliva testing will ever achieve the degree of standardization, reproducibility, and acceptance necessary to make it a valuable clinical tool (with lithium or any other drug). In fact, it is difficult to understand the continued fascination that this subject holds for both researchers and editors.

### Urine Lithium

Once absorbed, lithium is excreted almost entirely in the urine. Since lithium preparations differ in bioavailability, a variable portion may be lost in the feces and urine recovery may be as low as 85% of a dose. While the amount of lithium excreted in the urine over 24 hours approximates the amount taken in, there is a considerable variation in urine lithium concentration during a 24 hour period. Consequently, the monitoring of urine lithium concentration has no role in routine patient management [17].

At one time, it was suggested that an excretion test might be of value in predicting the anti-manic effect of lithium. Serry reported that, based on the amount of lithium excreted in the urine following a single dose of lithium, the extent of lithium retention would predict responsiveness [69,70]. Subsequent attempts to replicate the test were unsuccessful and it currently has no established value (summarized in [49,50]).

At times it may be useful to determine renal lithium clearance (which ranges between 10–40 ml/minute in the presence of normal renal function [11]) and in such instances determination of urine lithium concentration would be necessary.

While the procedure is not difficult, special considerations are necessary to avoid introducing substantial error and invalidating results [71,72].

### Cerebrospinal Fluid Lithium

While lithium is easily measured in cerebrospinal fluid (CSF) [15,73], the test has little clinical utility, even in monitoring intoxication. The CSF/plasma lithium ratio is less than 0.5, does not seem to correlate with diagnosis or therapeutic response and is not altered by hemodialysis [17,38,74].

### Fecal Lithium

When reference is made to fecal lithium loss, the presence of lithium in feces is usually estimated by the difference between the amount ingested and amount excreted in the urine rather than by direct measurement [13]. Hullin et al, in a metabolic study, did measure the lithium content of fecal homogenates and found that the amount excreted was "very small" (less than 0.2 mEq/day) [75]. It is unlikely that direct measurement of fecal lithium concentration will ever play a role in lithium monitoring (and it is unlikely that anyone would ever want it to).

### Tear Lithium

As might be expected, lithium is excreted in tears. When Brenner et al [76] found in 7 patients a tear/plasma ratio approaching unity, they stated "we consider the evaluation of lithium tear levels a practical and viable alternative to evaluating plasma lithium levels when clinicians have difficulty obtaining blood samples from their patients." These results, however, were not supported by our study (as yet unpublished) of 13 volunteers who after ten days on lithium had a mean tear/serum lithium ratio of 0.77 (±0.10).

Little is known about the excretion of drugs in tears and still less about tear lithium excretion. Many unstudied factors such as the method used to stimulate tear flow, collection procedure, flow rate, influence of other drugs, and sample timing could have a major influence on tear drug concentrations. In addition, the number of patients in whom blood collection is impractical or impossible is very few. Hence the use of tear lithium levels to monitor therapy is neither practical nor necessary. Hopefully, there will be no further research done to achieve this goal.

### Ejaculate Lithium

Lithium is present in ejaculate in concentrations approximating twice those of serum [77]. The use of ejaculate lithium levels to monitor therapy, while pleasurable for some, would be distasteful to others and limited to males. It will never be of any practical use.

### Sweat Lithium

Lithium is excreted in sweat in concentration 1.2-4.6 (mean 2.3) times higher than serum [78]. While sweat has not been suggested as an alternative to blood for monitoring lithium treatment, under certain conditions it may be a vehicle by which substantial lithium loss occurs [79].

### Breast Milk Lithium

Lithium is present in breast milk in concentrations 30–100% of the mother's serum and nursing infants will have serum levels between 10–50% of the mother [80]. Not only is there no role for measuring breast milk lithium concentration in order to monitor therapy, but breast feeding by "lithium mothers" is generally discouraged.

## THE FUTURE

Monitoring lithium therapy by laboratory procedures is currently limited to the measurements of serum lithium concentration. Despite considerable research, no other monitoring techniques have been more successful and none show great promise in replacing serum lithium levels in the future. At present, monitoring techniques could be most improved by stricter attention to the basics of serum level determination such as strict adherence to sampling interval (12 hours), understanding the concept of steady state, and promoting ways to insure compliance.

Hopefully, future research will answer questions about minimum effective therapeutic levels and how to predict them for given individuals; prediction of lithium responsiveness both acutely and long-term; the relative merits of divided versus single daily dose; and the use of laboratory testing for diagnostic purposes. Further pursuit of the use of other body fluids (saliva, CSF, tears) to monitor therapy seems pointless.

All in all, we are fortunate to have a drug as effective as lithium yet so simple in structure that it is not protein-bound, has no metabolites, and can be simply, inexpensively, and accurately measured by readily available clinical procedures.

## REFERENCES


1. Cade JFJ: Lithium salts in the treatment of psychotic excitement. Med J Aust 2:349–352, 1949
2. Strobusch AD, Jefferson JW: The checkered history of lithium in medicine. Pharmacy in History 22:72–76, 1980
3. Talbott JH: Use of lithium salts as a substitute for sodium chloride. Arch Intern Med 85:1–10, 1950
4. Cade JFJ: The story of lithium. In Ayd FJ, Blackwell B (eds): Discoveries In Biological Psychiatry. Philadelphia, JB Lippincott, 1978, pp. 218–229.
5. Corcoran AC, Taylor RD, Page IH: Lithium poisoning from the use of salt substitutes. JAMA 139:685–688, 1949
6. Amdisen A: Monitoring of lithium treatment through determination of lithium concentration. Dan Med Bull 22:277–291, 1975
7. Noack CH, Trautner EM: The lithium treatment of maniacal psychosis. Med J Aust 38:219–222, 1951
8. Schou M, Jeul-Neilsen N, Stromgren E, et al: The treatment of manic psychoses by the administration of lithium salts. J Neurol Neurosurg Psychiatry 17: 250–260, 1954
9. Schou M: Lithium in psychiatric therapy: Stock-taking after ten years. Psychopharmacologia 1:65–78, 1959
10. Amdisen A: Clinical and serum-level monitoring in lithium therapy and lithium intoxication. J. Anal Toxicol 2:193–202, 1978
11. Amdisen A: Serum level monitoring and clinical pharmacokinetics of lithium. Clin Pharmacokinet 2:73–92, 1977
12. Amdisen A: Serum concentration and clinical supervision in monitoring of lithium treatment. Ther Drug Monit 2:73–83, 1980
13. Amdisen A: Lithium. In Evans WE, Schentag JJ, Jusko WJ (eds): Applied Pharmacokinetics: Principles of Therapeutic Drug Monitoring. San Francisco, Applied Therapeutics, 1980, pp. 586–617
14. Amdisen A: Monitoring lithium dose levels: clinical aspects of serum lithium estimation. In Johnson FN (ed): Handbook of Lithium Therapy. Lancaster, England, MTP Press Limited, 1980, pp 179–195
15. Coombs HI, Coombs RRH, Mee UG: Methods of serum lithium estimation. In Johnson FN (ed): Lithium Research and Therapy. New York, Academic Press, 1975, pp. 165–179
16. Maessen FJMJ: Atomic spectrometric methods and techniques for the determination of lithium in biological materials: Fundamental principles and recent advances. In Johnson FN (ed): Handbook of Lithium Therapy. Lancaster, England, MTP Press Limited, 1980, pp 205–218
17. Cooper TB, Carroll BJ: Monitoring lithium dose levels: estimation of lithium in blood and other body fluids. J Clin Psychopharmacol 1:53–58, 1981
18. Cooper TB: Monitoring lithium dose levels: estimation of lithium in blood. In Johnson FN (ed): Handbook of Lithium Therapy. Lancaster, England, MTP Press Limited, 1980, pp. 169–178
19. Ehrlich BE, Diamond JM: Ultra micro method for analysis of lithium and other biologically important cations. Biochim Biophys Acta 543:264–268, 1978
20. Lehmann WD, Bahr U, Schulten HR: Quantitative field desorption mass-spectrometry: 10. Determination of lithium in microliter amounts of human

body fluids at therapeutic and normal levels by stable isotope dilution and field desorption mass-spectrometry. Biomed Mass Spectrom 5:536–539, 1978
21. Lloyd JR, Field FH: Analysis of lithium using a commercial quadrupole mass spectrometer. Biomed Mass Spectrom 8:19–24, 1981
22. Khandelwal SK, Khare CB, Raghavan KS, et al: Stability of serum lithium levels. Am J Psychiatry 139:1377, 1982
23. Lippmann S, Regan W, Manshadi M: Plasma lithium stability and comparison of flame photometry and atomic absorption spectrophotometry analysis. Am J Psychiatry 138:1375–1377, 1981
24. Hisayasu GH, Cohen JL, Nelson RW: Determination of plasma and erythrocyte lithium concentrations by atomic absorption spectrophotometry. Clin Chem 23:41–45, 1977
25. Cooper TB, Simpson GM: The 24-hour lithium level as a prognosticator of dosage requirements: A 2-year follow-up study. Am J Psychiatry 133:440–443, 1976
26. Cooper TB, Simpson GM, Allen D: Rapid direct micro method for determination of plasma lithium. Atomic Absorption Newsletter 13:119–120, 1974
27. Grof P: Lithium treatment and management: Introduction. In Cooper TB, Gershon S, Kline NS, et al (eds): Lithium: Controversies and Unresolved Issues. Amsterdam, Excerpta Medica, 1979, pp. 265–281
28. Kocsis JH: Lithium in the acute treatment of mania. In Johnson FN (ed): Handbook of Lithium Therapy. Lancaster, England, MTP Press Ltd, 1980, pp 9–16
29. Hullin RP: Minimum serum lithium levels for effective prophylaxis. In Johnson FN (ed): Handbook of Lithium Therapy. Lancaster, England, MTP Press Limited, 1980, pp 243–247
30. Lauritsen BJ, Mellerup ET, Plenge P, et al: Serum lithium concentrations around the clock with different treatment regimens and the diurnal variation of the renal lithium clearance. Acta Psychiatr Scand 64:314–319, 1981
31. Schou, M: Lithium Treatment of Manic-Depressive Illness: A Practical Guide. Basel, New York, S. Karger, 1980
32. Plenge P, Mellerup ET, Bolwig TG, et al: Lithium treatment: Does the kidney prefer one daily dose instead of two? Acta Psychiatr Scand 66:121–128, 1982
33. Schou M, Amidsen A, Thomsen K, et al: Lithium treatment regimen and renal water handling: The significance of dosage pattern and tablet type examined through comparison of results from two clinics with different treatment regimens. Psychopharmacology 77:387–390, 1982
34. Perry PJ, Dunner FJ, Hahn RL, et al: Lithium kinetics in single daily dosing. Acta Psychiatr Scand 64:281–294, 1981
35. Bohn J, Jefferson JW: Lithium and Manic Depression: A Guide. Madison, Board of Regents of the University of Wisconsin System (Lithium Information Center), 1982
36. Jefferson JW, Greist JH: Lithium intoxication: Psychiatric Annals 8:458–465, 1978
37. Schou M: The recognition and management of lithium intoxication. In Johnson FN (ed): Handbook of Lithium Therapy. Lancaster, England, MTP Press Limited, 1980, pp 394–402
38. Hansen HE, Amdisen A: Lithium intoxication (report of 23 cases and review of 100 cases from the literature). Q J Med 47:123–144, 1978

39. Cooper TB, Bergner PE, Simpson GM: The 24-hour serum lithium level as a prognosticator of dosage requirements. Am J Psychiatry 130:601–603, 1973
40. Cooper TB, Simpson GM: Issues related to the prediction of optimum dosage. In Cooper TB, Gershon S, Kline NS, et al (eds): Lithium: Controversies and Unresolved Issues. Amsterdam, Excerpta Medica, 1979, pp. 346–353
41. Chang SS, Pandey GN, Dysken M, et al: Predicting the optimal lithium dosage–prospective study. Clin Pharmacol Ther 25:217, 1979
42. Tyrer SP, Kalvar M, Shopsin B, et al: Prediction of lithium dose requirement: Comparison of renal lithium clearance and serum lithium estimation. In Grof P, Saxena B (eds): Recent Advances in Canadian Neuropsychopharmacology. Basel, New York, S Karger, 1980, pp 172–181
43. Gengo F, Timko J, D'Antonio J, et al: Prediction of dosage of lithium carbonate: use of a standard predictive method. J Clin Psychiatry 41:319–321, 1980
44. Tyrer SP, Grof P, Kalvar M, et al: Estimation of lithium dose requirement by lithium clearance, serum lithium, and saliva lithium following a loading dose of lithium carbonate. Neuropsychobiology 7:152–158, 1981
45. Perry PJ, Alexander B, Dunner FJ, et al: Pharmacokinetic protocol for predicting serum lithium levels. J Clin Psychopharmacol 2:114–118, 1982
46. Davis RA, Taylor MA, Abrams R: Body fluid lithium measurements: Severity of illness and prediction of outcome. Biol Psychiatry 13:595–599, 1978
47. Naiman IF, Muniz CE, Stewart RB, et al: Practicality of a lithium dosing guide. Am J Psychiatry 138:1369–1371, 1981
48. Norman KP, Cerrone KL, Reus VI: Renal lithium clearance as a rapid and accurate predictor of maintenance dose. Am J Psychiatry 139:1625–1626, 1982
49. Carroll BJ: Prediction of treatment outcome with lithium. Arch Gen Psychiatry 36:870–878, 1979
50. Marini JL: Predicting lithium responders and non-responders: Physiological indicators. In Johnson FN (ed): Handbook of Lithium Therapy. Lancaster, England, MTP Press Limited, 1980, pp. 118–125
51. Rybakowski J: Red blood cell/lithium ratio in patients with affective disorders. In Cooper TB, Gershon S, Kline NS, et al (eds): Lithium: Controversies and Unresolved Issues. Amsterdam, Excerpta Medica, 1979, pp 218–225
52. Petursson H: Prediction of lithium response. Compr Psychiatry 20:226–241, 1979
53. Greil W, Becker BF, Duhm J: On the relevance of the red blood cell/plasma lithium ratio. In Cooper TB, Gershon S, Kline NS, et al (eds): Lithium: Controversies and Unresolved Issues. Amsterdam, Excerpta Medica, 1979, pp 209–217
54. Kocsis JH, Kantor JS, Lieberman KW, et al: Lithium ratio and maintenance treatment response. J Affective Disord 4:213–218, 1982
55. Smith JA, Branton LJ, Glass R, et al: The red blood cell lithium/plasma lithium ratio: significance in recurrent affective illness. Med J Aust 1:631–632, 1979
56. Del Vecchio M, Farzati B, Maj M, et al: Cell membrane predictors of response to lithium prophylaxis of affective disorders. Neuropsychobiology 7:243–247. 1981
57. Frazer A: Determination of the Li ratio of human erythroctyes in vivo. In Cooper TB, Gershon S, Kline NS, et al (eds): Lithium: Controversies and Unresolved Issues. Amsterdam, Excerpta Medica, 1979, pp 976–977

58. Ostrow DG, Southam AS, Davis JM: Lithium–drug interactions altering the intracellular lithium level: an in vitro study. Biol Psychiatry 15:723–739, 1980
59. Ayd FJ: Checking for compliance with lithium therapy. International Drug Therapy Newsletter 16:33–34, 1981
60. Sims A: Monitoring lithium dose levels: Estimation of lithium in saliva. In Johnson FN (ed): Handbook of Lithium Therapy. Lancaster, England, MTP Press Limited, 1980, pp 200–204
61. Bowden CL, Houston JP, Shulman RS, et al: Clinical utility of salivary lithium concentration. Int Pharmacopsychiatry 17:104–113, 1982
62. Ravenscroft P, Vozeh S, Weinstein M, et al: Saliva lithium concentrations in the management of lithium therapy. Arch Gen Psychiatry 35:1123–1127, 1978
63. Rosman AW, Sczupak CA, Pakes GE: Correlation between saliva and serum lithium levels in manic-depressive patients. Am J Hosp Pharm 37:514–518, 1980
64. Vlaar H, Bleeker JAC, Schalken HFA: Comparison between saliva and serum lithium concentrations in patients treated with lithium carbonate. Acta Psychiatr Scand 60:423–426, 1979
65. Ben-Aryeh H, Naon H, Szargel R, et al: Salivary lithium concentration–a tool for monitoring psychiatric patients. Oral Surg 50:127–129, 1980
66. Selinger D, Hailer AW, Nurnberger JI, et al: A new method for the use of salivary lithium concentrations as an indicator of plasma lithium levels. Biol Psychiatry 17:99–102, 1982
67. Guelen PJM: Clinical pharmacokinetics of lithium. In Merkus FWHM (ed): The Serum Concentration of Drugs. Amsterdam, Excerpta Medica, 1980, pp 106–113
68. Preskorn SH, Abernethy DR, McKnelly WV: Use of saliva lithium determinations for monitoring lithium therapy. J Clin Psychiatry 39:756–758, 1978
69. Serry M: The lithium excretion test: I. Clinical application and interpretation. Aust NZ J Psychiatry 3:390–394, 1969
70. Serry M, Andrews S: The lithium excretion test: II. Practical and biochemical aspects. Aust NZ J Psychiatry 3:395–397, 1969
71. Amdisen A: Quantitative determination of lithium in urine. In Vinar O, Votava Z, Bradley PB (eds): Advances in Neuropsychopharmacology. Amsterdam, North-Holland Publishing Company, 1971, pp 67–71
72. Amdisen A: The estimation of lithium in urine. In Johnson FN (ed): Lithium Research and Therapy. New York, Academic Press, 1975, pp 181–185
73. Anderson DK, Prockop LD: Lithium absorption and distribution in the body tissues. In Johnson FN (ed): Lithium Research and Therapy. New York, Academic Press, 1975, pp 267–280
74. White K, Cohen J, Boyd J, et al: Relationship between plasma, RBC, and CSF lithium concentrations in human subjects. Int Pharmacopsychiatry 14:185–189, 1979
75. Hullin RP, Swinscoe JC, McDonald R, et al: Metabolic balance studies on the effect of lithium salts in manic-depressive psychosis. Br J Psychiatry 114:1561–1573, 1968
76. Brenner R, Cooper TB, Yablonski ME, et al: Measurement of lithium concentrations in human tears. Am J Psychiatry 139:678–679, 1982
77. Kolomaznik M, Musil F, Suva J: Lithium level in some biological fluids at its prophylactic-therapeutic application. Act Nerv Super (Praha) 21:169, 1979

78. Miller EB, Pain RW, Skripal PJ: Sweat lithium in manic-depression. Br J Psychiatry 133:477–478, 1978
79. Jefferson JW, Greist JH, Clagnaz PJ, et al: Effect of strenuous exercise on serum lithium level in man. Am J Psychiatry 139:1593–1595, 1982
80. Weinstein MR: Lithium treatment of women during pregnancy and in the post-delivery period. In Johnson FN (ed): Handbook of Lithium Therapy. Lancaster, England, MTP Press Limited, 1980, pp 421–429

CHAPTER 7

# Blood Level Determinations of Commonly Prescribed Medical Drugs

ARTHUR M. FREEMAN III
and CARL B. SHORY

With the increasing number of pharmaceutical preparations becoming available each year, it is important for both the physician who prescribes the medication, and the patient who takes it, to be aware of the intended and adverse effects associated with the use and overuse of these compounds. Contrary to most popular opinion, the medications which are most likely to cause problems are not the newer exotic drugs but the older, more widely used "safe" medications. Before a physician can hope to deal with these side effects he must be certain what medication the patient is taking and how much he has consumed. Certainly a history from the patient is of greatest importance, but often the patient is unconscious, does not remember how much he has taken, or, in the case of attempted suicide, uncooperative. In such cases the toxicology laboratory is invaluable.

Each year ingenious new assay techniques are developed. Many of these are simply refinements of standard assay techniques. Although it is not necessary for the physician ordering the assay to understand the precise test which is being employed, he should have some knowledge of the basic mechanisms involved and the limitations which are inherent in each test.

*Handbook of Psychiatric Diagnostic Procedures,* vol. 1, edited by R. C. W. Hall and T. P. Beresford. 

Factors which are of importance to the pathologist in choosing a particular assay, and of importance to the physician when interpreting the results include (1) the length of time necessary to complete the assay, especially in emergency situations; (2) the availability of the test; (3) the expense to both the patient and the laboratory; and (4) the reproducibility of the test. An assay which has highly consistent results in one laboratory but cannot be reproduced with the same accuracy in other laboratories by different technicians is of limited usefulness. Also of importance are (5) accuracy, the ability of a test to give results which are as close to the actual blood level as possible; (6) sensitivity, the ability of a test to measure very low concentrations of drug with accuracy; and (7) specificity, the ability of a test to measure only the substance in question and not to include other interfering factors which may be present in the plasma.

In performing most assays, the first procedural step involves extraction of the drug from the plasma. This involves mixing the plasma or blood sample with a water insoluble organic solvent (e.g., hexane, benzene). The particular solvent chosen depends on its polarity and the polarity of the drug in question. In general, the least polar solvent in which the drug will dissolve is chosen. The ability of the drug to dissolve in these organic solvents can be altered by changing the pH of the plasma sample. For example, an acidic drug will be made less ionized if an acid is initially added to the plasma. This will make the drug less soluble in the plasma (i.e., water) and more soluble in the organic phase. This organic solvent can then be drawn off and either evaporated to leave the parent drug or alkalinized to cause precipitation of the drug from the solvent.

Following extraction, an assay technique is chosen. The most commonly employed of these is some form of chromatography: thin layer chromatography (TLC), gas chromatography (GC), or high pressure liquid chromatography (HPLC), also known as high performance liquid chromatography. The three chromatographic techniques have two components in common, a stationary phase and a mobile phase. In thin layer chromatography, the stationary phase is usually silica gel coated on a plate, and the mobile phase is a mixture of solvents. Following extraction of the drug to be assayed, the solvent extract is concentrated to a small volume and applied to one end of the TLC plate. The solvent is allowed to evaporate, and the plate is placed in a tank such that the bottom edge is in contact with solvent. The solvent will ascend the plate by capillary action sweeping the extract along with it. The different components of the extract move at different relative speeds thereby allowing them to come to rest at different points along the plate. When the solvent has reached the top of the plate, the plate is removed from the tank and dried. An appropriate reagent is sprayed on the plate, making the drug of interest visible. TLC is of greatest usefulness in drug screening and is not routinely used for therapeutic monitoring.

In gas chromatography the stationary phase is of a high molecular weight liquid coated on small particles of an inert solid support. The mobile phase is a gas, usually helium or nitrogen. With this method the extract is injected into the GC column, vaporized, and heated to the proper temperature. The gaseous mobile phase sweeps the components along the column at varying rates. As each component emerges from the end of the column, one of various types of detectors record its passing as a peak on a strip-chart recorder. The flame ionization detector consists of two charged electrodes and a hydrogen flame. As an extract component passes through the flame it is ionized generating a current between the electrodes which can be recorded. The electron capture detector is a more sensitive means and is selective only for electronegative groups such as halogen atoms. The nitrogen–phosphorus detector is also quite sensitive and responds only to organic nitrogen or phosphorus.

In high pressure liquid chromatography the stationary phase is a very fine polar solid packed into a column while the mobile phase is a relatively nonpolar organic solvent. More common in drug assays is the reversed-phase HPLC which involves a nonpolar stationary phase (long chain hydrocarbons bonded to silica) and a more polar mobile phase. The plasma extract is pumped through the column at high pressure. As in the previous methods the various components move at different relative rates, and emerge from the column one at a time. The drug of interest is detected and quantitated by ultraviolet absorbence. Each drug has a characteristic wavelength in the ultraviolet spectrum at which the ultraviolet radiation is maximally absorbed. An ultraviolet spectrophotometer is set at that wavelength and a beam is passed through a dissolved sample of the drug. Quantitation is derived through the relative absorption of the beam by the drug.

Colorimetric spectrophotometry, one of the oldest assay techniques used in toxicology, is the predecessor of ultraviolet spectrophotometry. Following extraction of the drug from the plasma, the reagent is added to the sample to produce a color. This color is characteristic for the drug, and its absorbence at a particular visible wavelength is then measured. Absorbence is proportional to the drug concentration. The biggest drawback to this technique is that it generally lacks specificity.

In recent years an entirely new class of assay techniques has been developed employing principles of immunology. The most widely used of these is radioimmunoassay or RIA. With this method, a drug, such as digoxin, is covalently bound to a protein such as albumin to produce an antigen. This antigen is then injected into a laboratory animal which responds by producing antibodies to the antigen. These antigen-specific antibodies are then extracted and purified. To assay the concentration of digoxin in a sample of plasma, a radioactively labeled analog of digoxin is added to the plasma. This is followed by the addition of the previously prepared antibody which combines with both labeled and unlabeled antigen. Competition for antibody binding sites means that the larger the amount of unlabeled digoxin in the sample, the less radioactive digoxin that will be bound. Free and antibody-bound antigen is then separated by one of a number of methods; the

**Table 1. Half-Lives and Dosage Levels of Some Commonly Prescribed Drugs**

| | | Dosage levels | | |
|---|---|---|---|---|
| | | Therapeutic | Toxic | Lethal |
| Aspirin | 2–3 hrs (15–30 hrs in overdose) | 150–300 μg/ml | 300–500 μg/ml | >500 μg/ml |
| Acetaminophen (Tylenol®) | 1–4 hrs (prolonged at toxic levels) | ≤40 μg/ml | >300 μg/ml at 4 hrs post ingestion or a $T_{1/2}$ > 12 hrs | – |
| Digoxin | 1.7 days | 0.5–2.2 ng/ml | 2.0–9.0 ng/ml | >10 ng/ml |
| Digitoxin | 7 days | 10–35 ng/ml | – | >50 ng/ml |
| Quinidine | 6–7 hrs | 2–5 μg/ml | – | >8 μg/ml |
| Propranolol | 3–5 hrs | 50–100 ng/ml | – | – |
| Theophylline | 1.4–8.0 hrs (children and young adults)<br>24–36 hrs (premature infants) | 6–20 μg/ml | 20–40 μg/ml | >40 μg/ml |
| Gentamicin | 2–3 hrs | 4–8 μg/ml (peak)<br>≤2 μg/ml (trough) | >10 μg/ml (peak)<br>>2 μg/ml (trough) | – |
| Tobramycin | 2–3 hrs | 4–8 μg/ml (peak)<br>≤2 μg/ml (trough) | >10 μg/ml (peak)<br>>2 μg/ml (trough) | – |
| Diphenhydramine (Bendaryl®) | 3.5 hrs | 25–50 ng/ml | >50 ng/ml | – |

level of radioactivity of the unbound antigen is measured, compared with standards, and a quantitative determination of plasma digoxin concentration is made.

Another new immunological technique is enzyme immunoassay or EIA. With this method there is no radioisotope used and there is no need to separate free and bound drugs [1]. The "label" is an enzyme covalently bound to the drug. When this enzyme–drug complex binds to antibody there is a reduction in enzyme activity. Since free drug in the specimen competes with enzyme–drug complex for binding sites on the antibody, the amount of enzyme–drug complex left free in solution is directly proportional to the concentration of drug in the specimen. When required substrate and cofactors are added the enzyme activity can be measured spectrophotometrically.

Of increasing use in the assay laboratory is the gas chromatograph mass spectrometer. The gas chromatograph functions to separate the components of the plasma extract as previously described. As each fraction emerges from the GC column it is fed into the mass spectrometer where the molecules are fragmented and ionized by heat or some other means. These particles are then quantitated and evaluated according to their mass-to-charge ratio. A computer analyzes the results and determines the most likely compound to fit that particular pattern. This method is highly specific and is an excellent tool for emergency drug screening, but at present is not widely used due to the expense and complexity of the instruments involved.

The following is a discussion of various commonly used medications both prescription and nonprescription which often cause toxic side effects. Most of these drugs are among the most commonly assayed medications, either in acute emergency situations, or as a routine prophylactic measure. Table 1 presents an outline of the drugs discussed at various dosage levels.

## ASPIRIN

For centuries, the medicinal effect of the bark of the willow has been known by various cultures. In 1827 the active ingredient, salicin, was discovered by Leroux, and in 1838 Piria synthesized salicylic acid from this substance. Aspirin (acetylsalicylic acid) was introduced into medicine in 1899 by Dresser for use as an antipyretic in the treatment of rheumatic fever, and to increase the urinary excretion of uric acid in the treatment of gout [2].

Aspirin is no longer used in the treatment of gout because of the large doses necessary to be effective. But it is still widely used today as an analgesic for mild to moderate pain relief, an antipyretic, and an anti-inflammatory medication especially effective in the treatment of arthritis. Aspirin and the other nonnarcotic analgesics are probably the most widely used medications in the world. They are also the most abused. According to the National Clearinghouse for Poison Control

Centers there were 1,067 deaths attributed to analgesics and antipyretics in 1976, accounting for 38% of all pharmaceutical related deaths. These figures have been somewhat modified more recently, however, by the increased usage of child resistant bottle caps and the limitation on the amount of aspirin allowable in bottles of children's aspirin.

The problem of aspirin abuse continues. Many physicians do not even ask their patients if they take aspirin. Others advise their arthritic patients to continue increasing their doses until they begin to experience tinnitus. If they then reduce the dose there are probably no permanent side effects, but some patients may be taking more than 20 aspirin (325 mg each) per day on a long term basis. This is almost one-half the minimum lethal dosage of 15 gm/70 kg person or about 45 aspirin [3].

Following ingestion of acetylsalicylic acid the drug is rapidly absorbed, primarily in the small intestine, and de-acetylated. The salicylate is metabolized to a variety of organic acids and their conjugates which follow a complex pattern of excretion primarily in the kidney. Secretion, conjugation, and reabsorption all takes place here [1]. Reabsorption can be blocked by alkalinization of the urine through administration of sodium bicarbonate. At therapeutic doses, salicylates have an excretion half-time of 2–3 hrs but this may be prolonged to 15 to 30 hrs in overdose cases due to saturation of enzyme pathways [2].

During the initial phase of salicylate intoxication there is a marked increase in both the rate and depth of respiration. This is due not only to a metabolic acidosis by the salicylic acid but is also due to direct stimulation of the central respiratory centers in the medulla. Carbon dioxide is blown off, blood pH increases, and a respiratory alkalosis ensues. As the intoxication progresses the salicylate will begin to depress the medullary centers, respiration will slow, and the pH will drop. At this point there is a condition of combined respiratory acidosis due to increased $CO_2$ in the blood, and metabolic acidosis secondary to the salicylic acid. If untreated, the condition progresses rapidly to coma and death [2].

Other symptoms of salicylate intoxication include nausea, vomiting, headache, fever, hypoglycemia, thirst, dizziness, irritability, cyanosis, brown-black urine, diaphoresis, dehydration, gastritis, peripheral vasodilation, weakness, delirium, and convulsions [3].

The most common assay for salicylates was developed by Trinder in 1954. An acidic solution of ferric nitrate and mercuric chloride is added to plasma resulting in an immediate and persistent purple color. The level is quantitated by decanting the supernatant and reading it in a spectrophotometer at 540 nm [4].

The test is sensitive enough to be positive following the ingestion of only a small amount of aspirin, but is not specific only to salicylate. The purple color will appear if there are any phenol derivatives in the blood (e.g., phenothiazines) [1]. Refinements of this technique have been developed by various laboratories [1,3,5] as well as an assay employing thin layer chromatography.

Treatment of aspirin overdose includes activated charcoal and milk, followed by gastric lavage with warm water. Alternatively, 15 ml of syrup of ipecac may be used to induce vomiting. Fluids may be given to increase urinary output and to correct dehydration due to vomiting and sweating. Body heat, glucose, and electrolyte balance are maintained. Alkaline drinks may be given in milder cases but in more severe cases intravenous sodium bicarbonate is necessary to reverse acidosis and sodium loss. Electrolytes and blood gases should be monitored periodically and hemodialysis may be necessary in severe cases. Vitamin K and vitamin C may be given if necessary for low prothrombin [3].

## ACETAMINOPHEN

Acetaminophen (Tylenol®), a coal tar derivative, is an effective analgesic-antipyretic alternative to aspirin; however, unlike aspirin it has little anti-inflammatory activity. A predecessor of acetaminophen, acetanilid, was introduced into medicine in 1886 as an antipyretic [1]. It was found to be excessively toxic and was replaced by phenacetin, one of its metabolites. Phenacetin is still used today in analgesic mixtures but has been largely replaced by the even less toxic acetaminophen. This compound is a metabolite of both acetanilid and phenacetin and has been available without a prescription in the United States since 1955.

Acetaminophen is rapidly and almost completely absorbed from the gastrointestinal tract with peak plasma concentrations occurring between 30 to 60 minutes. It is uniformly distributed throughout body fluids and has a half-life in plasma of 1 to 4 hours. Virtually all acetaminophen is conjugated in the liver prior to excretion. Sixty percent is conjugated with glucuronic acid while about thirty-five percent is conjugated with sulfuric acid. When large doses are ingested these pathways become saturated and more toxic alternative metabolites are formed which are hepatotoxic.

In adults, hepatotoxicity may occur after ingestion of a single dose of 10 to 15 g (200 to 250 mg/kg) of acetaminophen and a dose of 25 g or more is potentially fatal. Acetaminophen is often given to children because it may be better tolerated by them than aspirin. But children have less capacity for conjugation of acetaminophen than adults and it may be potentially more toxic.

Following ingestion of a toxic dose of acetaminophen, symptoms may be vague and nonspecific. Nausea, vomiting, anorexia, and abdominal pain occur during the first 24 hours and may persist for a week or more. Liver function tests begin to show abnormal values within 2 to 6 days. Plasma transaminases and lactic dehydrogenase activity may be elevated, but initially alkaline phosphatase activity and serum albumin may be normal. Jaundice and coagulation disorders may ensue and progress to encephalopathy, coma, and death.

Measurement of the half-life of acetaminophen in the plasma during the first day following poisoning provides the best indication of the extent of hepatic damage. Hepatic necrosis is likely if the half-life exceeds 4 hours and hepatic coma should be anticipated if it is greater than 12 hours. Single plasma concentration determinations are less helpful but if they exceed 300 μg/ml at 4 hours post-ingestion, extensive hepatic damage is likely.

Early diagnosis and treatment are imperative in cases of possible acetaminophen overdose. Induction of vomiting and gastric lavage should be performed to limit further absorption. Hemodialysis may be of use if initiated within the first 12 hours and especially if the patient has an acetaminophen plasma concentration greater than 120 μg/ml at 4 hours. But most promising of all in treatment of overdose is the administration of sulfhydryl compounds such as L-methionine, L-cysteine, and N-acetylcysteine, which act, at least in part, by replenishing stores of glutathione in the liver. N-acetylcysteine (Mucomyst®) appears to be particularly effective and well tolerated orally. This drug is recommended if the acetaminophen ingestion has occurred within the past 24 hours. A loading dose of 140 mg/kg is given, followed by 70 mg/kg every 4 hours for 17 doses. If assays determine that the risk of hepatotoxicity is low then the antidote is discontinued.

Because of the need for rapid diagnosis and treatment of acetaminophen overdosage, rapid and accurate assay methods are required. Two basic methods are presently employed, a colorimetric method [6,7], and a high pressure liquid chromatography method [8–11]. Both methods have recently been compared [11,12] with advantages found for both methods. The colorimetric method is currently more widely available and simpler to perform. It consists of extraction of the acetaminophen from plasma and addition of a color reagent. If acetaminophen is present, a color change occurs, the intensity of which is proportional to drug concentration. This method is not specific for acetaminophen and falsely elevated plasma concentrations are commonly reported due to interference from salicylamide, salicylates, and possibly cresol, the latter being a constituent of some heparinized syringes. The HPLC technique is not only more specific for acetaminophen but is also more sensitive, having an average variation from the actual plasma concentration of only 4.8% in a trial involving 20 plasma samples ranging from 1 to 100 μg/ml. The colorimetric test, being simpler and less expensive to perform is potentially an excellent screening test. Several batches of these tests can be run at once as compared to the HPLC method where tests must be run serially, one at a time. On the other hand the high sensitivity and specificity of the HPLC method makes it the procedure of choice in determining the elimination half-time of acetaminophen in an acutely toxic patient seen in the hospital emergency room.

## DIGITALIS

The term digitalis refers to the dried leaf of the foxglove plant, *digitalis purpurea.* The seeds and leaves of this plant and related species contain digoxin, digitoxin, and other glycosides which have a common, powerful effect on myocardial contractility. It has been mentioned in the writings of Welsh physicians as far back as 1250, and in 1785 William Withering published his book "An Account of the Foxglove and Some of Its Medical Uses: With Practical Remarks on Dropsy and Other Disease." Withering attributed the effectiveness of digitalis in the treatment of dropsy (edema) to its effect on the kidneys as a diuretic. In 1799 John Ferriar was the first to ascribe the primary action of digitalis on the heart [13].

There are various preparations of digitalis and related cardiac glycosides found in numerous plant species, but the most commonly prescribed forms in use today are digoxin and digitoxin. Both have the same basic steroid ring structure but vary primarily in their water and lipid solubility. Digitoxin is more lipid soluble and is therefore much more completely absorbed from the gastrointestinal tract (90 to 100%) [1]. Digoxin on the other hand is more water soluble and its absorption varies from 40 to 90%. This variability is most prominent with tablets from different manufacturers and is related to differences in the rate and extent of dissolution [14–16]. It is important for the physician to be aware of this, to use a preparation with which they are familiar, and to prescribe the preparation by its commercial name.

Following oral administration of digoxin, peak plasma levels are attained in 2 to 3 hours, but the maximal tissue effect is delayed, becoming apparent at 4 to 6 hours. Digitoxin is more slowly absorbed with peak levels and effects occurring at 3 to 6 hours, and 6 to 12 hours respectively. Digitoxin in plasma is more completely bound to circulating proteins (90% or more) as opposed to a plasma digoxin binding of only 25%. This fact in part, is responsible for the slower elimination of digitoxin which has a disposition half-time of 7 days as compared to 1.7 days for digoxin. Digitoxin is primarily eliminated by hepatic degradation to inactive metabolites which are excreted by the kidneys [13]. Digoxin on the other hand, is primarily excreted by the kidneys unchanged and dosage may require adjustment in patients with renal disease.

The cardiac glycosides are most frequently employed today in the treatment of patients with congestive heart failure. The main pharmacodynamic property of these substances is to increase the force of myocardial contraction. They have also been used to slow the ventricular rate in cases of atrial fibrillation or flutter. The effect on the myocardium is dose dependent but varies widely from patient to patient with respect to plasma drug levels. This therapeutic index is quite low and coupled with patient variability, the therapeutic and toxic levels in fact overlap.

Following oral administration of toxic doses of digitalis, symptoms may be delayed for hours. Clinically, these include nausea, abdominal pain, vomiting, drowsiness, slow irregular pulse, anorexia, salivation, cold extremities, giddiness, diarrhea, headache, and generalized weakness [3]. Delirium and hallucinations may be present with blurred vision, diplopia, and disturbed color vision. Bradycardia, heart block, and cardiac arrhythmias are common. Death is usually due to ventricular fibrillation or cardiac arrest.

Definite changes in the EKG are present with digitalis toxicity. The normally upright T-wave becomes diminished in amplitude, isoelectric, or inverted in one or more leads [13]. The S-T segment may also show depression when the QRS complex is upward. Later the P-R interval may become prolonged, although rarely greater than 0.25 seconds. The Q-T interval may also be shortened due to accelerated repolarization of the ventricles.

The overall incidence of digitalis toxicity is not established, but as many as 25% of hospitalized patients taking digitalis show some signs of toxicity [17,18]. The sensitivity of the heart to digitalis may be modified by plasma potassium concentrations. Potassium blocks the binding of digitalis to myocardium and hypokalemia may cause increased toxicity. This is of importance because many congestive heart failure patients receive diuretics. Dialysis is contraindicated in digitalis toxicity because it may deplete potassium. On the other hand, hyperkalemia in patients on maintenance doses of digitalis may result in complete A-V block [13]. Hypercalcemia or hypomagnesemia may contribute to toxicity in a manner similar to potassium depletion.

Various blood level determinations of digoxin and digitoxin have been developed. Chemical assay methods were explored but most lacked sensitivity or were too tedious and difficult to perform [19-23]. The first practical assay was developed by Lowenstein [24]. His method consisted of substituting $^{86}Rb^+$ for $K^+$ in a sample of plasma and observing the relative blockage of the active transport of the $^{86}Rb^+$ across the membrane of red blood cells. The degree of blockage is relative to the concentration of cardiac glycoside in the patient's plasma.

The assay methods in use today involve either radioimmunoassay (RIA) or enzyme immunoassay (EIA) [1,25-28]. The RIA method takes just over an hour to perform and has an accuracy of ±20 percent. It is important to stress that each test is specific only for either digoxin or digitoxin and the particular substance in question must be specified. Writing simply "digitalis" or "digoxin" when the ingested substance is digitoxin will yield false results.

Diagnosis and treatment of suspected or confirmed digitalis toxicity relies heavily on clinical evaluation of the patient's symptoms. Digitalis and potassium depleting diuretics should be withheld. Continuous EKG monitoring is imperative in treatment of arrhythmias with phenytoin, lidocaine, and potassium repletion. In severe cases of toxicity, experimental treatment with antibodies specific to the drug ingested has been successful [29].

## QUINIDINE

Quinidine is the dextrostereoisomer of quinine, the chief alkaloid of the bark of the cinchona tree of South America. Both share the same antipyretic, antimalarial, and oxytocic effects, however, quinidine has a much greater effect on cardiac muscle than quinine [30].

Quinidine is used today as a broad spectrum antiarrhythmic for acute and chronic treatment of supraventricular and ventricular arrhythmias. It is primarily used chronically in the treatment of paroxysmal supraventricular tachycardia (PSVT), particularly when seen in the Wolff-Parkinson-White syndrome, and as prophylaxis for recurrent episodes of premature ventricular contractions (PVC). Lidocaine is the first line drug for treatment of PVC's but since it cannot be used orally, quinidine is preferred for chronic treatment.

From the outset of quinidine therapy plasma drug level monitoring is imperative to detect toxic reactions. This is important because the same dosage regimen will produce very different plasma concentrations in different patients and because the same arrhythmia will be more or less responsive to the same concentration in different individuals. The therapeutic index of quinidine is quite low and about one-third of patients who receive the drug will have immediate adverse effects that require discontinuation of therapy.

At high plasma concentrations of quinidine, a wide variety of arrhythmias appear. Ventricular tachycardia is especially life threatening and must be recognized as a toxic effect. It must be realized that the toxicity of the drug may mimic the disease that it is used to treat. Quinidine also causes vasodilatation and in the presence of other vasodilatory drugs (e.g., nitroglycerin) may produce a life threatening hypotension.

The most common untoward effects of quinidine are related to the gastrointestinal tract—nausea, vomiting, and diarrhea. These symptoms occur almost immediately following initiation of therapy, and warrant discontinuation of the medication. Other side effects include tinnitus, visual impairment, headache, flushing of skin, skin rash, low prothrombin blood levels, hypothermia, bradycardia, convulsions, and, of particular concern to the psychiatrist, mental confusion and delirium [3]. Death is usually due to respiratory collapse or asystole.

A number of important interactions occur between quinidine and other medications. Quinidine is metabolized in the liver and drugs such as phenobarbital or phenytoin which induce drug-metabolizing enzymes will shorten the duration of action of quinidine by increasing its rate of elimination [31]. Patients given quinidine who are already on digoxin often have a significant increase in digoxin plasma concentration [32]. Occasionally, patients who are taking oral anticoagulants such as warfarin will have an increase in prothrombin time following administration of quinidine [33]. Also, the effect of quinidine on the heart is increased when plasma concentrations of potassium are increased.

The single most important means of monitoring for acute quinidine toxicity is use of the EKG. Baseline electrocardiograms should be recorded before initiating therapy. As therapy progresses any arrhythmias should be noted. As plasma quinidine concentrations rise above 2 μg/ml the QRS complex and the $Q\text{-}T_c$ interval (corrected Q-T interval) will widen progressively [34]. This plasma concentration is well within the therapeutic range of zero to 4 μg/ml. The $Q\text{-}T_c$ interval can be calculated as the Q-T interval divided by the square-root of the average number of QRS complexes per second.

$$Q\text{-}T_c = \frac{Q\text{-}T}{QRS/sec}$$

If the heart rate is equal to 60 then the $Q\text{-}T_c$ interval will be equal to the Q-T interval. A 25% increase in the duration of the QRS complex, or a $Q\text{-}T_c$ interval greater than 0.44 seconds is cause for concern. A 50% increase in the QRS complex duration or a $Q\text{-}T_c$ interval greater than 0.50 seconds warrants a prompt reduction in dosage. It is also of importance to note that patients who initially have a widened QRS complex or prolonged $Q\text{-}T_c$ interval are more susceptable to quinidine-induced arrhythmias at lower plasma concentrations.

Monitoring of quinidine plasma concentrations with serial EKGs is not without its limitations. Significant variability exists from patient to patient. The correlation of plasma quinidine concentrations is more statistically significant with changes in the QRS complex duration than with changes in the $Q\text{-}T_c$ interval. However, prolongation of the QRS complex is difficult to measure on a standard speed EKG and does not occur until higher plasma concentrations are achieved. For these reasons laboratory derived plasma concentrations are important.

Most laboratory assays of quinidine plasma concentrations employ spectrofluorometry [35-38]. Using this methodology, the plasma is first alkalinized and this drug extracted into an organic solvent. The extract is then irradiated with light which causes the compound to fluoresce at characteristic frequencies. Quantitation is derived by the intensity of the fluorescence at those frequencies. Variations in results depend on the type of extraction reagents, and older methods tend to include various inactive metabolic products yielding falsely elevated plasma concentrations. The method developed by Cramer and Isaksson [37] eliminates most of these and has an average error of about 1%. This assay is also simple, rapid, and inexpensive.

## PROPRANOLOL

Propranolol was the first β-adrenergic antagonist of wide clinical usage in humans, and remains the most important compound within this classification. Its uses include the treatment of hypertension, prophylaxis of angina pectoris, and control of certain cardiac arrhythmias [39]. It blocks both $\beta_1$ and $\beta_2$ receptors competitively and is chemically related to the other $\beta$-antagonists nadolol, timolol, and metoprolol.

The major clinical effects of propranolol are on the cardiovascular system where it decreases heart rate and cardiac output, prolongs systole, and slightly decreases blood pressure in resting individuals. The effects on heart rate and cardiac output are more dramatic during exercise. Peripheral resistance is increased as a result of compensation through sympathetic reflexes, and blood flow to all organs except the brain is reduced [40].

Propranolol is an effective antihypertensive agent which effects a slowly developing reduction in blood pressure with chronic use. This effect is probably due to multiple causes. Following the initiation of treatment with propranolol there is a mild drop in blood pressure which is probably due to the decreased heart rate and cardiac output. With prolonged use, the release of renin from the juxtaglomerular apparatus is blocked [41], resulting in a reduced angiotensin effect. Thus, patients with initially high renin activity and hypertension benefit from much lower doses of propranolol than those with normal plasma concentrations [42].

Propranolol is almost completely absorbed following oral administration, but as much as two-thirds of the dose is metabolized by the liver in its first passage through the portal circulation. This combined with other variations results in as much as a 20-fold difference in plasma concentrations between individuals administered comparable doses. The half-life of the initial oral dose is usually about 3 hours but tends to become more prolonged with chronic therapy. Plasma protein binding of propranolol is usually between 90 and 95% [43].

The most serious side effect of propranolol is acute heart failure. Fortunately this is rare and occurs primarily in patients who already have a severely compromised myocardium. Another important danger is an increase in airway resistance due to the blockage of $\beta_2$ adrenergic mediated bronchodilatation. In normal individuals this effect is small and of no clinical significance, but in the asthmatic this can be life threatening [44]. For this reason propranolol is contraindicated in asthmatics.

A third life-threatening side effect of propranolol involves acute withdrawal following chronic therapy. Patients may experience severe anginal attacks or rebound blood pressure levels which may exceed pretreatment levels. These effects occur within hours to 1 or 2 days after termination of the drug, and are theoretically due to the increased number of $\beta$ receptors induced by the blocking agent. If therapy is to be discontinued, doses should be tapered, and if prodromal symptoms such as nervousness, diaphoresis and tachycardia develop, treatment should be reinstituted.

Another effect of propranolol is its potentiation of the hypoglycemic effect of insulin. Special care must be taken when treating insulin-dependent diabetics and patients prone to hypoglycemic episodes because propranolol masks the tachycardia associated with hypoglycemia.

Of particular interest to the psychiatrist are such CNS side effects as hallucinations, nightmares, insomnia, lassitude, dizziness, and depression [45]. Other reported side effects of propranolol include nausea, vomiting, diarrhea, and constipation. Rash, fever, and purpura may be associated with an allergic response to the medication.

Because of the wide variability of plasma concentrations and the variability of response to propranolol between individuals, there is a growing demand for improved assays of plasma concentrations. Presently, the most widely used procedure involves spectrofluorometry [46]. The procedure is simple, rapid, and inexpensive but lacks specificity. Interference from procainamide, quinidine, and methaqualone occurs at normal therapeutic levels, and the method is not sensitive at plasma levels below 15 ng/ml [47]. Various other methods have been employed which involve the use of thin layer chromatography, gas chromatography, and radioimmunoassay [48-50], but the most popular recently devised method involves high pressure liquid chromatography [51-53]. This method is simple, rapid, inexpensive, and specific for propranolol. The average variability of results on samples analyzed the same day was 1.90%, while the between-day reproducibility for samples analyzed over a three week period was 4.5% [51].

## THEOPHYLLINE

Theophylline, caffeine, and theobromine, closely related derivatives of xanthine, are found in varying amounts in a number of plant species from around the world. Over half the population of the world consumes tea, a beverage prepared from the leaves of a bush native to southern China, which contains caffeine and smaller amounts of theophylline and theobromine. Coffee, a more important source of caffeine in the American diet, was discovered by ancient Arabian shepherds. Legend states that they observed that their goats would stay awake and play all night after eating the berries of the coffee plant [54].

Theophylline has been used for over 50 years in the treatment of various respiratory disorders. Because of its effect on relaxation of bronchial smooth muscle, it is important in the treatment of bronchial asthma. Theophylline also has a central nervous system stimulating effect which acts directly to enhance respiration [1]. For the past 10 years theophylline has been recognized as effective for control of apneic episodes in premature infants [55,56]. Aminophylline is a common dosage form of theophylline which is formed by amination of theophylline to form a more water soluble salt.

Theophylline is well absorbed orally, with peak plasma concentrations occurring within 2 to 4 hours. The intravenous route is often used in acute asthmatic attacks or to ensure uniform absorption and distribution in the premature infant. Plasma protein binding is between 36 and 59%. The elimination half time of theophylline is highly variable between age groups and individuals. In children the

$T_{1/2}$ averages 3.7 hours (range 1.4–7.8 hours) compared to 5.8 hours (range 3.5–8.0) for young adults [57]. Half-lives in premature infants range from 24 to 36 hours and in patients with cardiac failure and pulmonary edema, half-lives may vary as much as 20-fold. The liver is an important site of theophylline metabolism with only 10% of a dose being excreted in the urine unchanged.

Toxic effects of theophylline include tachycardia, hypertension, irritability, agitation, and tachypnea. In more severe cases vomiting, cardiac arrhythmias, hypotension, dehydration, mania, hallucinations, tremor, and hyperreflexia may result. The most serious toxic effect is seizures which may become continuous and are often refractory to anticonvulsant therapy. These convulsions usually occur at plasma theophylline concentrations above 40 μg/ml but have also been reported at levels below 20 μg/ml. If not controlled they may progress to coma and death.

Because of the low therapeutic index of theophylline, its highly variable half-life in plasma, and the fact that prodromal signs of impending seizures are rarely present, periodic assay of plasma concentrations should be routine. The most commonly employed assay involves the use of spectrophotometry and was developed by Schack and Waxler in 1949 [58]. Plasma caffeine or barbiturates interfere with this method and improved extraction methods have been developed [59]. Still, however, interference may be encountered with allopurinol and its metabolic product alloxanthine [60].

Other methods have been developed using gas chromatography [61,62] and gas chromatography–mass spectrometry [63]. These are both highly sensitive and highly specific but require extensive extractions and derivations which make them cumbersome in routine use. Radioimmunoassay [64] and enzyme immunoassay [65] methods have also been developed and appear promising, but the method of choice appears to be the high pressure liquid chromatography for which several assays have been developed [66–68]. The method is inexpensive and rapid, requiring only about 30 minutes to perform. It is simple, specific for theophylline and highly sensitive. Day-to-day variability from standards is between 1 and 5% compared to 18% for the original spectrophotometric procedure.

## AMINOGLYCOSIDES

Streptomycin, the forerunner of today's aminoglycosides was first isolated from the fungus *Streptomyces griseus* in 1943 by Schatz, Bugie, and Waksman [69]. It was found to be an effective inhibitor of the growth of many gram-positive and gram-negative organisms as well as the tubercle bacillus. It was effective against many of the gram-negative organisms which were penicillin-resistant. Unfortunately many streptomycin-resistant mutants emerged rapidly and limited its usefulness. Subsequently, related fungi yielded new aminoglycosides. Currently we have kanamycin, gentamycin, tobramycin, amikacin, and neomycin, of which gentamicin is the most popular. They all share the same limitations in clinical use, but to varying degrees. Of primary importance are their ototoxicity, nephrotoxicity, and limited absorption in the gastrointestinal tract.

Aminoglycosides are poorly absorbed across intestinal mucosa due to their highly polar nature. For this same reason they do not readily cross cell membranes and, therefore, have an effective volume of distribution equal to the extracellular fluid volume (about 25% of lean body mass) [70]. Absorption is rapid whether administered by intravenous, intramuscular, or subcutaneous injection with peak plasma concentration occurring at 30 to 90 minutes following either of the latter two. Most of the aminoglycosides have less than 10% plasma protein binding [71]. They are concentrated in the urine and excreted for the most part unchanged. The only tissues in which the aminoglycosides are concentrated above plasma level levels are the renal cortex, and vestibular and cochlear fluids.

The half-lives of aminoglycosides in otic fluids are five to six times longer than in plasma. Penetration occurs mainly when plasma concentrations are high and back diffusion occurs when plasma levels are low. For this reason aminoglycoside levels should be monitored both at peak levels (30 minutes after a dose) and at trough levels (immediately prior to a dose). An adequate peak is necessary for microbial killing while the trough must be low enough to present ototoxicity.

Ototoxicity is the result of destruction of the sensory hairs first, and later the death of the hair cells themselves in both the cochlear and vestibular aparati. The first change is partially reversible, but if the drug is not discontinued, permanent impairment results. Clinical symptoms include tinnitus, a sensation of pressure in the ears, high frequency hearing loss, deafness, nystagmus, vertigo, nausea, and vomiting. Drugs such as ethacrynic acid, furosemide, mannitol, and possibly other diuretics potentiate the ototoxic effects of aminoglycosides [72]. Overt ototoxicity is found in about 2% of patients treated with gentamicin for less than 2 weeks, and the incidence increases markedly with prolonged use.

Nephrotoxicity, like ototoxicity, appears to correlate with high trough levels of aminoglycosides. Elderly patients, as well as patients with shock, dehydration, or preexisting renal disease are particularly susceptible. The nephrotoxicity is essentially a form of acute tubular necrosis. It rarely occurs before 5 to 7 days of therapy and is initially manifested by an inability to concentrate the urine. With continued use of the drug, protein and tubular cell casts may be found in the urine, followed by a progressive reduction in glomerular filtration rate and an increase in the plasma level of the aminoglycoside. These changes are usually reversible if the drug is discontinued. Gentamicin appears to be particularly nephrotoxic [73] with the incidence of renal toxicity reported to be from 2 to 10%.

Various assay methods have been developed to monitor gentamicin levels which involve the use of enzymes [74] or radioimmunoassay [75,76]. Older methods involve observing the effect of gentamicin containing plasma on the growth of microbial cultures [77]. This method is time consuming and lacks sufficient sensitivity, whereas the radioimmunoassay is expensive and results may vary in the hands of inexperienced technicians. A rapid and inexpensive assay of gentamicin levels involves the use of high-pressure liquid chromatography [78]. This method can be performed in as little as one hour and also has the advantage of easily detecting any interfering substance. Finally, the assay has a high degree of accuracy with an inter-assay average variability of no greater than 6.1%.

## ANTIHISTAMINES–$H_1$ BLOCKERS

Histamine-blocking activity was first described by Bovet and Staub in 1937 as an effect of a phenolic compound 2-isoprophy-5-methyl-phenoxyethyldiethylamine. This original drug was too weak and too toxic for clinical use, but in the following years scores of histamine blocking drugs were developed. All of these were effective but no one compound offered a clear advantage over the others [79]. These drugs fit into the class of antihistamines known as $H_1$ receptor blockers, which is variously broken into a number of subclasses according to the basic structure of each compound. In 1972 a new class of antihistamines known as $H_2$ blockers was introduced. The first drug in this class was cimetidine which acts primarily to inhibit gastric acid secretion, an effect not shared by the $H_1$ blockers.

As mentioned previously, the numerous $H_1$ blockers have similar pharmacological action and therapeutic applications. These compounds antagonize the constrictor effect of histamine on bronchial smooth muscle. This is of some clinical benefit to patients with acute anaphylactic bronchospasm but is limited in that these drugs fail to block other bronchoconstrictors such as SRS-A.

$H_1$ blockers also act to antagonize the histamine-induced capillary permeability associated with "wheal and flare" reactions in the skin. Through this mechanism $H_1$ blockers effectively block histamine induced pruritus and are widely prescribed by dermatologists.

Various central nervous system effects are attributed to $H_1$ blockers. CNS stimulation has been reported in occasional patients at therapeutic doses resulting in restlessness, nervousness, and insomnia. Small doses can provoke epileptiform seizures in patients with focal CNS lesions. Central excitation and seizures are also commonly encountered in overdose situations. Central depression, however, is a much more common effect at conventional doses with somnolence reported in about 50% of patients taking diphenhydramine (benadryl) [80]. $H_1$ blockers have also been used effectively in the treatment of motion sickness.

The $H_1$ blockers are well absorbed from the gastrointestinal tract with maximal effects occurring within 1 to 2 hours. Diphenhydramine has an elimination half-time of about 3.5 hours, with excretion primarily in the urine. Little of the compound is excreted unchanged with the major site of metabolism being the liver.

The most common side effect of the $H_1$ blockers is sedation. This may be desirable for some hospital patients or individuals before bedtime, but it interferes with daytime activities and may impair ability to concentrate and work. Caffeine or a reduction in dosage may be all that is necessary, while alcohol will exacerbate this symptom. Other central effects include dizziness, tinnitus, lassitude, incoordination, fatigue, blurred vision, diplopia, euphoria, nervousness, and tremors. Common peripheral effects include nausea, vomiting, anorexia, constipation, diarrhea, dryness of the mouth and throat, urinary frequency, palpitations, hypotension, headache, tightness of the chest, and weakness and tingling of the hands. Some of these may be anticholinergic actions which are common in many of the $H_2$ blockers.

The $H_1$ blockers have a relatively high therapeutic index, but, due to easy availability, they are commonly implicated in accidental poisonings in children and in suicides in adults. In children 20 to 30 tablets is potentially lethal. Overdose presentation entails both central depressant and central stimulant effects including hallucinations, ataxia, incoordination, athetosis, and convulsions. Fixed, dilated pupils with a flushed face and fever are common. Deepening coma and cardiorespiratory collapse may result in death within 2 to 18 hours. Treatment is non-specific involving the use of respiratory support and anti-convulsants.

Diphenhydramine is possibly the most frequently prescribed and most extensively studied of the $H_1$ blockers. One of the earliest assay methods involved a fluorescent-dye technique that permitted determination of plasma levels in the range of 0.2-2 μg/ml, but lacked reproducibility, especially at lower concentrations [81]. More recently, two methods have been devised using gas chromatography [82,83]. These methods are sensitive to plasma concentrations as low as 5 ng/ml and have an average variation from standard means of less than 5.0% at measured levels between 10 and 100 ng/ml.

## CONCLUSION

This chapter is not intended to include all medications which may cause toxic symptoms. Rather, it is a guide to follow for the understanding of how and why patients develop symptoms with certain medications, for knowing which assay methods are available to the clinician for diagnosis and treatment of toxic situations, and for an understanding of the advantages and flaws inherent in each assay procedure. It is hoped that this chapter will be relevant to both emergency care and to the prevention of toxicity.

## REFERENCES


1. Kalman SM, Clark DR: Drug Assay: The Strategy of Therapeutic Drug Monitoring. New York, Masson Publishing, 1979
2. Flower RJ, Moncada S, Vane JR: Analgesic-antipyretics and anti-inflammatory agents; drugs employed in the treatment of gout. In Gilman AG, Goodman LS, and Gilman A (eds): The Pharmacological Basis of Therapeutics, 6th ed. New York, Macmillan, 1980
3. Kaye S: Handbook of Emergency Toxicology, 4th ed. Springfield, IL, Charles C Thomas, 1980
4. Trinder P: Rapid determination of salicylate in biological fluids. Biochem J 57:301–303, 1954
5. Sunshine I: Methodology for Analytical Toxicology. Cleveland, OH, CRC Press, 1975
6. Grings CS, Saloom JM: Coloimetric methods for quantitation determination of acetaminophen in serum. Clin Toxicol 15:67–73, 1979
7. Glynn JP, Kendal SE: Paracetamol measurement. Lancet 2:1147–1148, 1975
8. Blair D, Rumack BH: Acetaminophen in serum and plasma estimated by high-pressure liquid chromatography: A microscale method. Clin Chem 23:743–745, 1977
9. Horvitz RA, Jatlow PI: Determination of acetaminophen concentrations in serum by high pressure liquid chromatography. Clin Chem 23:1596–1598, 1977
10. Lo LY, Bye A: Rapid determination of paracetamol in plasma by reverse-phase high performance liquid chromatography. J Chromatogr 173:198–201, 1979
11. Duffy JP, Byers J: Acetaminophen assay: The clinical consequences of a colorimetric vs. a high-pressure liquid chromatography determination in the assessment of two potentially poisoned patients. Clin Toxicol 15:427–435, 1979
12. West JC: Rapid HPLC analysis of paracetamol (acetaminophen) in blood and postmortem viscera. J Anal Toxicol 5:118–121, 1981
13. Hoffman BF, Bigger JT Jr: Digitalis and allied cardiac glycosides. In Gilman AG, Goodman LS, Gilman A (eds): The Pharmacological Basis of Therapeutics, 6th ed. New York, Macmillan, 1980
14. Lindenbaum J, Butler VP, Murphy JE, et al: Correlation of digoxin-tablet dissolution rate with biological availability. Lancet 1:1215–1217, 1973
15. Lindenbaum J, Mellow MH, Blackstone MO, et al: Variability in biological availability of digoxin from four preparations. N Engl J Med 285:1344–1347, 1971
16. Wagner JG, Christensen M, Sakmar E, et al: Equivalence lack in digoxin plasma levels. JAMA 224:199–204, 1973
17. Beller GA, Smith TW, Abelman WH, et al: Digitalis intoxication. A prospective clinical study with serum level correlations. N Engl J Med 284:989–997, 1971
18. Smith TW: Digitalis toxicity: Epidemiology and clinical use of serum concentration measurements. Am J Med 58:470–476, 1975
19. Watson E, Kalman SM: Assay of digoxin in plasma by gas chromatography. J Chromatogr 56:209–218, 1971
20. Okarma TB, Tramell P, Kalman SM: The surface interaction between digoxin and cultured heart cells. J Pharmacol Exp Ther 183:559–576, 1972
21. Watson E, Tramell P, Kalman SM: Identification of submicrogram amounts of digoxin, digitoxin, and their metabolic products. J Chromatogr 69:157–163, 1972

22. Watson E, Clark DR, Kalman SM: Identification by gas chromatography-mass spectroscopy of dihydrodigoxin—a metabolite of digoxin in man. J Pharmacol Exp Ther 184:424–431, 1973
23. Clark DR, Kalman SM: Dihydrodigoxin: A common metabolite of digoxin in man. Drug Metab Dispos 2:148–150, 1974
24. Lowenstein JM: A method of measuring plasma levels of digitalis glycosides. Circulation 31:228–233, 1965
25. Oliver GC Jr, Parker BM, Brasfield DL, et al: The measurement of digitoxin in human serum by radioimmunoassay. J Clin Invest 47:1035–1042, 1968
26. Smith TW, Butler VP Jr, Haber E: Determination of therapeutic and toxic serum digoxin concentrations by radioimmunoassay. N Engl J Med 281:1212–1216, 1969
27. Horgan ED, Riley WJ: Radioimmunoassay of plasma digoxin, with use of iodinated tracer. Clin Chem 19:187–190, 1973
28. Cerceo E, Elloso CA: Factors affecting the radioimmunoassay of digoxin. Clin Chem 18:539–543, 1972
29. Ochs HR, Smith TW: Reversal of advanced digitoxin toxicity and modification of pharmacokinetics by specific antibodies and Fab fragments. J Clin Invest 60:1303–1313, 1977
30. Bigger JT JR, Hoffman BF: Antiarrhythmic drugs. In Gilman AG, Goodman LS, Gilman A (eds): The Pharmacological Basis of Therapeutics, 6th ed. New York, Macmillan 1980
31. Data JL, Wilkinson GR, Nies AS: Interaction of quinidine with anticonvulsant drugs. N Engl J Med 294:699–702, 1976
32. Leahey EB, Reiffel JA, Drusin RE, et al: Interaction between quinidine and digoxin. JAMA 240:533–534, 1978
33. Koch-Weser J: Quinidine-induced hypothrombinemic hemorrhage in patients on chronic warfarin therapy. Ann Intern Med 68:511–517, 1968
34. Heissenbuttel RH, Bigger JT Jr: The effect of oral quinidine on intraventricular conduction in man. Correlation of plasma quinidine with changes in intraventricular conduction time. Am Heart J 80:453–462, 1970
35. Brodie BB, Udenfriend S: The estimation of quinine in human plasma with a note on the estimation of quinidine. J Pharmacol Exp Ther 78:154, 1943
36. Brodie BB, Udenfriend S, Baer JE: The estimation of basic organic compounds in biological material. J Biol Chem 168:299, 1947
37. Cramer G, Isaksson B: Quantitative determination of quinidine in plasma. Scand J Clin Lab Invest 15:553–556, 1963
38. Edgar AL, Sokolow M: Experiences with the photofluorometric determination of quinidine in blood. J Lab Clin Mcd 36:478, 1950
39. Weiner N: Drugs that inhibit adrenergic nerves and block adrenergic receptors. In Gilman AG, Goodman LS, Gilman A (eds): The Pharmacological Basis of Therapeutics, 6th ed. New York, Macmillan, 1980
40. Nies AS, Evans GH, Shand DG: Regional hemodynamic effects of beta-adrenergic blockade with propranolol in the unanesthetized primate. Am Heart J 85:97–102, 1973
41. Ganong WF: Biogenic amines, sympathetic nerves, and renin secretion. Fed Proc 32:1782–1784, 1973
42. Esler M, Zweifler A, Randall O, et al: Pathophysiologic and pharmacokinetic determinants of the antihypertensive response to propranolol. Clin Pharmacol Ther 22:299–308, 1977

43. Evans GH, Nies AS, Shand DG: The disposition of propranolol. III. Decreased half-life and volume of distribution as a result of plasma binding in man, monkey, dog, and rat. J Pharmacol Exp Ther 186:114–122, 1973
44. Nicolaescu V. Manicatide M, Stroescu V: β-Adrenergic blockade with practolol in acetylcholine-sensitive asthma patients. Respiration 29:139–154, 1972
45. Greenblatt DJ, Shader RI: On the psychopharmacology of beta adrenergic blockade. Curr Ther Res 14:615–625, 1972
46. Shand DB, Nuckolls EM, Oates JA: Plasma propranolol levels in adults, with observations in four children. Clin Pharmacol Ther 11:112, 1970
47. Vasiliades J, Turner T, Owens C: A modified sensitive spectrofluorometric method for the determination of propranolol in serum. Am J Clin Pathol 70:793–799, 1978
48. Hadzija BW, Mattocks AM: Quantitative TLC determinations of propranolol in human plasma. J Pharm Sci 67:1307–1309, 1978
49. Walle T: GLC determination of propranolol, other β-blocking drugs, and metabolites in biological fluids and tissues. J Pharm Sci 63:1885–1891, 1974
50. Kawashima K, Levy A, Spector S: Stereospecific radioimmunoassay for propranolol isomers. J Pharmacol Exp Ther 196:517–523, 1976
51. Jatlow P, Bush W, Hochster H: Improved liquid-chromatographic determination of propranolol in plasma with fluorescence detection. Clin Chem 25: 777–779, 1979
52. Nygard G, Shelver WH, Wahba Khalil SK: Sensitive high-pressure liquid chromatographic determination of propranolol in plasma. J Pharm Sci 68:379–381, 1979
53. Rosseel MT, Bogaert MG: High-performance liquid chromatographic determination of propranolol and 4-hydroxypropranolol in plasma: J Pharm Sci 70:688–689, 1981
54. Rall TW: Central nervous system stimulants. In Gilman AG, Goodman LS, Gilman A (eds): The Pharmacological Basis of Therapeutics, 6th ed. New York, Macmillan, 1980
55. Kuzemko JA, Paala J: Apnoeic attacks in the newborn treated with aminophylline. Arch Dis Child 48:404–406, 1973
56. Shannon DC, Gotay F, Steim IM, et al: Prevention of apnea and bradycardia in low-birthweight infants. Pediatrics 55:589–594, 1975
57. Rane A, Wilson JT: Clinical pharmacokinetics in infants and children. Clin Pharmacokinet 1:2–24, 1976
58. Schack JA, Waxler SH: An ultraviolet spectrophotometric method for determination of theophylline and theobromine in blood and tissues. J Pharmacol Exp Ther 97:283–291, 1949
59. Jatlow P: Ultraviolet spectrophotometry of theophylline in plasma in the presence of barbiturates. Clin Chem 21:1518–1520, 1975
60. Woodman TF, Canada AT, Seidman J: Interference of allopurinol and alloxanthine in ultraviolet theophylline assay. Am J Hosp Pharm 34:984–985, 1977
61. Johnson GF, Dechtiaruk WA, Solomon HM: Gas-chromatographic determination of theophylline in human serum and saliva. Clin Chem 21:144–147, 1975
62. Least CJ Jr, Johnson GF, Solomon HM: Gas-chromatographic micro-scale procedure for theophylline with use of a nitrogen-sensitive detector. Clin Chem 22:765–768, 1976

63. Sheehan M, Hertel RH, Kelly CT: Gas-chromatography mass-spectrometric determination of theophylline in whole blood. Clin Chem 23:64–68, 1977
64. Neese AL, Soyka LF: Development of a radioimmunoassay for theophylline. Application to studies in premature infants. Clin Pharmacol Ther 21:633–641, 1977
65. Gushaw JB, Hu MW, Singh P, et al: Homogeneous enzyme immunoassay for theophylline in serum. Clin Chem 23:1144, 1977
66. Nelson JW, Cordry AL, Aron CG, et al: Simplified micro-scale procedure for preparing samples for theophylline determination by liquid chromatography. Clin Chem 23:124–126, 1977
67. Ovcutt JJ, Kozak PP Jr, Gillman SA, et al: Micro-scale method for theophylline in body fluids by reversed-phase, high-pressure liquid chromatography. Clin Chem 23:599–601, 1977
68. Adams RF, Vandemark FL, Schmidt GJ: More sensitive high-pressure liquid chromatographic determination of theophylline in serum. Clin Chem 22:1903–1906, 1976
69. Sande MA, Mandell GL: Antimicrobial agents: The aminoglycosides. In Gilman AG, Goodman LS, Gilman A (eds): The Pharmacological Basis of Therapeutics, 6th ed. New York, Macmillan, 1980
70. Barza M, Brown RB, Shen D, et al: Predictability of blood levels of gentamicin in man. J Infect Dis 132:165–174, 1975
71. Barza M, Scheife RT: Antimicrobial spectrum, pharmacology, and therapeutic use of antibiotics. J Maine Med Assoc 68:194–210, 1977
72. Mathog RH, Capps MJ: Ototoxic interactions of ethacrynic acid and streptomycin. Ann Otol Rhinol Laryngol 86:158–163, 1977
73. Gary NE, Buzzeo L, Solaki J, et al: Gentamicin-associated acute renal failure. Arch Intern Med 126:1101–1104, 1976
74. Sabath LD, Casey JI, Rich PA, et al: Rapid microassay for circulating nephrotoxic antibiotics. Antimicrob Agents Chemother 83–90, 1970
75. Lewis JE, Nelson JC, Elder HA: Radioimmunoassay of an antibiotic, gentamicin: Nature New Biol 239:214–216, 1972
76. Smith DA, Van Otto B, Smith AL: Rapid chemical assay for gentamicin. New Engl J Med 286:583–596, 1972
77. Alcid DV, Seligman SJ: Simplified assay for gentamicin in the presence of other antibiotics. Antimicrob Agents Chemother 3:559–561, 1973
78. Peng GW, Gadalla MAF, Peng A et al: High-pressure liquid-chromatographic method for determination of gentamicin in plasma. Clin Chem 23:1838–1844, 1977
79. Douglas WW: Histamine and 5-hydroxytryptamine (serotonin) and their antagonists. In Gilman AG, Goodman LS, and Gilman A (eds): The Pharmacological Basis of Therapeutics, 6th ed. New York, Macmillan, 1980
80. Carruthers SG, Shoeman DW, Hignite CE, et al: Correlation between plasma diphenhydramine level and sedative and antihistamine effects. Clin Phrmacol Ther 23:375–382, 1978
81. Glazko AJ, Dill WA, Fransway RL: Determination of diphenhydramine blood levels using a new fluorescent dye-salt procedure generally applicable to basic organic compounds. Fed Proc 21:269, 1962

82. Albert KS, Sakmar E, Movais JA, et al: Determination of diphenhydramine in plasma by gas chromatography. Res Commun Chem Pathol Pharmacol 7: 95–103, 1974
83. Bilzer W, Gundert-Remy V: Determination of nanogram quantities of diphenhydramine and orphenadrine in human plasma using gas-liquid chromatography. Eur J Clin Pharmacol 6:268–270, 1973

CHAPTER 8

# Blood Level Monitoring of Antiepileptic Drugs


## B.J. WILDER and ROBERT J. PERCHALSKI


This chapter is concerned with antiepileptic drug monitoring, seizure control, and central nervous system drug toxicity. Particular emphasis is placed on the subtle toxicity of these agents that sometimes produces profound effects on behavior and higher cortical or cognitive functioning. The neurologist and the psychiatrist should be versed in the use of drug monitoring not only to effect seizure control but also to minimize the risk of undiagnosed drug toxicity.

A part of the chapter is devoted to the basic methodologies and techniques currently used for the quantitative analysis of the antiepileptic drugs.

### ANTIEPILEPTIC DRUG MONITORING AND SEIZURE CONTROL

With the development of modern analytical techniques, the monitoring of plasma concentrations of antiepileptic drugs has become part of routine management of the patient with seizures. The clinician is better able to choose a drug dosage that will achieve an optimum therapeutic response with minimum risk of dose-related toxic effects. The monitoring of plasma antiepileptic drug levels has


*Handbook of Psychiatric Diagnostic Procedures,* vol. 1, edited by R. C. W. Hall and T. P. Beresford.

helped prevent the consequences of adverse drug interactions and has reduced the use of multiple drug therapy.

The biological effect of an antiepileptic drug is proportional to the amount of drug that reaches the central nervous system, which in turn is in dynamic equilibrium with the amount of drug in the circulatory system. Thus, the antiepileptic effect of a drug is best estimated by the blood plasma concentration and not by the dosage.

Antiepileptic drug monitoring is helpful to the clinician in determining patient compliance, preventing dose-related toxic effects, prescribing individual therapy, and achieving a "therapeutic range" of plasma drug levels for each patient. The therapeutic range is a statistical concept, representing the range of plasma drug concentrations that gives optimum clinical control without adverse effects in the majority of patients. Patients whose seizures are well controlled in spite of subtherapeutic plasma drug concentrations should not have their dosage adjusted to increase, or "treat," the plasma level. In some patients, toxic effects may occur at low or even subtherapeutic drug concentrations because of individual differences in susceptibility to adverse effects. Table 1 gives the therapeutic ranges of the major and the minor antiepileptic drugs.

Although a correlation exists between dosage and plasma drug level in individual patients, interindividual correlation may be lacking because of multiple factors [1]. These include:

1. variable compliance;
2. time of plasma sampling in relation to previous dose;
3. individual differences in absorption, volume of distribution and elimination;
4. bioavailability differences due to the nature of drug formulation (e.g., capsule versus suspension);
5. environmental factors that may influence drug metabolism;
6. presence of diseases that may alter absorption, metabolism, or excretion of antiepileptic drugs (e.g., gastrointestinal, cardiac, hepatic, or renal diseases, abnormal protein binding);
7. drug interactions;
8. unknown genetic factors;
9. saturation (zero-order) kinetics of some antiepileptic drugs (e.g. phenytoin plasma concentration increases disproportionately with increasing dose);
10. alterations in plasma proteins and drug binding.

Therapeutic plasma concentrations have been defined for most antiepileptic drugs, so that seizure control can be achieved with little risk of toxicity. The effective plasma level may vary from patient to patient because the severity of seizures may be different, which may explain why seizures in some patients are well controlled at subtherapeutic plasma drug levels [2]. The usefulness of antiepileptic

**Table 1. Therapeutic Plasma Concentrations of the Antiepileptic Drugs**

| Nonproprietary name | U.S. trade name | Normal range (μg/ml) |
|---|---|---|
| Phenytoin | Dilantin | 9–21 |
| Phenobarbital | Luminal | 20–50 |
| Primidone | Mysoline | 4–14 |
| Ethosuximide | Zarontin | 45–90 |
| Carbamazepine | Tegretol | 2–10 |
| Clonazepam | Clonopin | 0.04–0.1 |
| Valproic acid | Depakene | 40–100 |
| Diazepam | Valium | 0.2–0.5 |
| Nitrazepam | Mogadon | 0.04–0.09 |
| Mephenytoin (measured as N-desmethylmephenytoin) | Mesantoin | 12–25 |
| Methsuximide (measured as N-desmethylmethsuximide) | Celontin | 12–25 |
| Mephobarbital (measured as phenobarbital) | Mebaral | 20–50 |
| Chlorazepate (measured as desmethyldiazepam) | Tranxene | 0.6–1.5 |
| Trimethadione | Tridione | 20–40 |
| Dimethadione | Paradione | 700–1400 |

drug monitoring in achieving optimum seizure control has been supported by many clinical studies [1,3,4–7]. It is important, however, that laboratories offering determination of antiepileptic drugs participate in a quality control program to establish interlaboratory reproducibility [8]. Commercial laboratories report total plasma drug levels at the current time.

Many drugs are bound to plasma protein to a variable extent, and the physician should be aware that the bioactive portion of drug in the plasma is the unbound or free fraction (Table 2). Some specialty laboratories are reporting free drug concentrations; however, the necessary correlations between free plasma drug levels and therapeutic and toxic free levels have not been made by clinical pharmacologists. The clinician should be aware that unexplained toxicity, drug interactions, and therapeutic effect may reflect changes in free drug concentrations that are not apparent when total levels are monitored [9]. For example, an important drug interaction occurs when phenytoin and valproate are given concurrently. Valproate significantly displaces phenytoin from protein binding sites, and free phenytoin may

**Table 2. Percentage of Drug Bound to Protein in Plasma**

| | |
|---|---|
| Phenytoin | 90 |
| Valproate | 95 (concentration-dependent) |
| Carbamazepine | 80 |
| Phenobarbital | 50 |

transiently increase and induce central nervous system toxicity that is not indicated by the total plasma phenytoin concentration.

The protein binding of valproate also depends on concentration. At high total valproate levels the ratio of free to total valproate concentration may be four or five times as high as when the total valproate level is lower [10,11]. Similar changes in the pharmacologic effects of the psychotropic drugs can be anticipated for those drugs that have a high affinity for protein binding sites. Table 2 gives the protein binding percentages of some commonly used antiepileptic drugs.

Administration of antiepileptic drugs with other agents used routinely in psychiatric treatment may result in drug interactions and possible increases in the pharmacologic actions and toxic effects of both classes of compounds. A predictable metabolic interaction occurs when a patient receiving phenytoin (Dilantin), a barbiturate, or a succinamide (Celontin) is given disulfiram (Anabuse) in an alcoholic rehabilitation program. Disulfiram inhibits the metabolism of the anticonvulsant, and plasma levels gradually increase. The clinical signs and symptoms of intellectual deterioration or lethargy, or both, often occur before the more recognizable signs of antiepileptic drug toxicity–nystagmus, ataxia, and incoordination. If the interaction is unrecognized, a diagnosis of chronic brain syndrome or presenile dementia may be made. Similarly, interactions between phenothiazines and phenytoin may result in a clinical picture of disturbed higher cortical or cognitive function without overt phenytoin intoxication.

Ideally plasma drug concentrations should be monitored when the plasma concentration is at steady state, and at fixed times in relation to drug administration. This is particularly important in the case of the antiepileptic drugs that have short half-lives (e.g., valproic acid, primidone, carbamazepine). Further information on antiepileptic drug monitoring may be found in the articles by Bruni and Wilder and Richens and Warrington and in Table 3 [12,13].

Although not done routinely, salivary monitoring of antiepileptic drugs can be performed and has the advantage of simplicity of sample collection [14]. The salivary concentration of most drugs corresponds to the that of the free, biologically active portion of the drug in the plasma. Constant saliva-to-plasma ratios have been obtained for phenobarbital, phenytoin, ethosuximide, carbamazepine, primidone, and diazepam. Salivary determinations may be useful when abnormalities of protein binding (e.g., uremia, hypoproteinemia) are suspected. The transport mechanisms

**Table 3. Indications for Antiepileptic Drug Monitoring**

| | |
|---|---|
| 1. | At initiation of therapy, to determine whether a satisfactory plasma drug level has been achieved; |
| 2. | when seizures are uncontrolled, to determine compliance, rapid drug metabolism, or seizure resistance to a specific drug; |
| 3. | when drug dosage is changed and a new steady-state concentration is achieved; |
| 4. | during development of intercurrent illness (e.g., hypoproteinemia; gastrointestinal, hepatic, or renal disease); |
| 5. | when drug interaction is suspected; |
| 6. | when toxic symptoms occur; |
| 7. | when unexplained behavioral changes are noted; |
| 8. | during pregnancy, when alterations in drug absorption and metabolism may occur; |
| 9. | during prepuberty or puberty, when changes in drug metabolism may require dosage adjustment; |
| 10. | when new drugs are added to treatment regimen. |

into saliva and cerebrospinal fluid are similar, and a correlation exists between drug concentration in the saliva and in the cerebrospinal fluid which is in equilibrium with brain drug concentrations [15,16].

## NEUROLOGICAL TOXICITY

### Disturbances of Higher Cortical Functions

Adverse effects of the antiepileptic drugs on cerebral function include behavioral and psychological aberrations, memory and cognitive disturbances, abnormal sensorimotor performance, seizure exacerbation, and electroencephalographic changes. These aspects of antiepileptic drug toxicity have received relatively little attention because of the difficulty in distinguishing drug-related mental symptoms from symptoms caused by brain injury or seizures themselves. In addition, this aspect of drug toxicity is difficult to analyze quantitatively.

It has long been recognized that mental symptoms may occur in epileptic patients. Lennox [17], for example, proposed the following possible causes for mental deterioration in epilepsy: (1) heredity, (2) psychological handicaps, (3) brain injury that precedes the seizure disorder, (4) epilepsy itself, and (5) drugs. The concurrent administration of multiple antiepileptic drugs theoretically could contribute a greater prevalence of toxic neurological effects. Monitoring of antiepileptic drugs, however, can help to avoid toxic plasma concentrations of drugs, although mental aberrations may occur with therapeutic or even subtherapeutic plasma drug concentrations.

It has been known for some time that phenytoin can cause an encephalopathy and seizure exacerbation [18-27]. The syndrome of chronic phenytoin encephalopathy is characterized by insidious deterioration of intellect and behavior with or without seizure exacerbation, mild cerebrospinal fluid pleocytosis, and a moderate increase in cerebrospinal fluid protein; the plasma phenytoin concentration may be in the therapeutic or toxic range [27]. The encephalopathy is rare and is probably more common in epileptic patients with underlying brain damage [22].

Decreased intellectual performance as a complication of long-term phenytoin use has been reported by numerous investigators [23-26]. Epileptic patients with drug toxicity have been shown to have a greater decrease in cognitive and sensorimotor performance than do those without toxicity [27]. Trimble [28] concluded with regard to effects on cognitive abilities that the antiepileptic drugs in general impair performance on psychological tests and some are associated with a progressive decline in intellectual ability that is often insidious and unrecognized.

The cause of these effects on higher cortical function is not definitely known, but a direct depressant effect on central nervous system function and an effect on folate metabolism are probably important. The cerebrospinal fluid folate concentration is normally three times higher than the serum folate concentration, and folate has a major role in central nervous system function. Long-term folate deficiency associated with antiepileptic drug therapy has been reported to cause mental slowing and apathy, lack of drive, organic brain syndrome, and psychosis, all of which develop in some epileptic patients. Reynolds reported that treatment with folic acid improves mental functioning in these patients at the possible expense of increasing seizures [29,30].

Phenytoin therapy, especially in doses that yield toxic plasma concentrations, may result in significant electroencephalographic abnormalities [31,32]. These abnormalities are most frequent in mentally retarded epiletic patients and are more prominent with toxic plasma phenytoin concentrations. Electroencephalographic effects include an increase in paroxysmal discharges, slowing of the background activity, impaired reaction to alerting procedures, diffuse slow wave abnormalities, abnormal fast activity, and asymmetries of the background activity.

Experimentally, phenobarbital has been associated with brain growth retardation in animals [33,34] and neuronal deficits after prenatal drug exposure [35]. The significance of these findings in relation to phenobarbital therapy for children and pregnant epileptic women is unknown. In children phenobarbital therapy may be associated with hyperactivity and irritability, and elderly patients may experience paradoxical excitation. Several studies have suggested that behavioral changes, decreased intellectual performance, and disturbed sensorimotor functions may accompany the use of phenobarbital [36-39]. It has also been shown that high plasma phenobarbital concentrations can slow short-term memory scanning without impairing long-term memory [39]. Since a significant portion of primidone is metabolized to phenobarbital, the expected side-effects are probably similar, although primidone itself and its second most abundant metabolite, phenylethylmalonamide, may be contributory.

Depression, personality changes, hysteria, hallucinations, delusions, and schizophreniform psychosis are also reported as consequences of anticonvulsant drug therapy [28]. Most reports are anecdotal; however, in patients receiving these drugs, the possibility of drug toxicity should be considered and plasma values obtained. Elderly patients and children are often more susceptible to the subtle toxic effects of the hydantoins than are adults. However, antiepileptic drug toxicity may be difficult to recognize in patients of any age. Wilder and Ramsay [40], in conjunction with a psychologist and a psychiatrist, examined adolescent and adult patients who had a presumptive diagnosis of acute psychosis, aggressive behavior, mental retardation, and dementia. All of these patients were found to have anticonvulsant drug intoxication with no underlying affective or structural brain disorders.

Of the major antiepileptic agents effective against generalized tonic-clonic seizures, carbamazepine has been suggested to have the least effect on intellectual and sensorimotor performance. Although a direct psychotropic effect of carbamazepine is unproved, it has a close chemical relationship to the tricyclic antidepressants. In a double-blind study, primidone caused a greater impairment of cognitive function than carbamazepine [41]. A psychometric evaluation by Dodrill and Troupin [42] comparing phenytoin and carbamazepine showed lesser impairment with carbamazepine. In a recent study of 20 epileptic patients with behavioral disorders, carbamazepine reportedly lessened excitement, irritability, hostility, and uncooperativeness [43].

The effects of ethosuximide therapy on mental function are not clearly defined, and controversies exist as to whether it impairs intellectual function. No adverse effects occurred in a controlled study of 37 patients [44], but earlier studies showed deleterious effects [45,46]. It has also been reported that ethosuximide therapy may exacerbate generalized nonconvulsive seizures [48].

Clonazepam has been implicated in behavioral abnormalities such as irritability, aggression, hyperactivity, and difficulty with concentration [29]. In the treatment of 22 children with intractable epilepsy, clonazepam therapy was associated with hyperactivity in four children, aggression in two, and depression in two others. A large-scale controlled study on the effects of clonazepam on intellectual function has not been performed.

The long-term effects of valproic acid therapy have not been fully established. One study, however, has shown psychomotor deterioration [48].

The effects of antiepileptic drugs on mental function have been comprehensively reviewed [28,49,50].

The importance of plasma level monitoring of antiepileptic drugs in epileptic patients and more particularly in those receiving psychotropic drugs cannot be overemphasized. A first rule should be to suspect toxicity in any patient who is receiving antiepileptic drugs and has a recent history of progressive personality change, behavioral aberration, or deterioration of intellectual function.

## QUANTITATIVE DETERMINATION OF ANTIEPILEPTIC DRUGS

In the last 15 years the reliability of the analytical methods for quantitation of drugs in biological fluids has changed the task of prescribing medicine from an art to a science. The confidence that physicians have in these methods is a result of constant and conscientious practice by laboratory personnel of inter- and intralaboratory quality control procedures that have been stressed almost from the outset of the modern-methods development era that began in the early 1970s. This confidence has caused an expansion of the role of the laboratory from a maintenance–diagnostic tool to a valuable therapeutic aid that few doctors today would neglect. Most would agree that the initial impetus for this expansion was the search for faster, more reliable methods of quantitative determination of antiepileptic drugs in plasma.

The basic methods that are commonly used for quantitation of anticonvulsants include spectrophotometry, immunoassay, and chromatography. Of these, only the chromatographic methods are versatile, specific, and sensitive enough to be applied to all the currently used drugs and their metabolites over the full concentration range of interest for each. However, because only a research laboratory or a laboratory specializing in antiepileptic drug analysis would be concerned with this capability, the more limited techniques have a definite place. Two major reference works that cover the use and analysis of antiepileptic drugs are available [51,52]. Two recent reviews summarize almost all of the pertinent literature and include recommendations based on the authors' personal experience in the field [53,54]. Pippenger et al [55] have also compiled a list of 470 references on quantitation of anticonvulsants for the Food and Drug Administration. Johannsen [56] has reviewed the pharmacokinetic and clinical considerations that are relevant to therapeutic drug monitoring.

The primary techniques can be divided into absorption and fluorescence spectrophotometry; radioimmunoassay and homogenous immunoassay; and thin-layer gas–liquid, and high-performance liquid chromatography. Of these, the most reliable, sensitive, versatile and selective methods are homogeneous immunoassay, gas–liquid chromatography, and high-performance liquid chromatography. Although successful spectrophotometric, radioimmunoassay, and thin-layer chromatographic methods are available, they have generally failed to provide rapid, reliable determination of all drugs of interest. Adequate treatment of these less-used techniques has been given in the aforementioned reviews. Interested readers should refer to the articles of Fellenberg and Pollard [57] on spectrophotometry, Felber [58] on radioimmunassay, and Wad and Rosenmund [59] on thin-layer chromatography, for references and information on the best methods available. The remainder of this chapter deals with the three primary methods.

Immunoassays in general are based on a competitive binding reaction between the analyte (drug of interest) and an analyte-macromolecule complex for an antibody that has been produced specifically for the system. Typically, the drug or hapten is made immunogenic (capable of stimulating antibody production) by covalently bonding it to a protein or polysaccharide. The resulting antigen is injected into an animal (sheep or rabbit) with the hope of producing antibodies that will bind specifically to the antigen and to the original hapten. If this occurs, the animal serum then becomes an analytical reagent. The second reagent is the antigen solution, which is adjusted to the approximate concentration of the drug in the sample. The activity of the antibody reagent is adjusted to bind 20 to 70 percent of the antigen in the absence of hapten. In the actual sample, a competition between the antigen and hapten results in an increase in unbound antigen proportional to the concentration of hapten. A measurement of unbound antigen is translated into the value of interest. In the *homogeneous* immunoassays no separation of bound and unbound antigen is necessary because only the unbound form produces a measurable response.

Three homogenous systems are currently used. The enzyme multiplied immunoassay technique (EMIT®; available from Syva Corporation, Palo Alto, California, 94394) is a versatile, mature method that allows rapid determination of the six major anticonvulsants–phenobarbital, primidone, phenytoin, carbamazepine, valproic acid, and ethosuximide. The method, based on the original morphine assay of Rubenstein et al [60], has been adapted for use in most automated kinetic analyzers. The reaction that is monitored is the increase of NADH that accompanies the enzymatic oxidation of glucose-6-phosphate, which is catalyzed by unbound antigen. Each molecule of antigen (enzyme) catalyzes many reactions, producing a chemical amplification effect that greatly increases sensitivity. With appropriate adjustment of standard concentrations, free drug levels can be measured. A review of EMIT has been published [61], and assays for other drugs and drug classes are available or under development.

The other two homogeneous systems are relatively new; however, they have the same potential for development as EMIT and offer such advantages as increased sensitivity and decreased reagent cost. These are the substrate-labeled fluorescent immunoassay and the fluorescence polarization immunoassay (FPIA). Soini and Hemmila [62] have written an excellent general review of fluoroimmunoassay. Wong et al [63] have described the substrate-labeled fluorescent immunoassay for phenytoin in which the enzyme substrate (antigen) is fluorogenic but is only free to react (become fluorescent) in the unbound state. Reagents are commercially available for phenobarbital, phenytoin, and carbamazepine (Ames Division, Miles Laboratories, Elkhart, Indiana). The fluorescence polarization assay [64–66] is not an enzyme technique but takes advantage of a change in the degree of polarization of fluorescence that occurs when the antigen is not bound to the antibody. If a rigid fluorescent chemical system is excited with horizontally or vertically polarized light, the light emitted as fluorescence will be similarly polarized. However, if the fluorescent molecule can rotate in its environment, the emitted light will be depolarized. The unbound antigen is relatively small in comparison with the antigen-antibody complex and is therefore much freer to rotate during the time between absorption and fluorescence. The system is commercially available with reagents for the six major anticonvulsants and many other drugs that are routinely monitored. Calibration curves are stable for a week or more, reducing calibration costs and making emergency testing economically feasible. Correlations with chromatographic methods are better than those of the enzyme methods.

With proper care and quality control, the chromatographic procedures are the most accurate and precise techniques for drug analysis. They are also the most versatile, allowing analysis of any sample for drugs and metabolites over the full concentration range of interest. Rambeck and Meijer [67] have reviewed the gas chromatographic methods with respect to internal standards, prechromatographic procedures, derivatization, and chromatography. Rambeck et al [68] have applied chromatographic theory of resolution and analysis time to the development of an optimized high-performance liquid chromatography method [69]. Both GLC and HPLC are mature techniques widely used in research and specialized clinical laboratories; however, most of the routine clinical testing is and will continue to be done by the immunoassays that require less time and technical skill to perform. The higher precision that the chromatographic techniques afford is not clinically significant. The cost of reagents, miniscule compared with that for the immunoassays, is somewhat offset by the more stringent personnel requirements and longer sample handling times; however, gas-liquid chromatography and high-performance liquid chromatography are still the least expensive methods of analysis [70].

Chromatographic techniques have the advantage of allowing the use of internal standards. These are compounds that are added to all standards and samples at the same concentration, and are chemically and chromatographically similar to the compounds of interest. Dudley [71] has reviewed the use of internal standards in determination of antiepileptic drugs. An internal standard is chosen that can be chromatographically separated from the analyte, but will otherwise undergo the same chemical reactions and behave like the analyte during sample preparation. The ratio of detector response of the analyte to that of the internal standard is the measurement used for calibration and quantitation. Articles that are representative of the most successful gas-liquid chromatographic procedures for the various anticonvulsants include those of Dudley et al [72], on column methylation of barbiturates, hydantoins, and succinimides; Vandemark and Adams [73], off-column alkytion of barbiturates, hydantoins, and succinimides; Godolphin and Thoma [74], underivatized analysis of most anticonvulsants; Kupferberg [75], derivatized analysis of valproic acid and ethosuximide; Bius et al [76], underivatized analysis of trimethadione and dimethadione; Perchalski and Wilder [77], derivatized analysis of carbamazepine and phenylethylmalonamide; Solow and Kenfield [78], electron capture determination of clonazepam.

The high-performance liquid chromatographic determination of all anticonvulsants and their metabolites except valproic acid and the benzodiazepines is generally carried out on a 5-μm particle octadecyl or octyl reversed phase with a phosphate-buffered acetonitrile mobile phase after solvent extraction [79], simple deproteinization [80], or a combination of the two [81]. This chromatographic system can be used to obtain free drug levels by direct injection of plasma ultrafiltrates (Centrifree Micropartition System; Amicon Corp., Danvers, Massachusetts). Westenberg and DeZeeuw [82] developed an excellent procedure for carbamazepine, and Perchalski and Wilder [83] developed a procedure for the benzodiazepine anticonvulsants that is easily adaptable to other benzodiazepines. Valproic acid can be determined by high-performance liquid chromatography after conversion to the p-bromophenyacyl ester [84].

Current advances in therapeutic drugs monitoring are generally being made in the electronics laboratory by electrical engineers rather than in the chemistry laboratory by chemists. The microprocessor has made automated instrumentation commonplace, and in many cases the chemist has little more to do than pipet samples. However, no computer can create accurate and precise results when accuracy and precision are lacking in the chemistry and quality control of the method. The research that has produced the current level of expertise and sophistication in the therapeutic monitoring of antiepileptic drugs can serve as a model for the future development and control of methods for other drug classes. Psychotropic drugs are a particular challenge because therapeutic concentrations are often measured in nanograms or picograms. Accurate determination of micrograms of anticonvulsants is simple by comparison.

## REFERENCES


1. Kutt H, Penry JK: Usefulness of blood levels of antiepileptic drugs. Arch Neurol 31:283–288, 1974
2. Feldman RG, Pippenger CE: The relation of anticonvulsant drug levels to complete seizure control. J Clin Pharmacol 16:51–59, 1976
3. Lascelles PT, Kocen RS, Reynolds EH: The distribution of plasma phenytoin levels in epileptic patients. J Neurol Neurosurg Psychiatry 33:501–505, 1970
4. Kutt H: Diphenylhydantoin. Relation of plasma concentration to seizure control. In Woodbury DM, Penry JK, Pippenger CE (eds): Antiepileptic Drugs, 2nd ed. New York, Raven Press, 1982
5. Sherwin AL: Ethosuximide: Relation of plasma concentration to seizure con-

trol. In Woodbury DM, Penry JK, Rippenger CE (eds): Antieplieptic Drugs, 2nd ed. New York, Raven Press, 1982
6. Cereghino JJ: Serum carbamazepine concentration and clinical control. Adv Neuro 11:309–330, 1975
7. Eadie MJ: Plasma level monitoring of anticonvulsants. Clin Pharmacokinet 1: 52–66, 1976
8. Pippinger CE, Penry JK, White BG, et al: Interlaboratory variability in determination of plasma antiepileptic drug concentrations. Arch Neurol 33:351–355, 1976
9. Booker HE, Darcy B: Serum concentrations of free diphenylhydantoin and their relationship to clinical intoxication. Epilepsia 14:117–184, 1973
10. Cramer JA, Mattson RH: Valproic acid: In vitro plasma protein binding and interactions with phenytoin. Ther Drug Monit 1:105–116, 1979
11. Wilder BJ, Karas BJ: Valproate: Relation of plasma concentration to seizure control. In Woodbury DM, Penry JK, Pippenger CE (eds): Antiepileptic Drugs, Second Edition, New York, Raven Press, 1982, pp 591–600
12. Bruni J, Wilder BJ: Antiepileptic drug monitoring. J Fla Med Assoc 66:697–699, 1979
13. Richens A, Warrington S: When should plasma drug levels be monitored? Drugs 17:488–500, 1979
14. Mucklow JC: The use of saliva in therapeutic drug monitoring. Ther Drug Monit 4:229–247, 1982
15. Anavekar SN, Saunders RH, Wardell WM, et al: Parotid and whole saliva in the prediction of serum total and free phenytoin concentrations. Clin Pharmacol Ther 24:629–637, 1978
16. DiGregorio GJ, Piraino AJ, Ruch E: Diazepam concentrations in parotid saliva, mixed saliva, and plasma. Clin Pharacol Ther 24:720–725, 1978
17. Lennox WG: Brain injury, drugs and environmental causes of mental decay in epilepsy. Am J Psychiatry 99:174–180, 1942
18. Gruber CM, Haury VG, Drake ME: The toxic actions of sodium diphenylhydantoinate (Dilantin) when injected intraperitoneally and intravenously in experimental animals. J Pharmacol Exp Ther 68:433–436, 1940
19. Levy LL, Fenichel GM: Diphenylhydantoin activated seizures. Neurology (Minneap) 15:716–722, 1965
20. Glaser GH: Dipehnylhydantoin: Toxicity. In Woodbury DM, Penry JK, Schmidt RP (eds): Antiepileptic Drugs. New York, Raven Press, 1972, pp 219–226
21. Rawson MD: Diphenylhydantoin intoxication and cerebrospinal fluid protein. Neurology (Minneap) 18:1009–1011, 1968
22. Reynolds EH, Travers R: Serum anticonvulsant concentrations in epileptic patients with mental symptoms. Br J Psychiatry 124:440–445, 1974
23. Rosen JA: Dilantin dementia. Trans Am Neurol Assoc 93:273, 1968
24. Idestrom CM, Schalling D, Carlquist U, et al: Acute effects of diphenylhydantoin in relation to plasma levels: Psychological studies. Psychol Med 2:111–120, 1972
25. Vallarta JM, Bell DB, Reichert A: Progressive encephalopathy due to chronic hydantoin intoxication. Am J Dis Child 128:27–34, 1974
26. Stores G: Behavioral effects of anticonvulsant drugs. Dev Med Child Neurol 17:647–658, 1975
27. Matthews CG, Harley JP: Cognitive and motor sensory performance in toxic

and non-toxic epileptic subjects. Neurology (Minneap) 25:184--188, 1975
28. Trimble M: Anticonvulsant Drugs, Behavior And Cognitive Abilities, New York, Spectrum Publications, 1981, pp 65–92
29. Reynolds EH: Chronic antiepileptic toxicity: A review. Epilepsia 16:319–352, 1975
30. Reynolds EH: Diphenylhydantoin: Hematological aspects of toxicity. In Woodbury DM, Penry JK, Schmidt RP (eds): Antiepileptic Drugs. New York, Raven Press, 1972, 247–262
31. Iivanainen M, Viukari M: Serum phenytoin, seizures and electroencephalography. Lancet 1:860–861, 1977
32. Iivanainen M, Viukari M, Seppalainen AM et al: Electroencephalography and phenytoin toxicity in mentally retarded epileptic patients. J Neurol Neurosurg Psychiatry 41:272–277, 1978
33. Schain RJ, Watanabe K: Origin of brain growth retardation in young rats treated with phenobarbital. Exp Neurol 50:806–809, 1976
34. Diaz J, Schain R, Baily BG: Phenobarbital induced brain growth retardation in artificially reared rat pups. Biol Neonate 32:77–82, 1977
35. Yanai J, Rosselli-Austin L, Tabakoff B: Neuronal deficits in mice following prenatal exposure to phenobarbital. Exp Neurol 64:237–244, 1979
36. Hutt SJ, Jackson PM, Belsham A, et al: Perceptual-motor behavior in relation to blood phenobarbital level: A preliminary report. Dev Med Child Neurol 10:626–632, 1968
37. Tchicaloff M, Gaillard F: Quelques effects indesirables des medicaments anti-epileptiques sur les rendements intellectuals. Rev Neuropsychiatr Infant 18: 599–602, 1970
38. Holdsworth L, Whitmore K: A study of children with epilepsy attending ordinary schools. Dev Med Child Neurol 16:747–758, 1974
39. MacLeod CM, Dakaban AS, Hunt E: Memory impairment in epileptic patients: Selective effects of phenobarbital concentration. Science 202:1102–1104, 1978
40. Wilder BJ, Ramsay RE: Psychological aberrations associated with antiepileptic drugs. Clin Electroencephalogr 5:199–200, 1974
41. Rodin EA, Rim CS, Kitano H, et al: A comparison of the effectiveness of primidone versus carbamazepine in epileptic outpatients. J Nerv Ment Dis 163:41–46, 1976
42. Dodrill CB, Troupin AS: Psychotropic effects of carbamazepine in epilepsy: A double-blind comparison with phenytoin. Neurology (Minneap) 27:1023–1028, 1977
43. Singh AN, Saxena BM, Germain M: Anticonvulsive psychotropic effects of carbamazepine in hospitalized epileptic patients: A long-term study. In Penry JK (ed): Epilepsy: The Eighth International Symposium. New York, Raven Press, 1977, pp 47–56
44. Browne TR, Dreifuss FE, Dyken PR, et al: Ethosuximide in the treatment of absence (petit mal) seizures. Neurology (Minneap) 25:515–524, 1975
45. Guey J, Charles C, Coquery C, et al: Study of psychological effects of ethosuximide (Zarontin) on 25 children suffering from petit mal epilepsy. Epilepsia 8:129–141, 1967
46. Soulayrol R, Roger J: Effects psychiatriques defavorables des medications anti-epileptiques. Rev Neuropsychiatr Infant 18:591–598, 1970
47. Todorov AB, Lenn NJ, Gabor AJ: Exacerbation of generalized nonconvulsive seizures with ehtosuximide therapy. Arch Neurol 35:389–391, 1978

48. Sommerbeck KW, Theilgaard A, Rasmussen KE, et al: Valproate sodium: Evaluation of so-called psychotropic effect. A controlled study. Epilepsia 18: 159–167, 1977
49. Trimble MR, Reynolds EH: Anticonvulsant drugs and mental symptoms: A review. Psychol Med 6:169–178, 1976
50. Trimble M: The effect of anticonvulsant drugs on cognitive abilities. Pharmacol Ther 4:677–685, 1979
51. Woodbury DM, Penry JK, Pippenger CE (eds): Antiepileptic Drugs, 2nd ed. New York, Raven Press, New York, 1982
52. Pippenger CE, Penry JK, Kutt H (eds): Antiepileptic Drugs: Quantitative Analysis And Interpretation. New York, Raven Press, 1978
53. Wilder BJ, Bruni J: Seizure Disorders: A Pharmacological Approach To Treatment. New York, Raven Press, 1981
54. Kumps AH: Therapeutic drug monitoring: A comprehensive review of analytical methods for anticonvulsive drugs. J Neurol 228:1–16, 1982
55. Pippenger CE, Hidman BE, Joseph K: Quantitative Determination Of Antiepileptic Drug Level. Report FDA/BMD-80-118: Order No. PB80-216088. Springfield, VA, National Technical Information Service, 1979
56. Johanssen SI: Antiepileptic drugs: Pharmacokinetic and clinical aspects. Ther Drug Monit 3:17–37, 1981
57. Fellenberg AJ, Pollard AC: A rapid and sensitive spectrophotometric procedure for the micro-determination of carbamazepine in blood. Clin Chim Acta 69: 423–438, 1976
58. Felber JP: Radioimmunoassay in the clinic chemistry laboratory. Adv Clin Chem 20:130–179, 1978
59. Wad NT, Rosenmund H: Rapid quantitative method for the simultaneous determination of carbamazepine, carbamazepine-10,11-epoxide, diphenylhydantoin, mephenytoin, phenobarbital and primidone in serum by thin-layer chromatography. J Chromatogr 146:167–168, 1978
60. Rubenstein KK, Schneider RS, Ullman EF: Homogeneous enzyme immunoassay. A new immunochemical technique. Biochem Biophys Res Commun 47: 846, 1972
61. Curtis EG, Patel JA: Enzyme multiplied immunoassay technique: A review. CRC Crit Rev Clin Lab Sci 9:303–320, 1978
62. Soini E, Hemmila I: Fluoroimmunoassay: Present status and key problems. Clin Chem 25:353–361, 1979
63. Wong RC, Burd JF, Carrico RJ, et al: Substrate-labeled fluorescent immunoassay for phenytoin in human serum. Clin Chem 25:686–691, 1979
64. Popelka SR, Miller DM, Holen JT, et al: Fluorescence polarization immunoassay. II. Analyzer for rapid, precise measurement of fluorescence polarization with use of disposable cuvettes. Clin Chem 27:1198–1201, 1981
65. Jolley ME, Stroupe SD, Schwenzer KS, et al: Fluorescence polarization immunoassay. III. An automated system for therapeutic drug determination. Clin Chem 27:1575–1579, 1981
66. Lu-Steffes M, Pittluck GW, Jolley ME, et al: Fluorescence polarization immunoassay. IV. Determination of phenytoin and phenobarbital in human serum and plasma. Clin Chem 28:2278–2282, 1982
67. Rambeck B, Meijer JWA: Gas chromatographic methods for determination of antiepileptic drugs. Ther Drug Monit 2:385–396, 1980
68. Rambeck B, Riedmann M, Meijer JWA: Systematic method of development in liquid chromatography applied to the determination of antiepileptic drugs. Ther Drug Monit 3:377–395, 1981

69. Riedmann M, Rambeck B, Meijer JWA: Quantitative simultaneous determination of eight common antiepileptic drugs and metabolites by liquid chromatography. Ther Drug Monit 3:397–413, 1982
70. Meijer JWA, Rambeck B, Riedmann M: Antiepileptic drug monitoring by chromatographic method and immunotechniques–Comparison of analytical performance, practicability and economy. Ther Drug Monit 5:39–53, 1983
71. Dudley KH: Internal standards in gas-liquid chromatographic determination of antiepileptic drugs. In Pippinger CE, Penry JK, Kutt H (eds): Antiepileptic Drugs: Quantitative Analysis and Interpretation. New York, Raven Press, 1978, pp 19–34
72. Dudley KH, Bius DL, Kraus, et al: Gas chromatographic on-column methylation technique for the simultaneous determination of antiepileptic drugs in blood. Epilepsia 18:259–276, 1977
73. Vandemark FL, Adams RF: Ultramicro gas chromatographic analysis for anticonvulsants with use of a nitrogen selective detector. Clin Chem 22:1062–1065, 1976
74. Godolphin W, Thoma J: Quantitation of anticonvulsant drugs in serum by gas chromatography on the stationery phase SP-2510. Clin Chem 24:483–485, 1978
75. Kupferberg HJ: Gas liquid chromatographic quantitation of valproic acid. In Pippenger CE, Penry JK, Kitt H (eds): Antiepileptic Drugs. New York, Raven Press, 1978, pp 147–151
76. Bius DL, Teague BL, Dudley KH: Simultaneous gas chromatographic determination of trimethadione and dimethadione in human plasma. Ther Drug Monit 1:495–506, 1979
77. Perchalski RJ, Wilder BJ: Gas-liquid chromatographic determination of carbamazepine and phenylethylmalonamide in plasma after reaction with dimethylformamide dimethylacetal. J Chromatogr 145:97–103, 1978a
78. Solow EB, Kenfield CP: A micro method for the determination of clonazepam in serum by electron-capture gas-liquid chromatography. J Anal Toxicol 1: 155–157, 1977
79. Adams RF, Schmidt GJ, Vandemark FL: A micro liquid column chromatography procedure for twelve anticonvulsants and some of their metabolites. J Chromatogr 145:275–284, 1978
80. Kabra PM, Stafford BE, Marton LJ: Simultaneous measurement of phenobarbital, phenytoin, primidone, ethosuximide, and carbamazepine in serum by high pressure liquid chromatography. Clin Chem 23:1284–1288, 1977
81. Perchalski RJ, Bruni J, Wilder BJ: Simultaneous determination of the anticonvulsants, cinromide (3-bromo-n-ethyl-cinnamamide),3-bromocinnamamide, and carbamazepine in plasma by high-performance liquid chromatography. J Chromatogr 163:187–913, 1979
82. Westenberg HGM, DeZeeuw RA: Rapid and sensitive liquid chromatographic determination of carbamazepine, suitable for use in monitoring drug anticonvulsant therapy. J Chromatogr 118:217–224, 1976
83. Perchalski RJ, Wilder BJ: Determination of benzodiazepine anticonvulsants in plasma by high-performance liquid chromatography. Anal Chem 50:554–557, 1978b
84. Moody JP, Allen SM: Measurement of valproic acid in serum as the 4-bromophenacyl ester by high performance liquid chromatography. Clin Chem Acta 127:263–269, 1983

CHAPTER 9

# Stimulant Challenge Tests


## JAN FAWCETT, HOWARD M. KRAVITZ, and HECTOR C. SABELLI


### INTRODUCTION

In our chapter on "CNS Amine Metabolites" (chapter 3), we focused on the importance of different monoamine systems in the pathophysiology of psychiatric disorders. Over the past decade stimulants have emerged as useful tools for studying alterations in monoamine function because of their effects on these systems. In addition to biochemical measurements, response to various drugs with selective effects on neurotransmitter processes may serve to elucidate the disorders of central synaptic transmission that underlie psychiatric illnesses. Thus, the mood elevating effects of amphetamines and their ability to induce manic-like and schizophrenic-like symptoms has been important in the development of the hypotheses than an excess and a deficit in brain adrenergic amines underlie mania and depression respectively, and that dopaminergic hyperactivity plays a major role in schizophrenia. In addition, the study of such pharmacological responses has practical clinical value. Thus, amphetamines (AMPH) and methylphenidate have been widely used as diagnostic aids for subclassifying depressive disorders as well as predictors of response to treatment [1-7]. More recently, there is some evidence that amphetamines may also be useful in determining the diagnosis and treatment of schizophrenia [8] and attention deficit disorder [9,10]. It seems that patients with different illnesses show a qualitatively different response to AMPH. With the


*Handbook of Psychaitric Diagnostic Procedures,* vol. 1, edited by R. C. W. Hall and T. P. Beresford.

availability of a complex array of therapeutic agents to choose from, it has become more imperative to choose the agent most likely to be therapeutically efficacious. Further, because of the novel effects of some of these drugs, we have become even more inquisitive and curious to know the mechanism of action of this diverse array of drugs [11], and even more so, the underlying pathophysiology of the disorders we treat with these agents. Thus the "Stimulant Challenge Test" has acquired an important place both in terms of fostering basic research into the mechanisms of both drug action and the pathophysiology of psychiatric disorders, as well as enhancing practical clinical psychopharmacotherapeutics. We review the current status of stimulants in challenge studies and propose some hypotheses regarding the biochemical and neuroendocrine mediation accounting for affective response to stimulants.

## PSYCHOBIOLOGICAL EFFECTS OF AMPHETAMINES

The behavioral effects of AMPH are clearly dose-dependent. In most but not all normal subjects, AMPH induce mood elevation at low doses and displeasurable hyperactivity and anxiety at high doses [12]. In addition, normal as well as depressed individuals exhibit a wide range of individual differences to amphetamines [13], not accounted for by differences in blood levels.

AMPH-like stimulants are phenylethylamines and are thus structurally and pharmacologically related to 2-phenylethylamine (PEA) and the catecholamines (CA). As PEA, and in contrast to CA, they cross the blood brain barrier and produce behavioral stimulation. The addition of hydroxyl groups decreases their stimulant effects while increasing their CA-releasing action; ephedrine is weaker than amphetamine in producing central stimulation but stronger than amphetamine in releasing CA and in activating CA receptors. As congeners of the CA, amphetamines bind to most of the tissue receptors for CA including the active receptor substances, the CA storage sites, the amine uptake pump of norepinephrine (NE) neurons, etc., but not to catechol-O-methyltransferase because AMPH lack hydroxyl groups in their phenyl ring. Through these direct and indirect activities, amphetamine is an agonist of NE and DA. This appears to be the major but not exclusive mode of action of amphetamines. CA release clearly mediates the sympathomimetic effects of amphetamines, which are fully prevented by reserpine-induced depletion of CA or by imipramine (IMI)-induced inhibition of amine uptake by NE neurons. In contrast, amphetamine-induced behavioral stimulation is not prevented by reserpine-induced CA depletion and is enhanced by IMI-like antidepressants. Clearly the central effect to AMPH cannot be due to the same processes operating in the periphery. Yet, CA mechanisms must be important because alpha-methyl-para-tyrosine, a specific NE and dopamine (DA) synthesis inhibitor, blocks the activating effects of amphetamines [14]. Amphetamines appear to release and subsequently enhance the synthesis of another central adrenergic neuroamine, PEA [15,16]. In addition, AMPH may also act as agonists of serotonin (5-HT) receptors [17]. AMPH also demonstrate effects on the acetylcholine (ACh) system [18]. Other amphetamines, the chloroamphetamines (4-chloramphetamine and 4-chloro-N-methylamphetamine) and the trifluoromethyl-substituted amphetamine (fenfluramine), apparently have more specific effects on central 5-HT systems and processes [19-22]. Since all of the above neurotransmitter mechanisms are important in the brain, it is in our view illogical to attribute the behavioral effects of AMPH to its action upon only one of them. Yet, different neurotransmitters may be involved in the various central actions of amphetamine. Thus, neuroendocrine responses appear to involve primarily noradrenergic transmission [23] while the altering effects may involve less hydroxylated amines such as DA [24] or PEA [25].

Methylphenidate is similar but weaker than AMPH in its neuropharmacologic effects [26], but it may affect preferentially central DA systems [27-29]. It may also affect the cholinergic system [30].

Acute AMPH administration can relieve symptoms of depression and fatigue in many normal subjects as well as in a subgroup of depressed patients, but such effect is not therapeutically useful because chronic AMPH administration can induce a depressive syndrome, presumably by depleting brain neuroamines [31,32]. The observation of the acute antidepressant effect and the chronic depressogenic effect of AMPH is one of the empirical bases for the neuroamine theories of depression. Note, however, that the failure of AMPH to improve mood in many depressives points out the heterogeneity of depressions (see later). In our experience, AMPH increase energy and motor activity even in patients whose depression is *not* ameliorated.

Checkley [33] made a distinction between the euphoric and the antidepressant effects of methylamphetamine in depressed patients. Following its intravenous administration there were immediate endocrine and mood changes, but relief from depression was delayed for one to three hours, and lasted for as long as thirty-six hours. This study opens to question the role of acute NE release in the antidepressant action of amphetamines; AMPH rapidly releases PEA, reducing its brain levels to one-third of its normal content, while four to twenty-four hours after its administration, brain PEA levels increase up to ten times [15,16]. Checkley's observations are also of practical significance regarding the time at which psychological testing should be employed in the antidepressant prediction test. In our clinical experience, the delayed and overall effects of AMPH and methylphenidate administered orally over a period of at least two days are better predictors of antidepressant response to treatment than are the short-lasting mood changes.

Van Kammen and associates [34] demonstrated that d-AMPH was 2 to 2.3 times more effective in producing activation, euphoria and antidepressant effects than comparable doses of l-AMPH; l-AMPH is more powerful than d-AMPH as a CA releaser and hence in producing sympathomimetic effects. On the other hand, d-AMPH is more powerful than l-AMPH in releasing PEA, pointing to a possible contribution of this amine to the central actions of AMPH. Because it has been proposed that an excess in brain neuroamines is involved in the pathogenesis of mania and a DA excess in the pathogenesis of schizophrenia, the behavioral effects of d-AMPH, which releases DA as well as other neuroamines, has been taken as a model for either mania or schizophrenia. Co-administration of lithium carbonate attenuates these responses in depressives administered d-AMPH, while l-AMPH responses were almost completely abolished [34]. These data suggest the possible efficacy of treating amphetamine-toxic states with lithium and further, it relates AMPH central effects to mania rather than to schizophrenia, because lithium is effective in acute manic states but generally ineffective in schizophrenia. These studies, however, do not assist us in analyzing the contribution of different neuroamines to AMPH central actions because lithium affects catecholaminergic [35], serotonergic [36,37], and PEA [38,39] mechanisms. Thus, lithium treatment causes increased uptake and decreased release of CA, altered CA metabolism, and decreased receptor response; all of these effects are in the opposite direction from amphetamine's effects, possibly resulting from antagonism produced at CA synapses [40]. In addition, lithium prevents the effects of both amphetamine and reserpine upon PEA metabolism and reduces their respective stimulant and depressant, behavioral effects.

High doses of AMPH can induce a schizophrenic-like psychosis in apparently normal subjects, supporting the view that DA or related amines are involved in the schizophrenic process. As a group, schizophrenics may respond to stimulants differently from normals or depressives [41]. Amphetamines and methylphenidate reportedly may precipitate or exacerbate psychotic symptoms in schizophrenics, but not in patients with affective disorders [42-45] although we have observed manic episodes precipitated by the administration of d-AMPH to bipolar depressed patients. Further, schizophrenic patients are heterogeneous in their response to AMPH. Van Kammen and associates [8] reported on a double-blind placebo controlled study of change in psychotic symptoms in schizophrenics following d-AMPH infusions. Thirteen of forty-five patients demonstrated an acute reduction in their psychotic symptoms while eighteen subjects became more psychotic. Upon rechallenge with d-AMPH at a later date, it was found that some patients varied in their response, suggesting that vulnerability to d-AMPH-induced changes in psychotic symptomatology is state-dependent in schizophrenia. These phenomena appear to relate to NE rather than to DA mechanisms. Thus, the authors did not observe any relation between behavioral response to AMPH and pre-infusion CSF homovanillic acid (HVA) and dihydroxyphenylacetic acid (DOPAC), but higher CSF MHPG levels were noted in those patients who worsened. Note that depressives with high urinary MHPG also fail to improve following AMPH (see later).

Van Kammen and associates [8] found that AMPH also induces euphoria and activation in schizophrenics. The activating and psychotogenic effects of d-AMPH appear to be unrelated [42,43,45], and the duration of the euphoriant and activating responses post-AMPH are independent of the changes in psychotic symptomatology. Finally, in contrast to the state-dependent psychotogenic responses, the activation response seems to be trait-dependent. If DA is implicated in euphoria and activation, different DA systems must be involved in the psychotogenic effects of d-AMPH in schizophrenia.

Another group of patients who show atypical responses to amphetamines are those with attention deficit disorders. Sedating effects and lack of tolerance are observed not only in hyperkinetic children but also in the adult form of this disorder.

In summary, in addition to increased motor activity (which may itself be felt as helpful), increased energy, or dysphoric agitation, the possible responses to amphetamine-like stimulants are: (1) mood elevation, as observed in normal subjects and in some depressives; (2) manic-like states; (3) dysphoric anxiety, mainly in depressed and anxious subjects; (4) a lack of mood change; (5) calming, which we as well as others [9] have observed in patients with a history of attention deficit disorder, with little tolerance to chronic methylphenidate administration; and (6) psychotomimetic effects, observed mainly in schizophrenics. Obviously, (5) and (6) represent a qualitatively different response. When we use AMPH-like stimulants as a challenge test in depressives, we have considered (1) and (2) as positive responses, and (3) and (4) as negative ones.

AMPH and methylphenidate release both CA (DA and NE) and PEA. According to the PEA theory of depression [46,47] and the CA theory of anxiety [48, 49] mood elevation by stimulants would result from the ability of these agents to release PEA, while anxiety would be due to CA release. Thus, the presence or absence of CA-mediated anxiety would determine whether or not AMPH induced mood elevation or dysphoric anxiety during an episode of depression. The relative proportion of CA and PEA stores in brain would determine the preponderance of CA or PEA release by AMPH; when PEA stores are larger than CA stores, mood elevation would predominate, while if CA stores are larger, anxiety would occur. In support of this view, Fawcett and associates [50] have shown that depressives with low 3-methoxy-4-hydroxyphenylglycol (MHPG) excretion show mood elevation with AMPH, while patients with high or normal MHPG more frequently had dysphoric responses. On the other hand, lack of mood change with AMPH would reflect a more profound depletion of all amine stores. Another important effect of AMPH is its ability to decrease appetite. While amphetamine and other PEA characteristically decrease appetite, experimental studies indicate that NE enhances eating [51]. Recent studies indicate that the anorexogenic effect of AMPH is due to activation of non-CA receptors [52]. These are not PEA receptors, which in turn have been shown to differ from CA and amphetamine receptors in several different studies [53] (and see this reference for more extensive list of references). While monoamine oxidase inhibitors (MAOI) and many tricyclic antidepressants (TCA), particularly amitriptyline (AMI), increase appetite, AMPH, maprotiline (our clinical observations), maprotiline plus isocarboxazid (our clinical observations), and often also desipramine (DMI) decrease appetite. One can speculate that the anorexogenic effect of PEA is due to their ability to increase pleasure. On the one hand, pleasure is the mood correlate of consummatory acts such as the satisfaction of a need; consummation decreases appetite (drive). On the other hand, the experiencing of pleasure counterbalances and outweighs the suffering induced by hunger.

## STIMULANT CHALLENGE AND AFFECTIVE DISORDERS

Although the use of antidepressant drugs has drastically altered the course and prognosis of depressive episodes, prediction of individual response to specific antidepressants remains an unsolved and important question, particularly because their therapeutic effects are often slow in onset, with three to six weeks at a therapeutic blood level required to ascertain whether responsiveness will be forthcoming. Research and clinical experience suggest that there are several subtypes and symptomatologically similar depressive disorders which can be distinguished by the differential response to stimulant agents and to antidepressants, as well as by the pattern of associated neuroendocrine and neuroamine alterations. Many patients improve with one antidepressant, be it a TCA or MAOI, but not another, and some respond to electroconvulsive shock therapy, while some patients respond to neither [54]. This variability in responsiveness has been attributed to: (1) the existence of multiple forms of depressive illness; (2) the use in inadequate doses of medication; and (3) the existence of psychodynamic factors which sustain the depression in spite of adequate treatment of this biological component [55,56]. TCA blood level measurements have demonstrated that many "nonresponders" improve with proper dose adjustments, but other data support the hypothesis of biochemically heterogeneous depressive disorders with differential responsiveness to antidepressants [54,57-59].

Symptomatology alone has not been useful in predicting which depressives respond most optimally to which medication. This indicates a need to develop rational ways of predicting antidepressant efficacy, both from a clinical as well as an economic standpoint [60,61]. The importance of a rapid, safe and effective means to predict pharmacologic responsiveness to the various antidepressants (especially TCA, the more commonly used antidepressants) is understandable in terms of personal, social, and economic values and variables.

Our particular approach to this problem, the Stimulant (amphetamine and methylphenidate) Challenge Test is not new, but has been relatively untested,

**Table 1. The Stimulant Challenge Test in Depression**

"How We Do It"

This Table presents examples of schedules for stimulant (D-AMPH, methylphenidate) administration that we use in our clinical practice. Such obvious factors as age, cardiovascular status, general health, and the ready availability of D-AMPH for inpatients versus the lesser abuse potential of methylphenidate for outpatients determine (and may modify) the method and dose schedule employed.

1. D-AMPH orally at 8 AM and 1 PM, 5 mg at each dose on Day 1, 10 mg on Day 2, 15 mg on Day 3, up to the minimum dose required to produce mood elevation or dysphoria, or as tolerated; maximum 15 mg twice a day (30 mg per day).
2. Methylphenidate orally at 8 AM and 1 PM, starting with a dose of 5 mg and raising the dose by 5 mg increments at each time daily, as allowed by side effects, up to the minimum dose that produces clear stimulation (mood elevation) or dysphoria, or up to a maximum of 30 mg twice a day (60 mg per day).

Clinical evaluations of mood and behavioral change, both subjective and objective, are obtained pre- and post-dose, the latter on at least two occasions, 2 and 8 hours after the initial dose. (The PM dose is given to potentiate the AM dose and to maintain stimulant blood levels throughout the waking day, provided no significant untoward effects or other contraindications are detected after the initial dose.) We find that many patients experience delayed mood and behavioral responses which may persist 24 hours after the AM dose.

**Table 2. Effectiveness of non-MAOI Antidepressants Predicted by the Stimulant Challenge Test (D-Amphetamine, Methylphenidate)**

| I. Mood elevation | II. Dysphoria or no mood change |
|---|---|
| Imipramine | Amitriptyline |
| Desipramine | Nortriptyline |
| Maprotiline | Trazodone |
| | Amoxapine |
| | Doxepin |

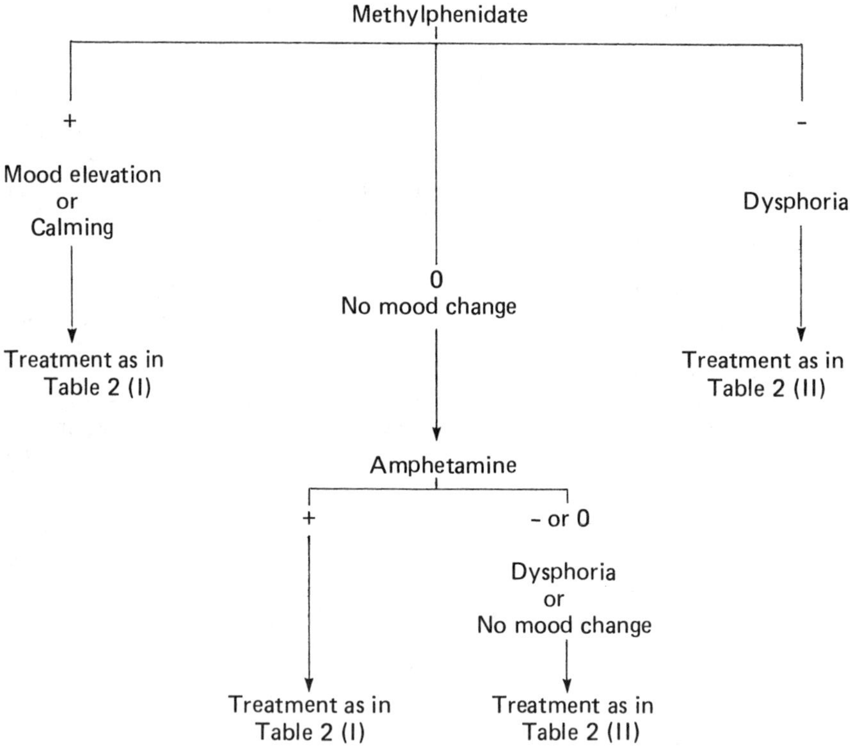


**Figure 1.** Possible responses to methylphenidate and dextroamphetamine.

despite its usefulness in our clinical experience. While previous studies [62,63] indicate that the Stimulant Challenge Test is a simple, rapid, noninvasive and safe procedure with possible clinical validity, which may serve to distinguish biochemically different types of depression, its primary significance is that it is clinically useful in predicting specific TCA response in *each individual patient.* This contrasts to tests of neuroamine metabolites which, because of overlap between depressive subtypes, are not useful in predicting response in individual cases. The applicability of the Stimulant Challenge Test under nonresearch conditions appears to be validated by our clinical experience. For many years we have given either d-AMPH or methylphenidate for one to three days and used the patient's self-report of presence or absence of mood elevation to choose between different TCA (see Table 1). In our experience, there is little difference between the two stimulants as clinical predictors, but pharmacological studies suggest that important differences might exist, and a comparative study should be carried out.

Table 2 and Figure 1 summarizes our current guidelines for selective tricyclic and tetracyclic antidepressants.

We do not have adequate data regarding responsiveness to MAOI, but in our experience, patients who require MAOI because of the ineffectiveness of any of the TCA show partial, small mood elevations with AMPH. Although at this point the observations of differential clinical response to various stimulants and antidepressant drugs seem more demonstrable than any of the current biochemical classifications, further studies using the double-blind technique are necessary.

In view of the latency to onset of the therapeutic action of TCA and lack of clinical predictors of responsiveness, Fawcett and Siomopoulos [62] developed a rapid pharmacological test to predict responsiveness to imipramine (IMI)-like TCA. d-AMPH, 10 to 15 mg twice a day, was administered double-blind, and responders and nonresponders were rated on the basis of both subjectively rated scales and objectively evaluated clinical interviews chosen for sensitivity to transient mood changes. Amphetamine produced a dramatic but time-limited mood elevation in a subgroup of depressives who subsequently responded to IMI or desipramine (DMI). Van Kammen and Murphy [63] reproduced these results and, by monitoring plasma levels, showed that behavioral responsiveness (acute activation, euphoria, and antidepressant response) was not simply dependent upon d-AMPH blood levels, despite other reports [12,64]. They [65] also observed that a euphoriant response to AMPH predicts some antidepressant response to lithium treatment, but only in female unipolar depressives, not in males or bipolar depressives.

We have recently found that mood elevation to stimulants also predicts a therapeutic response to maprotiline [66]. Clinical trials with amitriptyline [67] demonstrated its effectiveness in depressions resistant to IMI and vice versa. In 43 patients with primary, unipolar major depressive disorders, monitoring of tricyclic plasma concentration by gas-liquid chromatography indicated that some patients respond to IMI or DMI, but not to AMI or NT, or vice versa, even though plasma levels were within reported therapeutic range. Mood elevation by methylphendiate predicted marked improvement by subsequent treatment with IMI or DMI, but not with AMI or NT. It is noteworthy that the five patients who had panic attacks all showed mood elevation following methylphenidate. These results do not appear to be due to the therapist's expectations because negative results with NT were obtained in five patients by a clinician who expected its effectiveness when mood was elevated by methylphenidate. Further, these five patients improved after subsequent treatment with DMI. Such response to a second tricyclic after failure of the first one might be due to spontaneous recovery, but differential response to TCA may also be observed when two TCA were alternated in one patient. In the case of four patients with negative responses to methylphenidate who responded only partially to NT, the substitution of DMI for NT was followed by a worsening of the clinical picture, and return to NT restored the partial improvement. In five methylphenidate-negative patients, substitution of NT for AMI maintained therapeutic response.

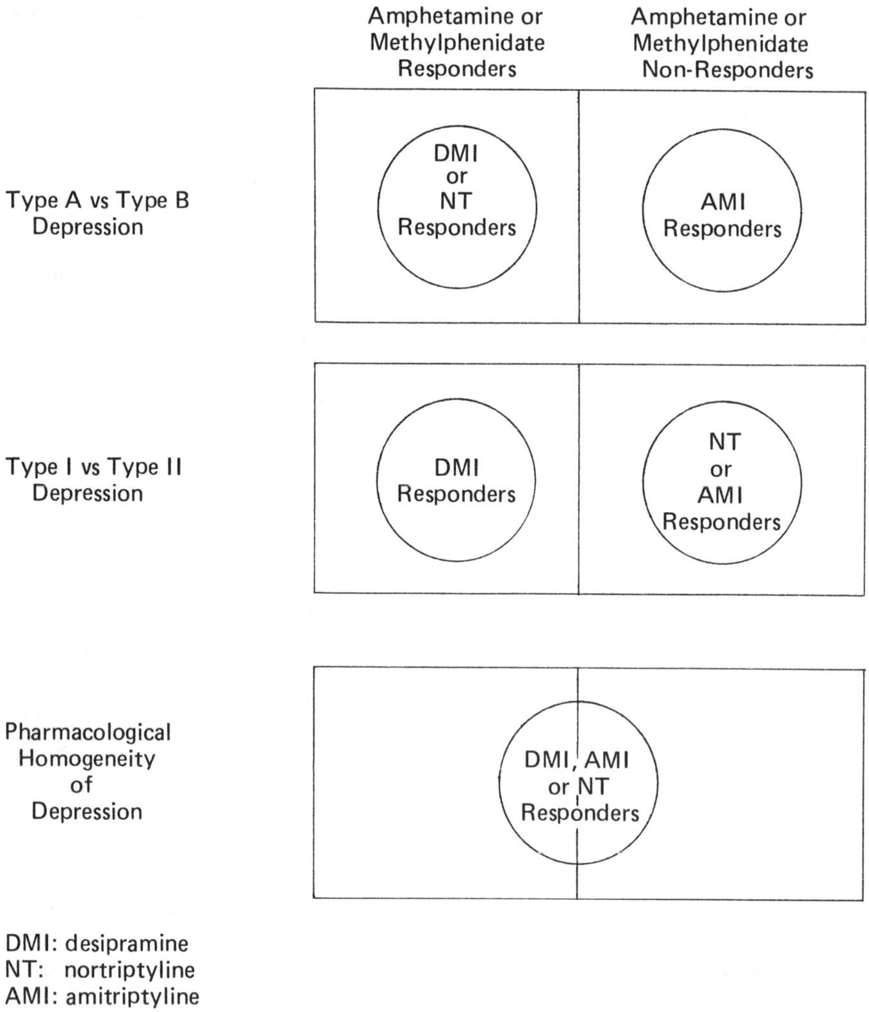


**Figure 2.** Predictions of tricyclic effectiveness on the basis of three different hypotheses.

In all except two cases, the subjective report of mood elevation by methylphenidate coincided with behavioral improvement as observed by the attending psychiatrist. In two patients with major depressive disorder and associated personality disorder, the mood elevation induced by methylphenidate was so ego-dystonic that the patients initially reported "dysphoria" but behavioral improvement was detected by the clinician. We have now observed that lack of mood change, or the induction of dysphoria, predicts a therapeutic response to AMI and nortriptyline (NT) [59]. In a crossover comparison [59], we have found that patients treated with AMI also respond to NT and vice versa, while DMI and NT were not interchangeable; patients responding to one failed to respond to the other (Figure 2). This point is important because both DMI and NT are assumed to act as "NE reuptake blockers" (see later). In our clinical experience, three patients who responded to trazodone had failed to show any significant mood elevation following stimulant administration. We have observed that amoxapine ameliorated depression in patients who responded to methylphenidate (N = 5) as well as among patients who did not (N = 6). However, methylphenidate responders did not maintain a therapeutic response to amoxapine, which often failed after approximately one month.

The Stimulant Test was originally based upon the hypothesis that both AMPH and DMI exert their effects by inhibiting NE reuptake. In our clinical experience there are patients who respond to stimulants, and whose depression is ameliorated by DMI but not by maprotiline and vice versa, or that fail to respond to either. In some cases, the response is incomplete. We are currently adding MAOI to maprotiline with subsequent enhanced responsiveness to this therapeutic regimen, although MAOI should not be combined with IMI or DMI. Similarly, patients who failed to respond to stimulants may or may not improve sufficiently on AMI-like antidepressants alone, sometimes requiring the addition of a MAOI. It should be noted that TCA should not be added to ongoing MAOI treatment.

We are currently accumulating a series of patients who in the course of their illness have responded to different TCAs. We have noted, for instance, patients who had a positive response to stimulants with subsequent improvement on DMI who later became depressed again and demonstrated no response to stimulants and improved upon the administration of NT. In three cases, we have observed several switches back and forth from one type of pharmacological responsiveness to the other.

Fawcett and his co-workers [50,68] correlated positive response to AMPH with a low MHPG urinary excretion and increased MHPG excretion post-AMPH; those patients responded to DMI. On the other hand, those patients whose initial MHPG was high tended to be nonresponders to both AMPH and DMI. Thus, AMPH-DMI responders may represent a subgroup of depressives with altered noradrenergic function. Beckmann and associates [40] confirmed that AMPH responders have low pre-treatment MPHG levels. In "CNS Amine Metabolites" (Chapter 3) we reviewed the literature demonstrating MHPG urinary excretion to be of limited value as a single predictor of TCA responsiveness, in part because the differences are small and the overlap between depressive subgroups is large, and in part because of contradictory results. Such contradictory findings may be in part due to the complicating issue of levels of anxiety (see later). In contrast, the significance of the Stimulant Challenge Test is that it is clinically useful in predicting specific TCA response in each individual patient. As described above, MHPG excretion may be valuable when utilized in conjunction with our Stimulant Challenge Test. At present, the Stimulant Test depends on subjective reports and behavioral observations. An objective biochemical or physiological response could serve to render the test more objective. Kadouch and associates [69] attempted to determine if a peripheral measure of receptor sensitivity could predict the central mood effects of stimulants. No correlation was found between plasma cAMP response and mood response to intravenous methylphenidate. Pharmacological studies indicate that AMPH and methylphenidate, as well as the TCA [70-72] affect brain PEA levels and clinical studies reveal that they increase the urinary excretion of PEA and of its main metabolite, phenylacetic acid (PAA). We are currently studying the correlation between behavioral responses to AMPH or to methylphenidate, the urinary excretion of PAA and its alteration by stimulant administration. We have found that methylphenidate reduces PAA excretion in patients who report behavioral stimulation as well as among those who do not. The ability of mood elevation by PEA (AMPH, methylphenidate) to predict antidepressant effects by IMI-like TCA must be considered in the light of animal experiments indicating a differential effect of TCA upon the sympathomimetic effects of these amines. TCA, including both IMI-like and AMI-like agents enhance the peripheral effects of NE [73,74]. Sigg [73] speculated that the antidepressant effects of IMI are thus due to NE potentiation, a hypothesis later reformulated in terms of inhibition of NE reuptake [75]. TCA also block completely the peripheral sympathomimetic effects of noncatecholic and particularly of nonhydroxylated phenylethylamines and enhance their central stimulant actions. In fact, AMI has now been shown to decrease the blood pressure elevating effect of tyramine in patients receiving a MAOI [76], supporting our clinical experience that it is safer to conjointly administer AMI and a MAOI than to give a MAOI alone. These results suggest to us that the mood elevating effect of AMPH is due mainly to its PEA-like actions rather than to CA release, which undoubtably mediate other CNS actions of AMPH [39,77]. In addition, IMI-like TCA increase brain PEA levels [70] (similar data is not available for AMI), and both IMI- and AMI-like TCA increase PAA urinary excretion (unpublished data), indirectly suggesting an increase in PEA production. In light of the fact that PEA is constantly produced but not stored and that PEA releases CA, we may speculate that there are two mechanisms for CA release: (1) phasic release due to action potentials, and (2) a tonic release due to humoral factors such as PEA. One of the mechanisms of the central action of TCA would be to block the tonic, PEA-mediated CA release. This could readily explain the antianxiety effect of TCA as well as their ability to reduce blood pressure. Likewise, ejaculation, which is adrenergically mediated, is reduced by TCA. Experimental studies indicate that NE can be released from nerve terminals by at least two mechanisms: (1) exocytosis, which is triggered following depolarization by action potentials [78, 79]; and (2) a carrier-mediated process, similar to the uptake mechanism [80] which mediates the release by PEA and other adrenergic amines. DMI inhibits the uptake by the nerve terminals of NE and related amines with phenolic hydroxyl groups (but not that of PEA, which readily cross plasma membranes). DMI also inhibits the NE release induced by PEA [81] without appreciable inhibition of adrenergic transmission.

## ENDOCRINOLOGICAL CORRELATES OF THE STIMULANT CHALLENGE TEST

There have been attempts to correlate the psychopharmacological response to these stimulants with observed neuroendocrinologic changes, especially because their secretion is regulated by central CA synapses, and possibly as well by serotonergic systems. These challenge studies have also been reviewed elsewhere [82, 83].

Cortisol dysregulation was one of the first biochemical abnormalities noted in depressives. Sachar and associates [84] noted that pulses of cortisol occur more frequently and with greater amplitude in depressives, while in a comparison of depressives and schizophrenics, Carroll [85] confirmed that this limbic system-hypothalamo-pituitary-adrenal dysfunction is specific for depressives. Fawcett and co-workers also established that cortisol secretion [86] as well as CA metabolism may be enhanced by stress [87].

Significant changes in plasma growth hormone (GH) as well as cortisol occur following the administration of AMPH. In man, methamphetamine, d-AMPH, and methylphenidate cause a prompt release of adrenocorticotropic hormone (ACTH), cortisol and GH [88-91]. While both AMPH and methylphenidate stimulate GH release, only the former stimulates cortisol release [90,91]. This is consistent with the preferential effects of methylphenidate on central DA systems and of AMPH on both DA and NE [92], and demonstrates the independence of the two neuroendocrine responses [91]. GH release induced by d-AMPH or methylphenidate has been found to be significantly deficient in endogenous depressives as compared with normal controls as well as schizophrenics [93]. However, Halbreich and associates [94,95] could not confirm that the GH response to d-AMPH either differentiates between endogenously depressed patients and age- and sex-matched normal controls or between depressive subtypes, in either morning or evening trials. Checkley [96,97] also could not discriminate the GH response to methamphetamine between endogenous depressives (pre- and post-recovery) [96] or between endogenous depressives, compared with other functional psychotic disorders, reactive depressives, and patients with nonpsychotic disorders [97], matched for variance caused by age and sex. It was suggested [94,98] that it is unclear whether hormonal responses to d-AMPH and methamphetamine are similar. Further, the response may be blunted in other psychiatric disorders [99]. While these effects of AMPH might be related to their actions on dopaminergic synapses, GH release by primarily dopaminergic agents such as L-DOPA and apomorphine in depressives does not differ from normals, if one controls for age and menopausal status [100]. Behaviorally, the GH response has been demonstrated to correlate with the euphoriant mood effect induced by both AMPH and methylphenidate [90,91]. Serum AMPH concentration correlates only with the degree of GH response and degree of euphoria [92]. These results certainly point out that in any endocrine study it is necessary to carefully control for variables such as age, estrogen status, and any other variable that may influence a hormonal response. Since both CA and corticosteroids are neurohormones involved in responses to stress, one could speculate that fear and other emotional activators may release brain NE which in turn releases ACTH (via CRF) thereby stimulating cortisol secretion by the adrenal gland. Endogenous cortisol or the exogenous administration of dexamethasone in turn reduce ACTH secretion. AMPH, by releasing NE, would elevate plasma cortisol levels. As expected, patients who suffer profound anxiety have high levels of cortisol in the blood [86,101-103] and excrete large amounts of 17-hydroxycorticosteroid [101-103]. Depressed patients, who characteristically are also anxious, likewise have high cortisol levels. Often, their endogenous activation of ACTH overcomes the inhibitory effect of low doses of dexamethasone (DST nonsuppressors), although higher doses are effective (in contrast to patients with Cushing's syndrome). This explanation is at variance with the assumption that there is a CA deficit in depression and that, in contrast to our hypothesis, such deficit is reflected by nonsuppression on the DST. To support the view that depressions can occur in the presence of CA deficit, it has been proposed that NE may inhibit cortisol release.

By repeated blood sampling, Sachar and associates [98,104] observed that intravenous d-AMPH induces a *rise* followed by a fall in plasma cortisol in normal subjects; in contrast, only a fall is observed in a population of endogenous depressives with high plasma cortisol levels, although it is unlikely that higher cortisol values per se accounted for the abnormal responses. This discrimination was greater on evening testing than following the morning d-AMPH infusion [98,105], possibly reflecting the loss of normal diurnal increase in brain noradrenergic activity in endogenous depressives. Similarly, an acute cortisol spike is observed in normal humans but not in depressives in response to methamphetamine [88,97], but for both drugs the degree of response appears to be dose dependent [98]. The neurotransmitter basis for the effects of AMPH on cortisol levels is still obscure. NE may have both acute phasic stimulatory and prolonged tonic inhibitory effects on cortisol secretion, the former via alpha-adrenergic receptor stimulation and the latter via beta-adrenergic receptor stimulation. Thymoxamine, an alpha-blocker, has been reported to block the cortisol release response to methamphetamine in humans, whereas GH release by methylphenidate is augmented by thymoxamine [106]. Propranolol, a beta-adrenergic blocker, augments both cortisol and GH release by amphetamine [106]. These findings suggest that cortisol release is mediated by NE release by methamphetamine [96]. Sachar and associates [98,104] suggested that cortisol suppression to normal levels by d-AMPH in depressives may be mediated by its noradrenergic effect, rather than by DA, and that a postsynaptic alpha-noradrenergic receptor is involved in the normal response (which exhibits subsensitivity in these depressives). Thus, the fact that depressives show both high resting cortisol levels and a failure to release cortisol acutely following the administration of amphetamines may *both* be explained by a deficit in NE transmission in some central synapses, either a deficit in the transmitter itself or in its receptive neurons. Brown and associates [91] found that this cortisol response to AMPH in normals was correlated with behavioral arousal. On the other hand, data from Halbreich and associates [107,108] found that AMPH induced a dysphoric reaction in a group of normal postmenopausal women, attributed to a decreased CA activity, possibly decreased dopaminergic activity, though the mechanism is not clear. They suggested that age and hypoestrogenism may alter the behavioral response [108].

Prolactin release may be inhibited by dopaminergic activity and enhanced by serotoninergic activity [109]. Since AMPH increase the release of both of these neurotransmitters, it is unclear which response should be expected from a stimulant challenge. Various investigators, studying different patient groups, reported either increase or no effect [110-113].

There is some evidence that the dexamethasone suppression test (DST) may predict early response to antidepressant pharmacotherapy [114-125]. Brown and co-workers [123-125] reported that nonsuppressors responded better than suppressors to antidepressants, preferably to IMI and DMI, while suppressors showed greater improvement with AMI and CMI. However, Brawley [117] studied 49 depressives with primary affective disorder and compared their response to the DST with their response to methylphenidate. He reported a significant negative correlation between their responses to the two challenges. Those with suppressed cortisol secretion had a positive mood change after the stimulant; nonsuppressors did not. Sternbach and associates [126] similarly studied fourteen inpatients with major depressive disorder and five with schizoaffective disorder, depressed type, and also found a significant negative correlation between responses to the two tests; eight of ten nonsuppressors had a negative stimulant response and seven of nine suppressors had a positive response. Thus, cortisol hypersecreters, defined by nonsuppression on the DST, do not have an antidepressant response to methylphenidate, while suppressors do.

As described earlier, methylphenidate responsiveness predicts TCA response to IMI-like antidepressants, whereas nonresponders (and negative responders, i.e., dysphoric responses or just increased motor activity) tend to respond to AMI.

The responses reported by Brawley and Sternbach are opposite to the hypothesis that nonsuppression on the DST indicates a central noradrenergic deficit state [98, 104,127]. The authors caution that their data need replication because only 4PM cortisols were obtained and the stimulant challenge was not double-blind. The interval between the two tests was not reported, only that the DST was done first. Another consideration is that two different neurotransmitter systems may be involved. Methylphenidate has been demonstrated to preferentially affect DA systems [90,91]. Perhaps d-AMPH, which is known to alter cortisol secretion as well as noradrenergic systems, produces different results. Studies involving more selective agents or concomitant use of antagonists are required before we can draw any definite conclusions from these studies with AMPH and its derivatives. Further, although CA synapses are believed to regulate (indirectly) cortisol secretion [98, 104], there have been no studies on other effects of dexamethasone administration on CA metabolites in normals as contrasted with depressed individuals.

## ANXIETY, DEPRESSION AND STIMULANTS

Cortisol and GH responses to stimulants may thus be useful in objectifying the Stimulant Challenge Test for prediction of antidepressant response, but needs to be studied within the larger context of the changes induced in these parameters by the depressive illness itself, as well as by accompanying anxiety. Both anxiety and depression markedly alter cortisol secretion, as expected from the role of this hormone in stress. Carroll [85] demonstrated that this increase in plasma cortisol in endogenous depressives may not simply be a stress response. Anxiety complicates the evaluation of depression and its biological correlates in a number of ways. Symptoms of anxiety may be crucial to differentiate subtypes of depression and to determine effectiveness of particular antidepressants. Further, anxiety as well as depression affect CA metabolism as well as cortisol levels. We need to clarify the interrelationship between anxiety and the various subtypes of depression, their differential responsiveness to amphetamines and TCA, and alterations in catecholaminergic mechanisms. Alterations in MHPG, cortisol, and other biochemical measures probably reflect anxiety levels in addition to depressive mood. The Stimulant Challenge Test may likewise depend significantly upon the ability of these drugs to affect not only depressive mood but also anxiety levels. AMPH induces anxiety in some depressives as well as in healthy controls. On the other hand, others report a "calming effect," or euphoria with anxiety reduction. The role of trait anxiety, pre-existing state anxiety, and drug-induced changes in anxiety levels upon the subjective and objective effects of AMPH on depressive mood have not been adequately evaluated in previous studies of this challenge test for prediction of TCA response.

## PEA THEORIES, ANXIETY AND DEPRESSION, AND STIMULANTS

Antidepressants increase the brain levels of PEA, an endogenous mood stimulant [70]. Animal studies suggest that amphetamines and methylphenidate initially release and subsequently enhance the synthesis of PEA [128,129]. Their mood stimulant effects may be due in part to CA and PEA release, while their delayed antidepressant effect (which is more important for prediction of TCA responsiveness) finds a temporal correlate in the augmentation of PEA levels. In human depressed subjects, methylphenidate reduces the urinary excretion of PAA, the main PEA metabolite, in both IMI and AMI responders, but there may be quantitative differences, currently under study. Amphetamine, on the other hand, has a differential effect, increasing PAA excretion in some subjects and lowering it in others. All antidepressants increase urinary PAA, but apparently only when they are effective (unpublished data). These results indicate that PEA mechanisms may be important (but not exclusively so) in the Stimulant Challenge Test, but research in this area has just begun.

## A NEW THEORY OF DEPRESSION: DIFFERENTIAL PREDICTORS AND SUBTYPES OF DEPRESSION

As described earlier, to account for the differential effectiveness of AMPH and TCA, Maas [57] proposed to distinguish between Type A depression, characterized by low pretreatment urinary MHPG excretion, a positive mood elevation response to stimulant challenge, and a favorable response to treatment with IMI, DMI or NT; and Type B; which demonstrates normal or high MHPG excretion, a poor response to stimulant challenge and a good response to AMI. NE deficit is held responsible for Type A depression, and a disorder of the serotonin (5-HT) system is thought to account for Type B. Such conclusions depend on attributing the antidepressant effects of AMI and DMI to their ability to inhibit amine uptake by NE neurons, and those of AMI to a selective inhibition of uptake by 5-HT neurons. The latter assumption is at variance with our study [59]. While this theoretical issue thus remains unsettled, the clinical distinction between Type A and Type B as the basis of their differential drug responsiveness remains generally valid. We have found [59] that depressives who responded to methylphenidate with mood elevation subsequently improved with IMI or DMI, whereas none improved with AMI or NT in spite of adequate plasma levels. In contrast, when mood was not elevated by methylphenidate, patients responded to AMI or NT; none responded to DMI. Further, crossover indicated that patients who did not respond on DMI improved on NT, and vice versa. This differential drug responsiveness cannot be accounted for by the NE–5-HT dichotomy. Thus, we have proposed a new pharmacological classification of depressive disorders. In fact, neither our own data nor

Maas' observations can be explained on the basis of biochemical and pharmacological studies involving amine uptake in rat brain slices. Contrary to popular lore, the pharmacological studies of Ross and Renyi [130] and Randrup and Braestrup [131] have not revealed the existence of selective 5-HT uptake inhibitors among the TCA, since for each of the drugs tested, uptake inhibition of NE was greater than 5-HT uptake inhibition. AMI is a highly effective potentiator of NE [130–133] and, in fact, this was the test used to select it as an antidepressant [132,133]. Chlorimipramine (CMI) although usually considered as a 5-HT reuptake blocker, also inhibits NE reuptake [134]. In light of the above findings, we speculated on the existence of at least two different types of depressions which can be differentiated empirically on the basis of their drug responsiveness: Type I, responsive to AMPH and IMI-like drugs, and Type II, responsive to AMI and NT. We speculated that Type I depression is due to monoamine depletion while Type II may not be. Thus, IMI and DMI have been found effective when urinary MHPG is low, while the related agent CMI was shown more effective when urinary MHPG was reduced or when urinary or CSF 5-hydroxyindoleacetic acid (5-HIAA) was reduced, suggesting depressions relieved by IMI-like antidepressants may be associated with a deficit of brain monoamines, including but perhaps not exclusively NE, 5-HT, and PEA. There is little evidence for NE or 5-HT depletion in depression responsive to AMI-like antidepressants (Type II). Thus, AMI has been shown effective when urinary MHPG is high and NT has been found therapeutic when CSF 5-HIAA is high or normal, although Hollister and associates [135] have found that patients with low urinary excretion of MHPG were more likely to respond to NT. We have found that urinary PAA is reduced in AMI responders, and in fact, AMI and NT raise urinary PAA levels (unpublished data).

## AMPHETAMINE AND SCHIZOPHRENIA

As alluded to earlier in this chapter, Van Kammen and co-workers have reviewed the literature and reported on their own series of studies on the use of amphetamine in prediction studies in schizophrenia [8,136–139]. They have studied "postpsychotic depressed" schizophrenics as well as psychotic schizophrenics. d-AMPH can increase psychosis in schizophrenia with or without long-term neuroleptic treament. Acute exacerbation of psychosis induced by intravenous d-AMPH (patients unmedicated for at least three weeks) predicted that lithium treatment would exert antipsychotic and antidepressant effects; the greater the increase in psychotic behavior induced by d-AMPH the greater the antipsychotic effect of lithium. However, lithium effects were small and observed in males only. This AMPH-induced increase in psychotic behavior is believed to confirm a diagnosis of schizophrenia [41,44]. This would suggest that a small part of the schizophrenic process is lithium-sensitive [136]. However, because a diagnosis of affective disorder or schizophrenia cannot be validated by independent biological parameters, the diagnostic implication of a minimal antipsychotic response to lithium in schizophrenia is unresolved. These lithium-induced changes seem to be drug-induced, not spontaneous fluctuations is behavior. The data suggest that affective disorders and schizophrenias share some common regulatory biochemical substrates but not necessarily the same etiology. DA, NE and more recently PEA have all been implicated in the action of lithium and d-AMPH and in schizophrenia. In another study, these investigators observed that the acute behavioral response to d-AMPH infusion predicted short-term treatment responsiveness to pimozide, a relatively specific DA blocker and antipsychotic [140,141]. Those who improved the most with the former drug improved the most with the latter drug, followed by those who worsened. Those who were unchanged did not respond to pimozide, though there were those who did not respond to d-AMPH and still responded to pimozide. In general, a change in psychosis in any direction with d-AMPH relates to improvement with pimozide, and the state-dependent factors, which can change over time, are important in the antipsychotic response to the latter group of drugs. However, because d-AMPH nonresponders also responded to pimozide, it is quite apparent that this prediction is not infallible. The d-AMPH challenge predicted the fourth week response to double-blind pimozide; the fifth week response was more accurately predicted by prepimozide psychosis ratings. In a retrospective study, they further found that a worsening of psychosis ratings during pimozide treatment following d-AMPH was associated with clinical relapse if the drug was withdrawn. Those schizophrenics in stable remission tended not to worsen with AMPH [142] or methylphenidate [41,42], suggesting a state-dependent phenomenon [138]. Thus there is a potential use for the Stimulant Challenge Test to provide an indication for risk of relapse upon neuroleptic withdrawal; neuroleptics seem to be protective against psychotic decompensation without changing the underlying vulnerability.

Possible explanations for these responses have been offered. A possible psychological explanation involves the role of stress. Biochemical mechanisms involved in the psychotropic response to d-AMPH may be associated with similar mechansims to those associated with postneuroleptic withdrawal relapse. Because of its relatively specific DA blocking actions, the fact that pimozide failed to block the psychotogenic effects of AMPH in six of thirteen patients indicates that other mechanisms besides DA may be involved in psychotic decompensation.

Lastly, Van Kammen and associates [139] examined the effect of AMPH on psychosis ratings after five weeks of treatment with pimozide. None of ten patients who did not change in psychosis following the pretreatment of d-AMPH infusion became worse or improsed following pimozide, suggesting that pimozide pretreatment did not induce functional DA receptor supersensitivity. Supersensitivity probably occurs after a much longer treatment time. They hypothesized that if d-AMPH effects are DA-mediated, then pimozide, as compared with placebo pretreatment, would either attenuate (through postsynaptic DA receptor blockade) or increase (through unmasking DA receptor supersensitivity) certain behaviors induced by d-AMPH. The stability of the preinfusion condition is more important to the type of response to d-AMPH than long-term receptor blocker pretreatment. However, with respect to all of their findings, they caution against clinical applications until studies with larger samples replicate their findings.

These data have etiopathogenetic implications for schizophrenia. Crow [143] has proposed two subtypes of schizophrenia: DA-sensitive (Type I) and DA-insensitive (Type II). The data on variable responses to d-AMPH questions this as well as the supersensitivity model of schizophrenia. If d-AMPH effects are DA-mediated, then pimozide should attenuate, via postsynaptic DA receptor blockade, or increase, through unmasking DA supersensitivity, certain behaviors induced by d-AMPH. DA responsiveness may change over time. Although prepimozide psychosis ratings correlated positively with the pimozide response, preamphetamine ratings did not correlate with AMPH-induced changes [138]. Thus, Van Kammen and associates' data support a mixed state- and trait-dependency (mainly the former) for DA involvement, as well as time-dependent changes in DA receptor responsiveness in different anatomical brain sites in schizophrenics. DA insensitivity seems to develop over time, and may or may not be associated with remissions. It may be that, over time, mechanisms other than DA blockade may play a role in the mechanism of antipsychotic efficacy and actions, as well as d-AMPH-induced change in psychosis. Postsynaptic DA receptor blockade may be involved only indirectly in long-term antipsychotic effects. If DA is involved, the possible biochemical bases of schizophrenia could include unstable regulatory mechanisms of the neuronal firing rate in a specific DA tract which may change over time, a disturbance of a certain type of DA receptor activity at different anatomic sites, or a membrane disorder responsive to d-AMPH.

Thus, changes in psychosis after d-AMPH could be an episode marker. Further, the activation-euphoria response to d-AMPH was unaffected by pimozide pretreatment, suggesting that the changes in psychosis and activation may be regulated by different (nondopaminergic) mechanisms. This emphasizes the dynamic aspects of neurotransmitter systems.

## CONCLUSIONS

Although current studies indicate that the Stimulant Challenge Test is a simple, rapid, noninvasive, and safe procedure with possible clinical validity, which presumably may serve to distinguish biochemically different types of depressions and schizophrenias, there are unresolved problems associated with the use of this test. First is the small number of patients with whom this test has been studied and shown effective. The finding, to be useful, requires confirmation in a larger group of carefully diagnosed patients studied under double-blind conditions. Second is the lack of objectivity in evaluations, a problem that potentially can be solved by measuring biochemical responses to amphetamine. Third, there is a deficient understanding of the meaning, in the study of depressives, of partial responses to stimulants, but our recent studies indicate that negative results predict responsiveness to AMI-like TCA, including NT. Fourth, many studies with AMPH and methylphenidate are incomplete in that TCA levels have not been measured, a major question in view of the dramatic difference in plasma levels observed using comparable doses in different patients. There is, however, recent evidence from our own studies that indicate that plasma levels alone do not account for differential drug sensitivity [59]. Further, the correlation of this Stimulant Challenge Test with extant diagnostic and biochemical procedures, including biogenic amine measurements and endocrinologic tests, may provide for a set of more precise tools to improve our diagnosis and treatment of various psychiatric disorders. Research with this test may also clarify the interrelationship between anxiety and various subtypes of depression, their differential responsiveness to AMPH and TCA, and alterations of catecholaminergic mechanisms. Alterations in MHPG, cortisol and biochemical measures probably reflect anxiety levels in addition to depressed mood. Lastly, and importantly, is that change may occur over time within a given individual in response to a stimulant challenge. Throughout the natural course of any psychiatric illness, the biochemical features of the illness may be as dynamic and variable as the clinical state. Therefore, the Stimulant Challenge Test is especially useful because it may predict treatment response as well as prognosticate course of the illness *in the individual patient.* In summary, the significance of these Stimulant Challenge Tests is two-fold: on the clinical side, to develop a rapid test for prediction of specific treatment response and to determine prognosis of treatment with various pharmacotherapeutic agents, and on the theoretical side, to further our understanding of various subtypes of depressions and schizophrenia on the basis of biological markers, as well as their relation to anxiety.

## ACKNOWLEDGMENT

Our grateful thanks and appreciation to June Ascareggi, for without her assistance and technical skills this manuscript could not have become a reality.

## REFERENCES

1. Simon SL, Taube H: A preliminary study of the use of methedrine in psychiatric diagnosis. J Nerv Ment Dis 104:593–596, 1946
2. Rudolph G de M: The treatment of depression with methylamphetamine. J Mental Sci 102:358–363, 1956

3. Leake CD: Therapeutic use of the amphetamines. In Leake CD (ed): The Amphetamines: Their Actions and Uses. Springfield, Illinois, Charles C Thomas, 1958
4. Robin AA, Wiseberg S: A controlled trial of methylphenidate (Ritalin) in the treatment of depressive states. J Neurol Neurosurg Psychiat 21:55–57, 1958
5. Roberts JM: Prognostic factors in the electro-shock treatment of depressive states. II. The application of specific tests. J Mental Sci 105:705–713, 1959
6. Wharton RN, Perel JM, Dayton PG, et al: A potential clinical use for methylphenidate with tricyclic antidepressants. Am. J. Psychiatry 127:1609–1625, 1971
7. Kiloh LG, Neilson M, Andrews G: Response of depressed patients to methylamphetamine. Brit J Psychiat 125:496–499, 1974
8. Van Kammen DP, Bunney WE, Docherty JP: d-Amphetamine-induced heterogeneous changes in psychotic behavior in schizophrenia. Am J Psychiatry 139:991–997, 1982
9. Wood DR, Reimherr FW, Wender PH, et al: Diagnosis and treatment of minimal brain dysfunction in adults. A preliminary report. Arch Gen Psychiatry 33:1453–1460, 1976
10. Wender PH: Diagnosis and treatment of adult minimal brain dysfunction: A replication. Presented at the American College of Neuropsychopharmacology, Maui, Hawaii, December, 1978
11. Zis AP, Goodwin FK: Novel antidepressants and the biogenic amine hypothesis of depression: The case for iprindole and mianserin. Arch Gen Psychiatry 36:1097–1107, 1979
12. Von Felsinger JM, Lasagna L, Beecher HK: Drug-induced mood changes in man. 2. Personality and reactions to drugs. JAMA 157:1113–1119, 1955
13. Lasagna L, Von Felsinger JM, Beecher HK: Drug-induced mood changes in man. 1. Observations on healthy subjects, chronically ill patients, and "post-addicts". JAMA 157:1006–1020, 1955
14. Johnsson L-E, Anggard E, Gunne L-M: Blockade of intravenous amphetamine euphoria in man. Clin Pharmacol Ther 12:889–896, 1971
15. Borison RL, Mosnaim AD, Sabelli HC: Biosynthesis of brain 2-phenylethylamine: Influence of decarboxylase inhibitors and D-amphetamine. Life Sci 15:1837–1848, 1974
16. Borison RL, Mosnaim AD, Sabelli HC: Brain 2-phenylethylamine as a mediator for the central actions of amphetamine and methylphendiate. Life Sci 17:1331–1344, 1975
17. Innes IR: Actions of dexamphetamine on 5-hydorxytryptamine receptors. Br J Pharmacol 21:427–435, 1963
18. Deffenu G, Bartolini A, Pepeu G: Effects of amphetamine on cholinergic systems of the cerebral cortex of the cat. In Costa E, Garattini S (eds): Amphetamines and Related Compounds. New York, Raven Press, 1970
19. Slater S, de la Vega CE, Skyler J, et al: Plasma prolactin stimulation by fenfluramine and amphetamine. Psychopharm Bull 12:26–27, 1976
20. Van Praag HM, Korf J: Chloramphetamines. In Usdin E, Forrest IS (eds): Psychotherapeutic Drugs, Part II—Applications. New York, Marcel Dekker, Inc., 1977
21. Murphy DL, Slater S, de la Vega CE, et al: The serotonergic neurotransmitter system in the affective disorders—A preliminary evaluation of the antidepres-

sant and antimanic effects of fenfluramine. In Deniker P, Radouco-Thomas, C, Villeneuve A (eds): Neuro-Psychopharmacology, Vol. 1. Proceedings of the Tenth Congress of the Collegium Internationale Neuro-Psychopharmacologicum. Oxford, Pergamon Press, 1978

22. Cole JO: Fenfluramine. In Cole JO (ed): Psychopharmacology Update. Lexington, Mass. The Collamore Press, 1980
23. Checkley SA: Neuroendocrine tests of monoamine function in man: A review of the basic theory and its application to the study of depressive illness. Psychol Med 10:35–53, 1980
24. Moore KE: The actions of amphetamines on neurotransmitters: A brief review. Biol Psychiatry 12:451–462, 1977
25. Sabelli HC, Giardina WJ, Bartizal F: Photic evoked cortical potentials: Interaction of reserpine, monoamine oxidase inhibition and DOPA. Biol Psychiatry 3:273–280, 1971
26. Scheel-Kruger J: Comparative studies of various amphetamine analogues demonstrating different interactions with the metabolism of the catecholamines in the brain. Eur J Pharmacol 14:47–59, 1971
27. Ferris R, Tang F, Maxwell R: A comparison of ten capacities of isomers of amphetamine, deoxypipradrol and methylphenidate to inhibit the uptake of tritiated catecholamines into rat cerebral cortex, hypothalamus and striatum and into adrenergic nerves of rabbit aorta. J Pharmacol Exp Ther 181:407–416, 1972
28. Ferris RM, Tang FLM: Comparison of the effects of the isomers of amphetamine, methylphenidate and deoxypipradrol on the uptake of 1-($^3$-H)norepinephrine and ($^3$H)dopamine by synaptic vesicles from rat whole brain, striatum and hypothalamus. J Pharmacol Exp Ther 210:422–428, 1979
29. Costall B, Naylor RJ: The involvement of dopaminergic systems with the stereotyped behavior patterns induced by methylphenidate. J Pharm Pharmacol 26:20–33, 1974
30. Janowsky DS, El-Yousef MK, Davis JM, et al: Antagonistic effects of physostigmine and methylphenidate in man. Am J Psychiatry 130:1370–1376, 1973
31. Schildkraut JJ, Watson R, Draskoczy PR, et al: Amphetamine withdrawal: Depression and MHPG excretion. Lancet 2:485–486, 1971
32. Watson R, Hartmann E, Schildkraut JJ: Amphetamine withdrawal: Affective state, sleep patterns, and MHPG excretion. Am J Psychiatry 129:263–269, 1972
33. Checkley SA: A new distinction between the euphoric and the antidepressant effects of methylamphetamine. Brit J Psychiat 133:416–423, 1978
34. Van Kammen DP, Murphy DL: Attenuation of the euphoriant and activating effects of d- and l-amphetamine by lithium carbonate treatment. Psychopharmacologia 44:215–224, 1975
35. Cooper JR, Bloom FE, Roth RH: Catecholamines II: CNS aspects. In Cooper JR, Bloom FE, Roth RH: The Biochemical Basis of Neuropharmacology. Fourth Edition. New York, Oxford University Press, 1982
36. Fyro B, Peterson U, Sedvall G: The effect of lithium treatment on manic symptoms and levels of monoamine metabolites in cerebrospinal fluid of manic depressive patients. Psychopharmacolugia 44:99–103, 1975
37. Bowers MB, Heninger GR: Lithium: Clinical effects and cerebrospinal fluid acid monoamine metabolites. Commun Psychopharmacol 1:135–145, 1977

38. Sabelli HC, Borison RL, Diamond BI, et al: 2-phenylethylamine as a neuromodulator of wakefulness, affect and extrapyramidal function: Recent advances. In Mosnaim AD, Wolf ME (eds): Noncatecholic Phenylethylamines: Part 1: Phenylethylamine: Biological Mechanisms and Clinical Aspects. New York, Marcel Dekker, Inc. 1978
39. Sabelli HC, Borison RL: Diamond BI, et al: Phenylethylamine and brain function. Biochem Pharmacol 27:1707–1711, 1978
40. Beckmann H, Van Kammen DP, Goodwin FK, et al: Urinary excretion of 3-methoxy-4-hydroxyphenylglycol in depressed patients. Modifications by amphetamine and lithium. Biol Psychiatry 11:377–387, 1976
41. Van Kammen DP, Bunney WE, Docherty, et al: Amphetamine-induced catecholamine activation in schizophrenia and depression: Behavioral and physiological effects. Adv Biochem Pharmacol 16:655–659, 1977
42. Janowsky DS, El-Yousef MK, Davis JM, et al: Provocation of schizophrenic symptoms by intravenous administration of methylphenidate. Arch Gen Psychiatry 28:185–191, 1973
43. Janowsky DS, Davis JM: Methylphenidate, dextroamphetamine and levamphetamine: Effects on schizophrenic symptoms. Arch Gen Psychiatry 33:304–308, 1976
44. Segal DS, Janowsky DS: Psychostimulant-induced behavioral effects: Possible models of schizophrenia. In Lipton MA, DiMascio A, Killam KF (eds): Psychopharmacology: A Generation of Progress. New York, Raven Press, 1978
45. Angrist B, Rotrosen J, Gershon S: Responses to apomorphine, amphetamine, and neuroleptics in schizophrenic subjects. Psychopharmacology 67:31–38, 1980
46. Fischer E, Ludmer RI, Sabelli HC: The antagonism of phenylethylamine to catecholamines on mouse motor activity. Acta Physiol Latinoam 17:15–21, 1967
47. Sabelli HC, Mosnaim AD: Phenylethylamine hypothesis of affective behavior. Am J Psychiatry 131:695–699, 1974
48. Everett GM, Toman JEP: Mode of action of Rauwolfia alkaloids and motor activity. In Messerman J (ed): Biological Psychiatry. New York, Grune and Stratton, 1959
49. Redmond DE: New and old evidence for the involvement of a brain norepinephrine system in anxiety. In Fann WE, Karacan I, Porkorny AD, et al (eds). New York, Spectrum Publications, Inc., 1979
50. Fawcett J, Maas J, Dekirmenjian H: Depression and MHPG excretion: Response to dextroamphetamine and tricyclic antidepressants. Arch Gen Psychiatry 26:246–251, 1972
51. Hopkinson G: A neurochemical theory of appetite and weight changes in depressive states. Acta Psychiat Scand 64:217–225, 1981
52. Paul SM, Hulihan-Giblin B, Skolnick P: (+)-Amphetamine binding to rat hypothalamus: Relation to anorexic potency of phenylethylamines. Science 218:487–490, 1982
53. Sabelli HC, Mosnaim AD, Vasquez AJ, et al: Biochemical plasticity of synaptic transmission: A critical review of Dale's principle. Biol Psychiatry 4: 481–524, 1976
54. Stern SL, Rush JA, Mendels J: Toward a rational pharmacotherapy of depression. Am J Psychiatry 137:545–552, 1980

55. Arieti S, Bemporad J: Severe and Mild Depression. New York, Basic Books, 1978
56. Keller MB, Shapiro RW: "Double depression": Superimposition of acute depressive episodes on chronic depressive disorders. Am J Psychiatry 139:438–442, 1982
57. Maas JW: Biogenic amines and depression: Biochemical and pharmacological separation of two types of depression. Arch Gen Psychiatry 32:1357–1361, 1975
58. Bielski RJ, Friedel RO: Prediction of tricyclic antidepressant response: A critical review. Arch Gen Psychiatry 33:1479–1489, 1976
59. Sabelli HC, Fawcett J, Javaid JI, et al: The methylphenidate test for differentiating desipramine-responsive from nortriptyline-responsive depression. Am J Psychiatry 140:212–214, 1983
60. Berk AA, Chalmer TC: Cost and efficacy of the substitution of ambulatory for inpatient care. N Engl J Med 304:393–397, 1981
61. Weissman MM, Meyers JK, Thompson WD: Depression and its treatment in a U.S. urban community—1975–1976. Arch Gen Psychiatry 38:417–421, 1981
62. Fawcett J, Siomopoulos V: Dextroamphetamine response as a possible predictor of improvement with tricyclic therapy in depression. Arch Gen Psychiatry 25:247–255, 1971
63. Van Kammen DP, Murphy DL: Prediction of imipramine antidepressant response by a one-day d-amphetamine trial. Am J Psychiatry 135:1179–1184, 1978
64. Ebert MH, Van Kammen DP, Murphy DL: Plasma levels of amphetamine and behavioral response. In Gottschalk LA, Merlin S (eds): Pharmacokinetics of Psychoactive Drugs: Blood Levels and Clinical Response. New York, Spectrum Publications, Inc., 1976
65. Van Kammen DP, Murphy DL: Prediction of antidepressant response to lithium carbonate by a 1-day administration of d-amphetamine in unipolar depressed women. Neuropsychobiology 5:266–273, 1979
66. Fawcett J, Sabelli H, Gusovsky F, et al: Phenylethylaminic mechanisms in maprotiline antidepressant effect. Fed Proc 42:1164, 1983
67. Kupfer DJ, Pickar D, Himmelhoch JM, et al: Are there two types of unipolar depression? Arch Gen Psychiatry 32:866–871, 1975
68. Maas JW, Fawcett JA, Dekirmenjian H: Catecholamine metabolism, depressive illness and drug response. Arch Gen Psychiatry 26:252–262, 1972
69. Kadouch R, Belmaker R, Ebstein RP, et al: The mood response and plasma cyclic-AMP response to intravenous methylphenidate. Neuropsychobiology 3:250–255, 1977
70. Mosnaim AD, Inwang EE, Sabelli HC: The influence of psychotropic drugs on the levels of endogenous 2-phenylethylamine in rabbit brain. Biol Psychiatry 8:227–234, 1974
71. Spatz H, Spatz N: Urinary and brain phenylethylamine levels under normal and pathological conditions. In Mosnaim AD, Wolf ME (eds): Non-catecholic Phenylethylamines: Part I: Phenylethylamine: Biological Mechanisms and Clinical Aspects. New York, Marcel Dekker, Inc., 1978
72. Fawcett J, Sabelli HC, Javaid JI, et al: Urinary phenylethylamine in affective disorders. Presented at the WPA/APA Regional Meeting, New York City, October 30–November 3, 1981

73. Sigg EB: Pharmacological studies with Tofranil. Canada Psychiat Assoc J (Suppl 4):S75–S85, 1959
74. Sabelli HC: Pressor effects of adrenergic agents and serotonin after the administration of imipramine. Arzneim-Forsch 10:935–936, 1960
75. Glowinski J, Axelrod J: Inhibition of uptake of tritiated-noradrenaline in the intact rat brain by imipramine and structurally related compounds. Nature 204:1318–1319, 1964
76. Pare CMB, Kline N, Hallstrom, et al: Will amitriptyline prevent the "cheese" reaction of monoamine oxidase inhibitors. Lancet 2:183–186, 1982
77. Fischer E, Ludmer LI, Sabelli HC: The antagonism of phenylethylamine to catecholamines on mouse motor activity. Acta Physiol Latinoam 17:15–21, 1967
78. Raiteri M, Levi G, Federico R: Stimulus-coupled release of unmetabolized 3-H-norepinephrine from rat brain synaptosomes. Pharmacol Res Commun 7:181–187, 1975
79. Colburn RW, Thoa NB, Kopin IJ: Influence of ionophores which bind calcium on the release of norepinephrine from synaptsomes. Life Sci 17:1395–1399, 1975
80. Bosdanski DF: Mechanisms of transport for the uptake and release of biogenic amines in nerve endings. Adv Exp Med Biol 69:291–305, 1976
81. Raiteri M, delCarmine R, Bertollini A: Effect of desmethylimipramine on the release of ($^3$H)norepinephrine induced by various agents in hypothalamic synaptosomes. Molecular Pharmacology 13:746–758, 1977
82. Risch SC, Kalin NH, Murphy DL: Neurochemical mechanisms in the affective disorders and neuroendocrine correlates. J Clin Psychopharmacol 1:180–185, 1982
83. Siever L, Insel T, Uhde T: Noradrenergic challenges in the affective disorders. J Clin Psychopharmacol 1:193–206, 1982
84. Sachar EJ, Hellman L, Roffwarg H, et al: Disrupted 24-hour patterns of cortisol secretion in psychotic depression. Arch Gen Psychiatry 28:19–24, 1973
85. Carroll BJ: Limbic system-adrenal cortex regulation in depression and schizophrenia. Psychosom Med 38:106–121, 1976
86. Davis J, Morrill R, Fawcett J, et al: Apprehension and elevated serum cortisol levels. J Psychosom Res 6:83–86, 1962
87. Maas J, Dekirmenjian H, Fawcett J: Catecholamine metabolism and stress. Nature 230:330–331, 1971
88. Besser GM, Butler PWP, Landon J, et al: Influence of amphetamines on plasma corticosteroid and growth hormone levels in man. Brit Med J 4:528–530, 1969
89. Brown WA, Williams BW: Methylphenidate increases serum growth hormone concentrations. J Clin Endocrinol Metab 43:937–939, 1976
90. Brown WA: Psychologic and neuroendocrine response to methylphenidate. Arch Gen Psychiatry 32:1103–1108, 1977
91. Brown WA, Corriveau DP, Ebert MH: Acute psychologic and neuroendocrine effects of dextroamphetamine and methylphenidate. Psychopharmacology 58:189–199, 1978
92. Frohman LA, Stachura ME: Neuropharmacologic control of neuroendocrine function in man. Metabolism 24:211–234, 1975
93. Langer G, Heinze G, Beim B, et al: Reduced growth hormone responses to amphetamine in "endogenous" depressive patients: Studies in normal, "re-

active" and "endogenous" depressive, schizophrenic, and chronic alcoholic subjects. Arch Gen Psychiatry 33:1471–1475, 1976
94. Halbreich U, Asnis GM, Halpern FS, et al: Diurnal growth hormone responses to dextroamphetamine in normal young men and postmenopausal women. Psychoneuroendocrinology 5:339–344, 1980
95. Halbreich, U, Sachar EJ, Asnis GM, et al: Growth hormone response to dextroamphetamine in depressed patients and normal subjects. Arch Gen Psychiatry 39:189–192, 1982
96. Checkley SA, Crammer JL: Hormone response to methylamphetamine in depression: A new approach to the noradrenaline depletion hypothesis. Brit J Psychiat 131:582–586, 1977
97. Checkley SA: Corticosteroid and growth hormone responses to methylamphetamine in depressive illness. Psychol Med 9:107–115, 1979
98. Sachar EJ, Halbriech U, Asnis GM, et al: Paradoxical cortisol responses to dextroamphetamine in endogenous depression. Arch Gen Psychiatry 38: 1113–1117, 1981
99. Feinberg M, Carroll BJ, Greden JF: Comparison of two neuroendocrine markers for endogenous depression. Presented at the Society of Biological Psychiatry 35th Annual Program, 1980
100. Gold PW, Goodwin FK, Wehr T, et al: Growth hormone and prolactin response to levodopa in affective illness. Lancet 2:1308–1309, 1976
101. Persky H, Grinker RR, Hamberg DA, et al: Adrenal cortical function in human subjects: Plasma level and urinary excretion of hydrocortisone. AMA Arch Neurol Psychiat 76:549–558, 1956
102. Sabshin M, Hamberg DA, Grinker RR, et al: Significance of preexperimental studies in the psychosomatic laboratory. AMA Arch Neurol Psychiat 78: 207–219, 1957
103. Rubin RT, Mandell AJ: Adrenal cortical activity in pathological emotional states: A review. Am J Psychiatry 123:387–400, 1966
104. Sachar EJ, Asnis G, Nathan RS, et al: Dextroamphetamine and cortisol in depression: Morning plasma cortisol levels suppressed. Arch Gen Psychiatry 37:755–757, 1980
105. Halbreich U, Sachar EJ, Asnis GM, et al: Studies of cortisol diurnal rhythm and cortisol response to d-amphetamine in depressive patients. Psychopharm Bull 17:114–116, 1981
106. Rees L, Butler PWP, Gosling C, et al: Adrenergic blockade and the corticosteroid and growth hormone responses to methylamphetamine. Nature 228: 565–566, 1970
107. Halbreich U, Asnis GM, Ross D, et al: The behavioral and mood response to d-amphetamine: Some possible physiological correlates. Psychopharm Bull 17:83–84, 1981
108. Halbreich U, Asnis GM, Ross D, et al: Amphetamine-induced dysphoria in postmenopausal women. Brit J Psychiat 138:470–473, 1981
109. Boyd AE, Reichlin S: Neural control of prolactin secretion in man. Psychoneuroendocrinology 3:113–130, 1978
110. Janowsky DS, Parker D, Leichner PP: Growth hormone and prolactin response to methylphenidate. Psychopharm Bull 12:27–28, 1976
111. Meltzer HY, Goode DG, Fang VS: The effect of psychotropic drugs on endocrine function. I. Neuroleptics, precursors and agonists. In Lipton MA, DiMascio A, Killam KF (eds): Psychopharmacology: A Generation of Progress. New York, Raven Press, 1978

112. Van Kammen DP, Docherty JP, Marder SR, et al: D-amphetamine raises serum prolactin in man: Evaluations after chronic placebo, lithium and pimozide treatment. Life Sci 23:1487–1492, 1978
113. Nurnberger JI, Gershon E, Sitaram N, et al: Dextroamphetamine and arecholine as pharmacogenetic probes in normals and remitted bipolar patients. Psychopharm Bull 17:80–82, 1981
114. Carroll BJ: The hypothalamic-pituitary-adrenal axis in depression. In Davies B, Carroll BJ, Mowbray RM (eds): Depressive Illness: Some Research Studies. Springfield, Thomas Publishing Company, 1972
115. McLeod WR: Poor responses to antidepressants and dexamethasone nonsuppression. In Davies B, Carroll BJ, Mowbray RM (eds): Depressive Illness: Some Research Studies. Springfield, Thomas Publishing Company, 1972
116. Brown WA, Johnston R, Mayfield D: The 24-hour dexamethasone suppression test in a clinical setting: Relationship to diagnosis, symptoms and response to treatment. Am J Psychiatry 136:543–547, 1979
117. Brawley P: Dexamethasone, methylphenidate, and depression. In Abstracts of the Scientific Proceedings of the 132nd Annual Meeting of the American Psychiatric Association. Washington, DC, APA, 1979
118. Greden J, Tarika J, DeVigne JP: Dexamethasone suppression test predicts treatment response. In Abstracts of the Scientific Proceedings of the 133rd Annual Meeting of the American Psychiatric Association. Washington, DC, APA, 1980
119. Carroll BJ: Clinical applications of the dexamethasone suppression test. Int Drug Ther Newsletter 16:1–4, 1980
120. Carroll BJ, Feinberg M, Greden JF, et al: Diagnosis of endogenous depression: Comparison of clinical, research and neuroendocrine criteria. J Affective Disord 2:177–194, 1980
121. Carroll BJ, Schroeder K, Mukhopadhyay S, et al: Plasma dexamethasone concentrations and cortisol suppression response in patients with endogenous depression. J Clin Endocrinol Metab 51:433–437, 1980
122. Greden JF, Albala AA, Haskett RF, et al: Normalization of dexamethasone suppression test: A laboratory index of recovery from endogenous depressive illness. Biol Psychiatry 15:449–458, 1980
123. Brown WA, Haier RJ, Qualls CB: Dexamethasone suppression test identifies subtypes of depression which respond to different antidepressants. Lancet 1: 928–929, 1980
124. Brown WA: Studies of response to dexamethasone in psychiatric patients. Psychopharm Bull 16:44–45, 1980
125. Brown WA, Haier RJ, Qualls CB: The dexamethasone suppression test in the identification (of) subtypes of depression differentially responsive to antidepressants. Psychopharm Bull 17:88–89, 1981
126. Sternbach H, Gwirtsman H, Gerner RH: The dexamethasone suppression test and response to methylphenidate in depression. Am J Psychiatry 138:1629–1631, 1981
127. Carroll BJ, Feinberg M, Greden JF, et al: A specific laboratory test for the diagnosis of melancholia: Standardization, validation, and clinical utility. Arch Gen Psychiatry 38:15–22, 1981
128. Borison RL, Mosnaim AD, Sabelli HC: Biosynthesis of brain 2-phenylethylamine: Influence of decarboxylase inhibition and D-amphetamine. Life Sci 15:1837–1848, 1974

129. Borison RL, Mosnaim AD, Sabelli HC: Brain 2-phenylethylamine as a mediator for the central actions of amphetamine and methylphenidate. Life Sci 17:1331–1344, 1975
130. Ross SB, Renyi AL: Tricyclic antidepressant agents–I. Acta Pharmacol Toxicol (Copenh) 36:382–394, 1975
131. Randrup A, Braestrup C: Uptake inhibition of biogenic amines by newer antidepressant drugs: Relevance to the dopamine hypothesis of depression. Psychopharmacology 53:309–314, 1977
132. Toman JEP, Everett GM, Jeans RF: Seizure latency method and other procedures for antipsychotic drugs. In Himwhich HE (ed): Tranquilizing Drugs. Washington, Amer Associ Adv Sci., 1957
133. Sabelli HC: A pharmacological strategy for the study of central modulator linkages. In Wortis J (ed): Recent Advances in Biological Psychiatry, Vol. 6, New York, Plenum Press, 1964
134. Sulser F: Pharmacology: Current antidepressants. Psychiatr Ann 10(suppl): 381–386, 1980
135. Hollister LE, Davis KL, Berger PA: Subtypes of depression based on excretion of MHPG and response to nortriptyline. Arch Gen Psychiatry 37:1107–1110, 1980
136. Van Kammen DP, Docherty JP, Marder SR, et al: Acute amphetamine response predicts antidepressant and antipsychotic responses to lithium carbonate in schizophrenic patients. Psychiatry Res 4:313–325, 1981
137. Van Kammen DP, Docherty JP, Bunney WE: Prediction of early relapse after pimozide discontinuation by response to d-amphetamine during pimozide treatment. Biol Psychiatry 17:233–242, 1982
138. Van Kammen DP, Docherty JP, Marder SR, et al: Antipsychotic effects of pimozide in schizophrenia: Treatment response prediction with acute dextroamphetamine response. Arch Gen Psychiatry 39:261–266, 1982
139. Van Kammen DP, Docherty JP, Marder SR, et al: Long-term pimozide pretreatment differentially affects behavioral responses to dextroamphetamine in schizophrenia: Further exploration of the dopamine hypothesis of schizophrenia. Arch Gen Psychiatry 39:275–281, 1982
140. Pinder RM, Brogden RN, Sawyer PR, et al: Pimozide: A review of its pharmacological properties and therapeutic uses in psychiatry. Drugs 12:1–40, 1976
141. Denef C, van Neuten JM, Leysen JE, et al: Evidence that pimozide is not a partial agonist of dopamine receptors. Life Sci 25:217–226, 1979
142. Kornetsky C: Hyporesponsivitity of chronic schizophrenic patients to dextroamphetamine. Arch Gen Psychiatry 33:1425–1428, 1976
143. Crow TJ: Molecular pathology of schizophrenia: More than one disease process? Brit Med J 280:66–68, 1980

# Laboratory Evaluations in Specific Psychiatric Environments

CHAPTER 10

# Laboratory Evaluation of Newly Admitted Psychiatric Patients

RICHARD C. W. HALL
and THOMAS P. BERESFORD

The goal of this chapter is to define a useful, readily utilizable data base to assist the physician in the initial evaluation of severely disturbed psychiatric patients admitted to the hospital. The purpose of this initial laboratory workup is not to mindlessly suspend the physician's judgment nor to go on an unnecessary laboratory search for imaginary pathology, rather it is: (1) to provide a workable and useful data base for a patient likely to receive psychotropic medication, (2) to assist in defining unrecognized physical illness, and (3) to establish patient specific laboratory and physiologic norms which can subsequently be monitored for change, to provide a baseline for long term treatment.

This laboratory data base, when coupled with a careful history and physical examination, provides the information necessary to arrive at a correct diagnosis and undertake a safe and intelligent course of treatment.

*Handbook of Psychiatric Diagnostic Procedures,* vol. 1, edited by R. C. W. Hall and T. P. Beresford. 

## PSYCHIATRIC PATIENTS: A POPULATION AT RISK

An extensive literature exists supporting the fact that psychiatric symptoms are nonspecific in their nature and are often caused by a variety of unrecognized physical illnesses, intoxications, and aberrant metabolic states [1-85].

Our group and many others have demonstrated that psychiatric patients are at risk for the presence of unrecognized physical illnesses [1,7,20,21,38,48,53,54, 57,64,65,75,80,85-91]. Psychiatrically, these conditions are most likely to present as organic mental states, moderate to severe anxiety states, depressive disorders and acute psychotic reactions of various types [20,35,48,40,41,42,44,61]. The acutely psychotic patient admitted to a psychiatric facility is at particular risk for the presence of unrecognized physical illness [4,7,11,20,21,23-25,27,35,38,44,48,51, 54,57,64,65,86-101].

Several lines of inquiry support the association of physical illness and psychiatric symptoms. These include health surveys of general medical populations with independent assessment of their physical and psychiatric status [11,77] and studies showing increased rates of psychiatric symptoms in medical patients [6,10, 12, 13,15-20,25,26,29,34,36,53,55,59,63,66,69,70-72, 74,78,79,81,98,102-144]. Several authors report significant rates of unrecognized physical illness among psychiatric inpatients [38,48,65,87,89], psychiatric outpatients [4,7,21,57,86,88], psychiatric day-hospital patients [90], and psychiatric emergency patients [4,145-146].

Studies defining the incidence and prevalence of psychiatric symptoms in general medical populations form another source of such data. These studies include those of hospitalized patients [98,104-106] and those attending medical outpatient clinics [99,107-109,147,148]. Other studies deal with the development of specific psychiatric symptoms such as anxiety and depression in patients housed in special medical environments such as the burn, dialysis, spinal injury, and coronary care units of general hospitals [12,111,149-174].

Additional literature exists which defines the occurrence of psychiatric symptoms in patients with particular somatic disease states such as endocrine and gastrointestinal disease, cardiovascular disorders and cancer [2,12,15-17,25,26,55,59,63, 70,71,79,81,102,111-114,116-117,120,126,129,132,134,150,175-185]. There is an increased incidence of psychiatric symptoms in patients following the development of certain physical illnesses [55]. Other studies document an increased prevalence of personality disorders and behavioral disturbances in children following the development of chronic illness [71].

Extensive reviews of this literature are available in several recent textbooks [20,53,85] and journal articles [23,24,26,27,35,38]. Consequently, we do not attempt to reproduce them here. We do, however, discuss a few studies which are pertinent to the topic of laboratory evaluation. In a recent study of 215 patients referred to a specialized medical psychiatric inpatient unit, Hoffman [51] reports that a thorough neuropsychiatric evaluation resulted in a therapeutically important alteration of the referral diagnosis in 41% of cases. Particularly impressive in this study was the fact that of the patients referred with a tentative diagnosis of dementia, 63% were found to have treatable conditions.

Hoffman [51] calls attention to the process by which a physician should make a diagnostic formulation: first by applying a preliminary or informal diagnosis which is then confirmed or altered by the utilization of data obtained during the patient's workup (i.e., history, physical, laboratory evaluation). The physician then searches for a specific cause to explain the patient's abnormal findings. Hoffman suggests that if a primary physician makes a preliminary diagnosis of mental disorder, its inclusion as a diagnosis often alters his willingness to develop a subsequent data base and thus impedes the further workup of the patient. His study was designed to test the accuracy of the physician's initial impression that psychiatric disease produced psychiatric symptoms. His findings suggest that a substantial proportion of psychiatric diagnoses, whether applied by medical or psychiatric practitioners, are in error. He demonstrated that a thorough neuropsychiatric assessment resulted in 41% of patients having their diagnosis changed and that a careful physical and laboratory evaluation was essential in providing data which subsequently altered the entire diagnostic and treatment approach to the patient.

Hoffman's workup was "thorough but not exceptional." Initially all patients received a detailed history, physical examination, and separate neurological examination. Each patient also received a standard mental status examination and a routine admission laboratory evaluation which consisted of complete blood count, 18-factor automated chemical analysis, urinalysis, VDRL, ECG, and chest film. Physical exams were done by at least three different physicians and often more. If the initial mental status assessments were suspicious or indicated that an organic disease was present, a more detailed neuropsychiatric assessment was undertaken. This included blood and urine toxicology screens; a determination of plasma levels of current medications, if available; a sedimentation rate; thyroid function studies; B-12 and folate levels; FTA-ABS, stool test using the hemoccult slide method; tuberculin skin test; and EEG. Other laboratory tests were ordered as indicated. Wherever practical, therapy with any medication known to have psychotoxic potential was discontinued. If major depressive disorders were suspected, the dexamethasone suppression test was performed. If the aforementioned studies did not reveal a cause for a suspected organic mental disorder, a CT scan was obtained and followed in some cases by lumbar puncture. Finally, persistently unclear cases of dementia received a trial of psychoactive drugs to differentiate true dementia from depressive pseudodementia.

Of the 215 patients studied, 122 had an initial diagnosis of functional psychiatric disorder. Forty percent of these were changed as a result of the patient's workup; 6% changed within the functional category to an extent that appreciably altered treatment; 34% were changed to a diagnosis of organic mental disorder.

Ninety three patients had an initial admitting diagnosis of organic mental disorder. Fifty seven percent of these remained unchanged following workup, while 31% were changed within the organic category, that is, a different etiology than was initially suspected was discovered as a result of workup. Twelve percent of these patients were subsequently assigned a diagnosis of either pseudodementia or of a functional psychiatric disorder.

In considering all of these patients, a careful neuropsychiatric workup produced a 41% change across the functional–organic boundary in either direction. Particularly noteworthy was the fact that 24% of these patients were suffering from an unrecognized organic impairment.

Hoffman calls our attention to three important sub-findings of his study. First was the surprisingly high frequency by which behavioral symptoms were due to the prescription of nonpsychiatric medications that were not suspected at the time of referral. Most of these patients presented with either depression or delirium. In only three of the thirteen cases of toxic delirium produced by medications had medications been suspected as a causative factor. Secondly, of 35 patients who were referred with a diagnosis of dementia, careful neuropsychiatric and laboratory evaluation confirmed this diagnosis in only 22 cases (63%). Of the remaining 37%, 26% were found to be delirious and 11% to have a functional disorder presenting as dementia. Of the 44 patients where an extensive physical and laboratory workup confirmed the diagnosis of dementia, 41% (18 patients) were found to have a dementia that was treatable or potentially reversible.

Hoffman's comments on the findings of his study provide a compelling argument for the careful physical and laboratory evaluation of psychiatric patients: "Our major finding was that informal or tentative diagnoses in patients with behavioral disorders were frequently in error: 41% of our series, after thorough evaluation, received therapeutically important changes in diagnosis, with a change across the functional–organic boundary in 24%" [51].

Bunce, et al [186] studied 102 consecutive female patients admitted to an acute medical care unit of a large psychiatric hospital. These patients were transferred because of nonspecific changes in their physical condition or because of alterations in behavior. More than 70% of the patients were unable to communicate adequately with their physician. Ninety two percent of the sample were found to have at least one, with an average of three, previously undiagnosed physical diseases not predicted by their symptoms on referral. These findings prompted the authors to recommend a high index of suspicion for physical disease in psychiatric populations and to recommend an aggressive multidisciplinary diagnostic approach to their management.

The evaluation profile used by Bunce and his group included complete review of the patient's chart with detailed physical examination, EEG, CBC, urinalysis, SMA-18, chest x-ray, cytology screening, and thyroid profile. Electrocardiograms were obtained in all patients over the age of 30. Other diagnostic procedures, where indicated included x-ray examinations of the GI and GU tracts, CAT scans, ultrasonography, lumbar puncture, and sigmoidoscopy.

In reviewing the data from this study, Bunce points out several important findings: (1) The diagnostic impressions of the referring physician were confirmed in only 54% of cases. (2) An average of 2.7 unexpected diseases were found in each of these patients. (3) Infections accounted for the highest percentage of medical diseases encountered and were found in 55% of the population (GU infections being the most prevalent). (4) Degenerative diseases of the cardiovascular–renal axis and bone disease were also frequently seen. (5) Most of these patients had no specific medical complaints, they were chronically disabled, and complained of such things as "general weakness." (6) These patients had difficulty communicating, and were often confused, agitated, or delusional. These communication problems significantly complicated their diagnostic workup. In addition, many of these patients had atypical presentations of their medical illnesses.

Rabins, evaluating 41 demented patients admitted to the Henry Phipps Psychiatric Clinic during a one year period, found four of these patients to have a reversible etiology for their dementia. In addition, he found that sixteen elderly patients with an admission diagnosis of depression were in fact demented. Thirteen of these cases had a reversible etiology. He concluded that the percentage of patients with reversible dementia seen in a psychiatric facility was similar to that encountered on the neurological and medical services of a general hospital. His study demonstrated the value of a thorough psychiatric and neurological evaluation to determine whether the dementia of patients presenting to a psychiatric service was reversible [73].

The implications of this study take on increased meaning when one considers that 12% of all of the patients who were discharged from general hospital psychiatric units during the year 1970 to 1971 carried a diagnosis of organic brain syndrome [187]. The rate of organic mental disorders in patients over 65 years of age exceeded 30%.

An increased severity of psychiatric disease has been shown to be related to an increased tendency to suffer from multiple physical disorders. Eastwood and Trevelyan selected 124 psychiatric cases from a random sample of 1,471 persons registered with a London group practice. They matched these cases with a sample of psychiatrically well controls and carefully evaluated physical illness in both groups. The psychiatric patients had a significantly greater number of physical diseases of all kinds than did the nonpsychiatric controls. These investigators noted that the patients with the most severe psychiatric dysfunctions were also those who were most likely to suffer from multiple physical illnesses. The severely ill psychiatric patients comprised only 17% of the psychiatric sample but suffered from 52.4% of the diagnosed major physical illnesses.

Browning et al, in a study of psychiatric emergency patients confirmed that such patients are at high risk for unrecognized medical illness [4]. His group compared psychiatric emergency patients seen in a general hospital emergency room with patients seen in the same emergency room for nonpsychiatric reasons. They demonstrated that the psychiatric patients rate of medical hospital admissions was more than twice that of the control group during the succeeding six month period.

These studies suggest that the medical workup of severely ill psychiatric patients (i.e., those likely to be admitted to a psychiatric inpatient facility in an agitated, confused, or acutely psychotic state) will provide a high yield of positive medical findings. They argue that these patients represent a specific and appropriate sample for detailed laboratory study. Such patients do not represent a random general population to be screened, rather they are a population at high risk. This difference is critically important, since a variety of articles exist in laboratory journals which suggest that the biochemical laboratory evaluation of a healthy population is not cost effective. In fact, many insurance companies are currently refusing to pay for such routine laboratory evaluations in patients newly admitted to hospital [188-189]. We concur with these observations, but we do not concur that acutely psychotic patients should be included in this group.

A variety of studies link physical and mental symptoms by establishing that medically ill patients have a higher incidence of psychiatric symptoms than expected in the general population. For example, McKegney in a study of 144 patients referred from medical and surgical wards with "conversion symptoms" found 47% to suffer from coexistent organic disease [190]. Schwab in a study of 153 medical inpatients reported that approximately 20% suffered from significant depression [102]. Stewart, Drake, and Winokur also found 20% of severely ill medical inpatients to suffer from clinically significant depression. The depression in these cases followed the onset of illnesses that were likely to be either fatal or lead to severe disability. This study suggests that careful evaluation of these patients, if they presented psychiatrically, would be medically rewarding [103]. In a meticulous study of 80 patients hospitalized with advanced cancer or acute onset leukemia, Plumb et al demonstrated that 30% developed an affective disorder, while 12% became psychotic [191].

Other studies suggest that the medical illnesses present in psychiatric patients are often unknown to either the patient or his treating physician [38]. Koranyi studied 100 consecutive patients referred to his outpatient clinic and found that fully 50% suffered from a physical illness. Half of these illnesses had not been diagnosed prior to the referral of the patient [86]. In our own study of 658 consecutive outpatients, who were carefully evaluated using a detailed review of systems questionnaire, a biochemical laboratory screening, and physical examination, we were able to document a 9.1% incidence of psychiatric symptoms which we believed to be caused by previously unrecognized medical illness [44]. Other important studies in this area include those of Maguire and Granville-Grossman who found a 33.5% physical illness rate in 200 consecutive inpatients, 70% of which were "severe." Forty nine percent of these patients suffered from illnesses that were unknown to either them or their physician [64]. Koranyi, in an impressive study of 2,090 lower socioeconomic class outpatients, showed that 46% of these illnesses were undiagnosed by the referral source. In 69% of these cases, the patients medical illness strongly influenced his/her psychiatric state. Eighteen percent of these patients were thought to have experienced psychiatric symptoms purely on the basis of their underlying medical disorder [57].

Hall et al, in a study of 100 acutely ill, lower socioeconomic class patients admitted to a clinical research ward, found that 46% had medical illnesses which either directly produced or exacerbated their psychiatric symptoms and which were believed to have prompted or contributed to their admission [38]. An additional 34% of these patients were found to be suffering from some medical illness which required treatment. Careful evaluation of these patients suggested that a detailed psychiatric, neurological, and physical examination with repetitive mental status testing, SMA-34 biochemical analysis, CBC, urinalysis, electrocardiogram, and sleep deprived EEG were able to establish the presence and nature of the underlying medical disorder in 90% of cases. In looking at the relative yield of various diagnostic procedures we found that detailed evaluation of hearing and vision, a complicated computerized medical history, detailed social history, a life history questionnaire and psychological testing (MMPI, Wais, Graham-Kendell) were not specifically useful in assisting the diagnostic workshop.

The procedures that were useful, in order of their frequency of positive findings, were SMA-34 blood chemistries, complete physical examination, detailed psychiatric history, CBC and SMA-12 sub-panels of the SMA-34, sleep deprived EEG, electrocardiogram, and urinalysis [38].

Lishman [192] in citing the work of Macfie discusses the yield of various tests in 136 consecutive psychiatric inpatient admissions. The most important investigations in this series, in order of yield, were detailed mental status evaluation for organicity, evaluation of serum proteins and liver function tests, lumbar puncture, EEG, chest x-ray, serum electrolyte determinations, CBC, skull x-rays, urine drug screen, and serological test for syphilis.

Lishman suggests that a routine laboratory workup should be performed on all psychiatric inpatients and should include the following: hemoglobin, erythrocyte sedimentation rate, white blood cell count and differential. If anemia is present, more detailed hematologic studies are indicated. In addition, a serological test for syphilis, serum B-12 and folate, and laboratory investigations of BUN, electrolytes, calcium, phosphorus, serum proteins, liver function tests, and blood sugar should be obtained. Thyroid function tests, drug screens and on occasion, tests for LE cells or antinuclear antibodies were also felt to be of value. A routine urinalysis and "occasional" urine examinations where indicated, for porphyrins, catechols, and urinary steroids were considered useful, as was the selective search for heavy metals. Lishman believes routine chest x-rays are important for evaluating cardio-pulmonary status and for the detection of carcinoma of the lung and tuberculosis. He suggests electrocardiography as a useful routine component to provide evidence of dysrhythmia, cardiac ischemia, coronary thrombosis, or electrolyte abnormality. Finally, he suggests that EEG's are of considerable value.

Several conclusions can be drawn from this brief review:

1. Psychiatric patients of all types are at risk for the presence of physical illnesses.
2. Some sub-groups of psychiatric patients are particularly vulnerable to the presence of unrecognized physical illness, which in a significant number of cases may be either causally related to or exacerbate their psychiatric symptoms. High risk patients are those seen in psychiatric emergency facilities, and psychiatric inpatients admitted with diagnoses of acute psychotic or major depressive disorders and/or dementia.
3. A careful physical and laboratory examination of high risk patients is rewarding and does not represent the random laboratory screening of a healthy population; rather, it represents the appropriate study of a high risk group.
4. Since as many as 50% of the illnesses discovered by routine evaluation are previously unknown to either the patient or the patient's physician, a negative history of disease or a previously negative physical examination cannot be relied upon as a data base to rule out the presence of a current, unrecognized physical illness.
5. Tentative admission diagnoses have a high probability of being changed if detailed physical and laboratory evaluations are undertaken.
6. Conversely, admission misdiagnoses are likely to be confirmed if a detailed workup is not undertaken.
7. The routine evaluation of a high risk patient admitted to hospital must be meticulous and multifaceted. At a minimum it should include: (A) a complete review of systems, (B) a careful and detailed physical and neurological examination, (C) biochemical laboratory evaluation (to be described), (D) detailed mental status testing, (E) careful observational measurements of behavior made on the admission ward, (F) chest x-ray, (G) electrocardiogram, (H) some would argue, an electroencephalogram, and (I) where feasible, a urine drug screen.

## THE VALUE OF A LABORATORY EVALUATION

Careful laboratory evaluation is of value for several reasons. Laboratory testing is useful in assisting the physician to discover covert disease and in preventing the irreparable damage that might occur if some conditions persisted (i.e., hypothyroidism). Laboratory tests also permit the early diagnosis of specific conditions after the onset of a particular sign or symptom and assist in the differential diagnosis of possible disease states. They help the physician determine the stage or activity of a particular disease and provide a base line for a particular patient which may be useful in detecting the occurrence of relapse. A particular test may be useful in measuring the effect of a specific therapy or by providing information necessary for the genetic counseling of a relative, for example, Wilson's or Tay-Sachs disease. Laboratory base lines may also provide assistance in clarifying medical-legal issues and by protecting patients from the adverse effects of treatment with specific agents (i.e., urine drug screen for opiates or the detection of hyponatremia in individuals prior to the onset of lithium therapy).

These evaluations provide an important part of the data base from which decisions are made. For example, the evaluation of liver function tests can be of great diagnostic value in discriminating various types of underlying hepatic disease. Sher, in evaluating 175 patients, found that the study of total and direct bilirubin, alkaline phosphatase, lactate dehydrogenase, and aspartate aminotransferase, correctly classified up to 73% of cases of hepatic disease depending upon the homogeneity of the diagnostic group [193].

The multivariate analysis of other clinical laboratory patterns is of use in establishing the etiology of a variety of lipid disorders, endocrine disease states, pulmonary and cardiovascular degenerative diseases, and disorders of mineral metabolism. Renal, adrenal, and pancreatic functions are also readily assessed by these means [194–198].

Arguments that routine laboratory evaluation should not be undertaken in acutely ill psychiatric patients because of cost factors and inefficiency are incorrect and we believe potentially dangerous, since much of the initial diagnostic workup in psychiatry is predicated on symptom diagnosis. Psychiatrists who have widely divergent underlying assumptions about the nature of disease may have a very low concordance rate for arriving at the same conclusions, given particular symptoms. Since the psychiatric symptoms produced by underlying medical disorders are diverse, it is crucial that a concrete data base be derived if correct diagnoses are to be effected.

Psychiatry, perhaps more than any other medical specialty, has been accused of paying selective attention to particular signs and symptoms. The laboratory workup helps the psychiatrist to overcome this bias. Such evaluations provide readily accessible, clear information which is external to the problem solver and helps focus his attention in the correct area. It shifts his knowledge base from symptom centered knowledge to disease centered knowledge and thereby helps significantly to increase the accuracy of his diagnosis and treatment [199].

Working with a laboratory information system, the physician's training becomes useful in synthesizing the available facts into a workable diagnosis. Laboratory and physical findings, coupled with symptom patterns, provide a substantive data base upon which the physician can then formulate a diagnosis, define further needs for knowledge and finally structure a treatment plan which is rational, replicable, and which can be monitored. Within this model, "laboratory tests attain their greatest value when they are used to detect an organ-system abnormality not otherwise apparent, to define a disease process, to identify etiologic factors in the disease process, or to provide information at lower hierarchical levels that can elucidate observations at higher levels. These uses of laboratory tests apply to the detection of disease, differential diagnosis, and patient monitoring" [199].

The greatest dangers inherent in routine lab testing are: that (1) the information will be disregarded, and (2) it will be inappropriately interpreted. In the latter case, laboratory error or clinical naivety may lead to the follow up of simple screening tests with invasive or other potentially dangerous procedures (i.e., invasive studies). It becomes apparent, therefore, that if patients are routinely screened and evaluated, the data derived from these examinations must be carefully scrutinized and made relevant to the treatment process. Unfortunately this is not always done.

An excellent study by Fraser et al looked at what happened to 189 abnormal urine results obtained from 182 patients following routine screening. The results were translated into further diagnostic action or treatment in only 13 cases. These authors analyzed the action taken and placed the results in 5 discrete groups. They found that in 11 of the 182 patients no report of the results was ever entered into the patient's medical record. In 33 of the patients, an abnormal result was obtained and returned to the physician but was recorded as "no abnormality detected" in the medical record; i.e., the physician did not realize that the result was abnormal. In 106 patients, the abnormal result was obtained and documented in the medical record. However, these were unexpected and unexplained abnormalities which were not consistent with the physician's thinking and therefore were not commented on. It was noteworthy that further laboratory tests or investigational procedures were not ordered or embarked upon even though they were indicated. Nineteen of these patients had abnormalities that, in all probability, were related to the primary problem and so no new clinical or laboratory procedures were initiated as a direct result. In these cases none were indicated. In 13 cases, a new clinical decision was made or new laboratory investigations were ordered, in part directly owing to the results of the urinalysis [200].

Because of findings like these, we strongly encourage psychiatrists to build into their morning rounds a time at which all of the laboratory results obtained during the proceeding day can be discussed with the staff and appropriate follow-up instituted.

## CONDUCT OF EXAMINATION AND HANDLING OF SAMPLES

When a patient is admitted to a psychiatric facility his initial diagnostic evaluation should be completed, where possible, before the patient is medicated, since psychotropic drugs interfere with a variety of laboratory and electrophysiologic evaluations (i.e., electrocardiogram and EEG). A dietary history is important if tests of glucose metabolism are to be evaluated. If the patient has a poor dietary history, it is often wise to wait until he has been adequately nourished on a fixed caloric intake for three to seven days. Dehydration and intoxication with various substances can also affect workup values.

It is important that when blood is drawn or urine collected that the staff is sure of the source of the sample, and that such samples are gathered at the appropriate times and placed in proper containers. If 24 hour urine samples are to be attained, it is crucial that ward physicians instruct the nursing staff so that bathroom doors can be adequately secured and refrigeration facilities made available. It is also suggested that any individual test which is frequently reported as abnormal be checked with the laboratory to make sure that no procedural errors are inherent in the collection or processing of the samples. Finally, one needs to be sure that samples are quickly and appropriately delivered to the correct laboratory facility, as delays in sample processing often result in error.

## THE NORMATIVE RANGE—WHAT IT MEANS

It is crucial that the physician understand both the reliability and validity of the tests he is ordering and what their normative values mean. In the last decade, with the development of multi-element chemical testing (MET), laboratory normal ranges have been derived on larger samples of the population than was previously possible for any local laboratory to accomplish. These increased sample sizes, with their increased reliability of processing within any given automated multi-channel processor, have helped establish normal ranges in a more consistent fashion. When dealing with the clinical chemistry or urology laboratory one must remember what the definition of "normal range" means, since any deviation from normal may be taken as evidence that an abnormal state (i.e., disease) exists.

The normal range is derived by considering the 95% confidence interval for the healthy population. This usually means that "of all healthy individuals surveyed, 95% of them fall within the stated range. This type of definition permits any laboratory to establish its own method-dependent normal values. The introduction of reliable multi-channel auto-analyzers provided a large subject population with which to statistically define the normal range" [201].

The physician, however, must be aware of the potential problems which can be caused by using "normal range" values. First, by definition, 5% of all healthy individuals will have an abnormally high or low value thereby producing a "false positive test." Second, statistical concepts or normalcy are helpful for evaluating large numbers of people but may mislead the clinician concerning any individual at any moment in time. For example, one system's normal range of uric acid variance is from 1.5 mg/dl to 7.5 mg/dl. This 95% interval is composed of a large number of individual values which range from the low of 1.5 mg/dl to the maximum of 7.5 mg/dl, with each individual showing considerable fluctuation and variation over a narrower range. The change in concentration ($\Delta$) may be of considerably more import to a physician than the patient's actual serum level. Consider the individual whose normal uric acid is 1.5 mg/dl, who comes to hospital and has a single 7.5 mg/dl uric acid level reported, a fivefold increase from that individual's "normal" value but still within the "normal range." The change in level here would indicate to the physician that a significant problem might exist. Thus, the physician should, when possible, compare an individual's laboratory values to his own baseline when studying the long-term variations of any constituent biochemical level. This is the best way to establish the patient's own 95% confidence level, which is clinically much more relevant than those of the general population. Intrasubject comparative data, however, is only relevant if intra- and interlaboratory results are comparable and if the standardizations of analyses are correct.

The physician must be cautious of placing too much significance on any particular test. He must be cognizant of the expected laboratory changes that are likely to occur, for example with the administration of a particular drug or as the result of a particular physiologic state (see Table 1). For cxample, if a group of patients were playing tackle football or if the ward went on a three mile jog, one would expect to find changes in the patient's urinary catecholamines, creatine phosphokinase, WBC count, prolactin, and ornithine carbamyl transferase levels. Recent studies have suggested that thyroid function tests are altered in acutely psychotic patients. These alterations do not necessarily reflect hyper- or hypothyroidism, but seem to be a transient phenomenon associated with the development of agitated psychotic states. Spratt and colleagues found that of 645 patients admitted to an acute psychiatric unit, 33% had elevated serum thyroxin ($T_4$) levels while 18% had an elevated free $T_4$ index (FTI). Serum triiodothyronine ($T_3$) was low, normal, or minimally elevated in 77 patients who had a high initial free $T_4$ index. 22 patients with an initial elevation of their free $T_4$ index were serially followed. $T_4$, free $T_4$ index, and free $T_4$ fell in every patient.

Psychiatrists need to know that these thyroid function tests are likely to be abnormal in acutely psychotic patients. If a question of thyroid disease exists, the physician must be able to obtain additional physical and laboratory information to confirm or rule out this possibility. In such a case, a careful physical examination, with specific notation of the relaxation phase of deep tendon reflexes, altered voltage on electrocardiogram, evaluation of thyrotropin releasing hormone and thyroid stimulating hormone levels would all provide data useful in establishing a precise diagnosis. The assumption of thyroid disease, however, based on a transitory change of either $T_3$ or $T_4$ could produce significant diagnostic error [202].

**Table 1. Alteration of Laboratory Test Values by Selective Drugs**

| Test and how altered | Drug | |
|---|---|---|
| *Urine color altered* interfere with fluorometric, colorimetric, photometric determination | Methyldopa | Red darkens on standing, pink or brown |
| | Phenothiazines | Pink, red, purple, orange, rust |
| | Quinine and derivatives | Brown to black |
| *False positive test for urine protein* by causing false positive turbidity tests | Chlorpromazine, promazine | |
| *False positive test for urine glucose* by reducing action with Benedict's solution and Clinitest but not with Clinistix or Testape | Chloral hydrate | |
| *False negative test for urine glucose* by glucose oxidase method, e.g., Clinistix, Testape | Ascorbic acid | |
| | Levodopa (with Clinistix but not Testape) | |
| *False positive urine acetone* | Levodopa with Labstix | |
| *False positive urine diacetic acid test* | Chlorpromazine<br>Other phenothiazines<br>Levodopa<br>Salicylates | |
| *Positive test for urine amino acids* | ACTH and cortisone | |
| *Urine test for occult blood* | | |
| False positive by Guaiac | Bromides<br>Copper<br>Iodides<br>Oxidizing agents | |
| by Benzidine | Bromides<br>Copper<br>Iodides<br>Permanganate | |
| False negative | Ascorbic acid (high doses) | |
| *Positive tests for bile in urine* | Chlorpromazine and other phenothiazines–interfere with Bili-Labstix | |

*continued*

**Table 1.** (continued)

| Test and how altered | Drug |
|---|---|
| *Increased urine urobilinogen* | Chlorpromazine<br>Other phenothiazines<br>Tricyclic antidepressants which increase serotonin |
| *Positive fluorometric test for urine porphyrins* | Acriflavine<br>Ethoxazene<br>Phenazopyridine<br>Sulfamethoxazole<br>Tetracycline |
| *Drugs that may precipitate porphyria* | Antipyretics<br>Barbiturates<br>Phenylhydrazine<br>Sulfonamides |
| *Cause urine creatine to be* | |
| Increased | Caffeine |
| Decreased | Androgens and anabolic steroids |
| *Cause urine creatinine to be* | |
| Increased | Ascorbic acid<br>Corticosteroids<br>Levodopa<br>Methyldopa |
| Decreased | Androgens and anabolic steroids |
| *Cause urine calcium to be* | |
| Increased | Androgens and anabolic steroids<br>Corticosteroids |
| *Cause urinary 17-ketosteroids to be* | |
| Increased | Chlorpromazine<br>Other phenothiazines<br>Dexamethasone<br>Meprobamate<br>Quinidine<br>Secobarbital |
| Decreased | Chlordiazepoxide<br>Estrogens<br>Meprobamate<br>Promazine<br>Reserpine |
| *Cause urinary 17-hydroxy-corticosteroids to be* | |
| Increased | Chloral hydrate |

Table 1. (continued)

| Test and how altered | Drug |
|---|---|
| | Chlordiazepoxide<br>Chlorpromazine<br>Meprobamate<br>Paraldehyde<br>Quinine |
| Decreased | Estrogens and oral contraceptives<br>Phenothiazines<br>Reserpine |
| *Interfere with determination of urinary catecholamines* | Ascorbic acid<br>Chloral hydrate<br>Epinephrine<br>Methyldopa<br>Quinine<br>Vitamin B complex |
| *Urine vanillylmandelic acid (VMA)* | |
| Increased | Aspirin<br>Glyceryl guaiacolate |
| Decreased | Guanethidine<br>Imipramine<br>MAOIs |
| *Urine 5-hydroxyindoleacetic acid (5-HIAA)* | |
| Increased | Glyceryl guaiacolate<br>Reserpine |
| Decreased | Chlorpromazine, other phenothiazines<br>Imipramine<br>Isoniazid<br>MAOI's<br>Methyldopa<br>Promethazine |
| *Urine pregnancy test* | |
| False positive | Chlorpromazine, other phenothiazines (frog, rabbit, immunologic)<br>Promethazine (Gravindex) |
| False negative | Promethazine (DAP test) |
| *Erythrocyte sedimentation rate (ESR)* | |
| Increased | Methyldopa<br>Methysergide<br>Trifluperidol |

*continued*

**Table 1.** (continued)

| Test and how altered | Drug |
|---|---|
| Decreased | Quinine, salicylates, drugs that cause a high blood glucose level |
| *Cause positive direct Coomb's test* | |
| | Chlorpromazine |
| | Levodopa |
| | Phenytoin sodium |
| | Quinidine, quinine |
| *False positive test for lupus erythematosus cells and/or* antinuclear antibodies | Acetazolamide |
| | Aminosalicylic acid |
| | Birth control pills |
| | Chlorprothixene |
| | Chlorothiazide |
| | Griseofulvin |
| | Hydralazine |
| | Isoniazid |
| | Methyldopa |
| | Penicillin |
| | Phenylbutazone |
| | Phenytoin sodium |
| | Procainamide |
| | Streptomycin |
| | Sulfonamides |
| | Tetracyclines |
| | Thiouracil |
| | Trimethadione |
| *Drugs that regularly increase prothrombin time* | Chloral hydrate |
| | Phenytoin sodium |
| | Quinidine |
| | Salicylates |
| | d-Thyroxine |
| *Drugs that may increase prothrombin time* | Disulfiram |
| | Methyldopa |
| | Methylphenidate |
| | Thyroid drugs |
| *Drugs that regularly decrease prothrombin time* | Barbiturates |
| | Ethchlorvynol |
| | Glutethimide |
| | Heptabarbital |

**Table 1.** (continued)

| Test and how altered | Drug |
|---|---|
| *Drugs that may decrease prothrombin time* | Adrenocortical steroids |
| | Birth control pills |
| | Meprobamate |
| *Drugs that may inhibit heparin* | Antihistamines |
| | Phenothiazines |
| *Cause idiosyncratic thrombocytopenia* | |
| Anticonvulsant | Ethosuximide (Zarontin) |
| | Methylhydantoin |
| | Paramethadione |
| | Phenacemide |
| | Trimethadione |
| Tranquilizers | Chlordiazepoxide |
| | Chlorpromazine |
| | Meprobamate |
| | Promazine |
| *Cause allergic vascular purpura with normal platelet function and numbers* | Aspirin |
| | Chloral hydrate |
| | Chlorpromazine |
| | Diphenhydramine (Benadryl) |
| | Meprobamate |
| | Trifluoperazine |
| | Other phenothiazines |
| *Cause false negative test for occult blood in stool* | Vitamin C (usually $>$ 500 mg/day) |
| *Cause increased serum urea nitrogen by methodologic interference* | Chloral hydrate |
| *Cause increased serum uric acid* | Levodopa |
| | Phenytoin sodium |
| By methodologic interference | Ascorbic acid |
| | Levodopa |
| | Methyldopa |
| *Caused increased serum bilirubin due to* | |
| Methodologic interference on SMA 12/60 | Aminophenol |
| | Ascorbic acid |

*continued*

**Table 1.** (continued)

| Test and how altered | Drug |
|---|---|
| | Levodopa<br>Methyldopa |
| *Cause increased serum cholesterol due to* | |
| Hepatotoxic effect | Phenytoin sodium |
| Cholestatic effect | Androgens and steroids<br>Promazine |
| Hormonal effect | Corticosteroids<br>Birth control pills |
| Methodologic interference | Bromides<br>Chlorpromazine<br>Corticosteroids<br>Vitamin C<br>Vitamin A |
| *Cause decreased serum cholesterol due to* | |
| Hepatotoxic effect | MAO inhibitors |
| *Cause increased serum triglycerides* | |
| | Estrogens<br>Birth control pills |
| *Cause decreased serum triglycerides* | Ascorbic acid |

[a]This table is modified, adapted and reproduced with permission from Wallach J: Interpretation Of Diagnostic Tests. A Handbook Synopsis Of Laboratory Medicine. Third Edition, Little, Brown and Company, Boston, copyright 1978.

## ALTERATION OF LABORATORY TEST RESULTS BY MEDICATION

It is important that psychiatrists be aware of the possible effects that psychotropic and other drugs may have on influencing laboratory tests. The correct interpretation of laboratory tests requires that the physician be aware of all the drugs that a patient is taking and relate their ingestion to test outcome. The classes of drugs that are most often involved in altering laboratory results include oral hypoglycemics, hormones of various types, psychoactive agents, anticoagulants, anticonvulsants, antihypertensives, and anti-infectives [203].

Laboratory tests can be affected by a variety of mechanisms which may operate simultaneously. These include interference with the chemical reaction used in the testing procedure, damage to a specific organ such as the liver or kidney, development of specific metabolic alterations such as the enhanced or retarded formation of a particular chemical in the body, competition for binding sites, or stimulation or suppression of a particular enzyme system [203-204]. Table 1 illustrates some of the effects that commonly encountered medications can have on laboratory tests.

## WHAT TESTS TO ORDER AND HOW TO INTERPRET THEM

Cole, in an excellent article on biochemical test profiles [205] points out that no single automated process meets all needs. He emphasizes that it is always less expensive to order a single test than a profile; however, he makes very clear that if three or more tests are to be ordered, that the use of a profile is considerably less expensive for the patient. "In some situations a profile may contain a test or two not otherwise considered necessary. However, the cost and charge to the patient are less even though the number of tests is greater." Cole, in evaluating laboratory studies conducted on 2,871 patients admitted to the University of Alabama Hospitals, divided the tests ordered into a variety of specific uses.

Routine tests to assess the patient's nutritional status included glucose, urea/creatinine ratio, hematocrit, serum osmolality, sodium, potassium, chloride, bicarbonate, calcium, phosphorus, magnesium, protein, albumin, cholesterol, triglycerides, and uric acid.

Tests to monitor hemostasis and inflammation included hematocrit, hemoglobin, erythrocyte count, leukocyte count, leukocyte differential count, platelet count, prothrombin time, clotting time, or partial thromboplastin time, fibrinogen, immunoglobulins A, G, and M.

Tests helpful for evaluating organ injury, inflammation, growth and repair included: acid phosphatase, amylase, lipase, alkaline phosphatase, bilirubin fractions, gamma glutamyl transferase, SGOT, SGPT, LDH, and CPK, with their isoenzymes.

Cole felt the most important admission screening tests identified in this study were electrolytes (sodium, chloride, potassium and carbon dioxide content), creatine, glucose, calcium, phosphorus, SGOT, SGPT, LDH and CPK (both with isoenzymes), cholesterol, triglycerides, bilirubin fractions, and alkaline phosphatase.

He points out that simultaneous knowledge of serum protein and albumin levels are essential for proper interpretation of mineral concentration. Finally he stresses the fact that several of these determinations are useful when read as a pattern or combined to get appropriate ratios. For example, electrolytes provide information for the evaluation of the anion gap, where the number of cations should exceed the number of anions by an average of 1.5 mEq per liter. The urea/creatine ratio can be very helpful in evaluating water balance. By summating millimoles of sodium, urea and glucose, one can estimate serum osmolality. Various enzyme patterns permit the differentiation of specifically diseased organs, and so on. The point

| Chemistry | Normal range |
|---|---|
| Sodium | 135–145 meq/l |
| Potassium | 3.5–5.0 meq/l |
| Carbon dioxide | 22–32 meq/l |
| urea nitrogen | 7–21 mg/dl |
| Creatinine | 0.5–1.2 mg/dl |
| Glucose | 70–115 mg/dl |
| Calcium | 4.3–5.3 meq/l |
| Inorganic phosphate | 2.5–4.5 mg/dl |
| Uric acid | 2.5–5.7 mg/dl |
| Total protein | 6.0–8.5 g/dl |
| Albumin | 3.5–5.5 g/dl |
| SGOT (AST) | 0–40 U/l |
| Lactate dehydrogenase | 100–225 U/l |
| Creatine kinase | 0–110 U/l |
| SGPT (ALT) | 0–35 U/l |
| GGT | 2–30 U/l |
| Alkaline phosphatase | 30–100 U/l |
| Cholesterol | 120–250 mg/dl |
| Total bilirubin | 0.2–1.2 mg/dl |
| Direct bilirubin | 0.0–0.4 mg/dl |
| BUN/creat | 10–20 |

**Figure 1.** Hospital Biochemical Profile SMA-C21.

is that the clinician can use these tests to determine not only specific aberrant values, but also combinations and shifts in values to arrive at specific diagnostic conclusions.

No single screening battery has any particular advantage over others, once the basic 18 to 22 tests that are routinely examined by automated processing are evaluated. If these tests show changes, specific separate tests can be ordered to provide the additional diagnostic information necessary to sort out particular organ involvement or to monitor the progression of a disease. If the local laboratory uses an SMA-12/60 to provide its cheapest screening battery, that would be the most appropriate system to employ when screening patients. If, however, the hospital uses a Technicon SMACII to provide a SMA-21 for the most reasonable cost, that would be the best system (see Figures 1 and 2).

A recent inquiry of the actual costs incurred by various hospitals in our locality for automated batteries showed that a 24 test profile at one hospital cost $12.50 while a 20 test profile at another cost $8.50, while a 21 test profile at a third facility cost $59.05. These were hospital costs, not patient charges. The information

| | |
|---|---|
| *Glucose | SGPT |
| BUN | *LDH |
| Creatine | *Total Bilirubin |
| Sodium | Direct Bilirubin |
| Potassium | BUN Creatinine Ratio |
| Chloride | Complete Blood Count |
| $CO_2$ | White Cell Count |
| *Uric Acid | Red Cell Count |
| *Total Protein | Hematocrit |
| *Albumin | Hemoglobin |
| *Globulin | Differential |
| A/G Ratio | MCV |
| *Calcium | MCHC |
| *Phosphorus | Platelet Count |
| *Cholesterol | $T_3$ |
| Triglyceride | $T_4$ |
| *Alk. Phos | $T_7$ |
| *SGOT | |

*These are the tests which are run in SMA-12 series

**Figure 2.** Tests in one 34 analysis series.

that could be gained for this $8.50 to $60.00 is enormous, considering the fact that day costs often average between $120–300 per day in various facilities.

If one were ordering selected individual tests, i.e., automated batteries were not available, the yield/cost ratio for occult disease would be highest when ordering CBC, routine urinalysis, glucose, alkaline phosphatase, urea, bilirubin, electrolytes, and thyroid function screens [17,86].

As a routine admission laboratory evaluation, we would propose the following: 1. CBC; 2. urinalysis; 3. the automated admission battery which provides the best cost/test ratio, whether it be the SMA-12,18,20,21,34, or 36; 4. urine drug screen; 5. thyroid function studies; and 6. FTA. Further workup should be determined based on the results of the testing obtained. In patients with dementia, laboratory evaluation should include: CBC, sedimentation rate, major metabolic screen, thyroid function studies, vitamin B-12 and folate levels, STS, and in addition CT scan and electroencephalogram if the rest of the workup is negative [206]. See Popkin [207] for an excellent of this subject. The guidelines for interpretation and evaluation of other electrophysiological and chemical tests are provided in other chapters of this text.

Table 2 is provided to assist the reader in the interpretation of tests commonly

**Table 2. A Guide to the Interpretation of Screening Laboratory Tests[a]**

| Test | Indicates (or physiologic role) | Normal range | Increased in | Decreased in | Comments |
|---|---|---|---|---|---|
| Aldolase | If increased–tissue destruction | 4-14 Bruns units/ml | Mycoardial infarction<br>Hemolytic anemia<br>Muscular dystrophies<br>Metastatic prostatic carcinoma<br>Leukemia–also 20% of other cancer patients<br>Acute pancreatitis<br>Acute hepatitis | | In obstructive jaundice and cirrhosis is normal or only slightly elevated |
| Ammonia | Liver disease, ↑ protein metabolism | 80-110 $\mu$g/ml whole blood | Portacaval shunt<br>Hepatic insufficiency<br>Starvation<br>GI bleeding<br>Acute hepatic necrosis | | Decreased by MAOIs in cirrhosis. Blood ammonia may be increased after portacaval anastomosis. Not all cases of hepatic coma show increased blood ammonia |
| Amylase serum | Produced in pancreas and salivary glands, ↑ if these glands obstructed or inflammed | 80-180 Somogyi units/100 ml serum | Acute pancreatitis<br>Pancreatic obstruction by stone; stricture; CA; chlorothiazide, codeine, methylcholine, or morphine.<br>Drug induced spasm of sphincter of oddi.<br>Chronic pancreatitis (acute exacerbation)<br>Mumps<br>Perforating peptic ulcer | Extensive destruction of pancreas<br>Pancreatic insufficiency<br>Toxemia of pregnancy<br>Barbiturate poisoning<br>Severe liver damage<br>Advanced cystic fibrosis<br>Severe thyrotoxicosis<br>Severe burns | In acute pancreatitis level should be at least 500 Somogyi units/100 ml<br><br>May be increased by morphine, codeine, meperidine |

Renal insufficiency (occasionally)
Diabetic acidosis (occasionally)
Post-operative–especially post partial gastrectomy (level up to 2X normal in 1/3 of patients)
Acute pancreatitis may be induced by: indomethacin
  furosemide
  chlorthalidone
  ethacrynic acid
  corticosteroids
  histamine
  salicylates
  tetracyclines
Macroamylasemia
Acute alcohol ingestion or poisoning
Salivary gland disease such as supporative inflammation or duct obstruction due to calculus
May also be increased in acute cholecystitis
Intestinal obstruction with strangulation
  mesenteric thrombosis
  ruptured aortic aneurism
  ruptured tubal pregnancy
  viral hepatitis
  carcinoma of lung

*continued*

**Table 2.** (continued)

| Test | Indicates (or physiologic role) | Normal range | Increased in | Decreased in | Comments |
|---|---|---|---|---|---|
| Amylase urinary | If kidney intact—amylase is rapidly excreted | 40-250 Somogyi units/hr. | Acute pancreatitis—[urinary amylase] remains elevated for up to one week after serum amylase levels have returned to normal levels following an acute attack of pancreatitis | Renal insufficiency—an elevated or normal serum amylase associated with a low urine amylase excretion rate | A timed urine specimen (2,6 or 24 hr) should be collected and the rate of excretion determined |
| Bicarbonate serum or plasma | Acid-base balance—buffer capacity of body | 22-28 mEq/liter | Metabolic alkalosis [where arterial blood pH is increased]<br>A. ingestion of external sodium bicarbonate<br>B. protracted vomiting<br>C. accompanying potassium deficit | Metabolic acidosis [arterial blood pH decreased]<br>A. diabetic ketosis<br>B. persistent diarrhea<br>C. starvation<br>D. salicylate intoxication<br>E. renal insufficiency | Measured as $CO_2$ content |
| | | | Respiratory acidosis [arterial blood pH decreased]<br>A. $CO_2$ retention (elevated $P_{CO_2}$) secondary to emphysema, aveolar membrane disease, heart failure with pulmonary congestion or pulmonary edema<br>Ventilatory failure from<br>oversedation<br>narcotics<br>inadequate respiratory function | Respiratory alkalosis [arterial blood pH increased]<br>A. hyperventilation ($P_{CO_2}$ decreased) | |

| | | | | | |
|---|---|---|---|---|---|
| Bilirubin serum<br><br>Total<br>Direct<br>(conjugated)<br>Indirect<br>(unconjugated) | Increases indicate liver insufficiency, biliary obstruction, increased rate of hemolysis or hepatic enzyme deficiency | <br><br>0.2-1.2 mg/100ml<br>0.1-0.4 mg/100ml<br><br>0.2-0.7 mg/100ml | *Direct and indirect elevations*<br>A. acute-chronic hepatitis<br>B. biliary tract obstruction<br>C. toxic reactions-drugs. chemicals, etc.<br>D. Dubin-Johnson and Rotor's syndromes<br><br>*Indirect elevation* (unconjugated)<br>A. hemolytic disorders<br>B. Gilbert's disease<br>C. Crigler-Najjar syndrome<br><br>*Direct and total elevation*<br>A. 12-48 hr. fasts<br>B. prolonged caloric restriction | | Should be drawn fasting. Bilirubin is produced by the destruction of hemoglobin. Unconjugated bilirubin is conjugated in the liver and excreted in the bile<br><br>May be elevated by acetaminophen, chlordiazepoxide and other drugs. A 48 hour fast produces a mean increase of 240% in normal patients and 194% in those with hepatic dysfunction |
| Calcium serum | Affected by endocrine, renal, metabolic, gastrointestinal and nutritional factors | 8.5-10.5 mg/100ml<br>or<br>4.2-5.2 mEq/l | Hyperparathyroidism [hyperplasia or adenoma]<br>endocrinologically active tumors–ex: oat cell CA of lung<br>Vitamin D excess<br>Milk-alkali (Burnett's) syndrome<br>Osteolytic disease<br>1. multiple myeloma (some patients)<br>2. boney metastases of CA<br>3. Paget's disease<br>4. Boeck's sarcoid | Hypoparathyroidism<br>Vitamin D deficiency<br>1. rickets<br>2. osteomalacia<br>Renal insufficiency<br>Hypoproteinemia<br>Malabsorption syndrome<br>Starvation<br>Pregnancy–late<br>Pancreatic insufficiency<br>Ileitis<br>Pancreatitis with fat necrosis | Should be drawn fasting. Bound to serum albumin thus [serum albumin] is necessary to properly interpret results |

*continued*

**Table 2.** (continued)

| Test | Indicates (or physiologic role) | Normal range | Increased in | Decreased in | Comments |
|---|---|---|---|---|---|
| Calcium serum (continued) | | | 5. immobilization or long term bed rest-osteoporosis<br>Hyperthyroidism (occasional)<br>Hypothyroidism (occasional)<br>2° Ingestion thiazide diuretics<br>Lymphoma, leukemias<br>Metastatic carcinoma to bone (10% of patients)<br>Berylliosis<br>Cushing's syndrome (some patients)<br>Addison's disease (some patients) | Pseudohypoparathyroidism<br>Obstructive jaundice<br>Hypoalbuminemia secondary to:<br>cachexia<br>nephrotic syndrome<br>sprue<br>celiac disease<br>cystic fibrosis of pancreas | |
| Calcium urinary | | 50-150 mg/24 hr | Hyperparathyroidism (usually exceeds 200 mg/24 hrs.)<br>Usually elevated when serum calcium is high | | Should be on diet free of cheese or milk for 3 days prior to testing or on neutral ash diet for 3 days |
| Ceruloplasmin (CP) and serum copper (CU) | 5% of copper bound to albumin (loosely) remaining 95% to ceruloplasmin | 25-43 mg/100ml<br>70-200 μg/100ml | Pregnancy–CP<br>Hyperthroidism–CP & CU<br>Infection–CP & CU<br>Aplastic anemia–CP & CU<br>Acute leukemia–CU<br>Malignant lymphoma–CU<br>Hodgkin's disease–CP & CU<br>Cirrhosis of liver–CP | Wilson's disease [serum copper] and ceruloplasmin are low, urine copper is high<br>Nephrosis–CP & CU<br>Sprue–CP<br>Kwashiorkor–CP & CU<br>Normal infants | Ceruloplasmin is an $alpha_2$ globulin which is an oxidase enzyme. Ceruloplasmin may be normal in 2-5% of patients with Wilson's disease.<br>Ceruloplasmin should |

| | | | | | |
|---|---|---|---|---|---|
| | | | Oral contraceptives–CP<br>Rheumatoid arthritis–CP & CU<br>Cancer–CP<br>Estrogens–CP<br>Hemochromatosis–CU<br>SLE–CU<br>Acute rheumatic fever–CU<br>Glomerulonephritis–CU<br>Hypothyroidism–CU<br>Pernicious anemia–CU<br>megaloblastic anemia of pregnancy–CU<br>Iron deficiency anemia–CU | Acute leukemia in remission–CU<br>Iron deficiency anemia of childhood –CU | be measured in any patient under age 30 with hepatitis, hemolysis or neurological symptoms to insure early diagnosis of Wilson's disease |
| Chloride serum | Principal inorganic anion of extracellular fluid.<br>Maintains acid-base balance.<br>If chloride is lost → alkalosis.<br>Chloride retained → acidosis. Controls (with sodium) the osmolarity of body fluids | 96-106 mEq/l | Renal insufficiency<br>Nephrosis<br>Renal tubular acidosis<br>Dehydration<br>Overtreatment with saline solution | Gastrointestinal disease (diarrhea, vomiting, gastric suction)<br>Renal insufficiency with salt deprivation.<br>Overtreatment with diuretics<br>Emphysema (chronic respiratory acidosis)<br>Diabetic acidosis<br>Excessive sweating<br>Adrenal insufficiency<br>Hyperadrenocorticism (with chronic $K^+$ loss)<br>Metabolic alkalosis | |

*continued*

**Table 2.** (continued)

| Test | Indicates (or physiologic role) | Normal range | Increased in | Decreased in | Comments |
|---|---|---|---|---|---|
| Cholesterol | Levels affected by heredity, endocrine state, nutrition and liver and kidney function | 150-280 mg/100ml | Idiopathyic hypercholesterolemia<br>Chronic pancreatitis<br>Xanthomatosis<br>Hypothyroidism<br>Diabetes mellitus<br>Nephrotic syndrome<br>Chronic hepatitis<br>Biliary cirrhosis or obstruction<br>Obstructive jaundice<br>Hypoproteinemia such as occurs with<br>1. idiopathic hypoproteinemia<br>2. nephrosis<br>3. chronic hepatitis<br>Lipidemia<br>1. idiopathic<br>2. familial<br>Pregnancy<br>*Drugs*<br>bromides<br>anabolic steroids<br>oral contraceptives<br>other drugs | Hypo-beta and a-beta-lipoproteinemia<br>Acute hepatitis with severe liver cell damage<br>Gaucher's disease<br>Hyperthyroidism (occasionally)<br>Acute infections<br>Anemia (chronic)<br>Malnutrition<br>Tangier disease<br>*Drugs*<br>Haloperidol<br>nicotinic acid<br>salicylates<br>thyroid hormone<br>estrogens<br>cortisol and ACTH therapy<br>other drugs | Fasting sample preferred<br>In chronic hepatitis and chronic biliary obstruction the ratio of cholesterol ester to total cholesterol is less than 65% |
| Creatine phosphokinase (CPK) serum | Derived from skeletal and heart muscle and brain. | Varies with assay<br>10-50 IU/liter | Myocardial infarction<br>Muscle trauma–may last 14 days | | Levels raise within 3-5 hrs following myocardial infarction |

| | | | | |
|---|---|---|---|---|
| | elevated with muscle damage or destruction of nervous tissue–50% of patients with extensive brain infarction show elevations with maximum levels at 3 days returning to normal by 14 days. Levels exceeding 300 IU associated with high mortality | Intramuscular injection–<br>returns to normal in 48 hrs<br>Strenuous exercise<br>Muscular dystrophies<br>Polymyositis<br>Parturition and last few weeks of pregnancy<br>Hypothyroidism<br>Cerebral infarction with necrosis<br>Von Gierke's disease<br>Nephrosis 2° to<br>renal vein thrombosis<br>post operative state<br>myoglobinuria<br>amyloidosis<br>systemic lupus erythematosus<br>periarteritis<br>diabetic glomerulosclerosis<br>Pregnancy<br>Status epilepticus | | and remain elevated for only 2-3 days–no change with pulmonary infarction or liver disease (parenchymal)<br><br>3 isoenzymes localize damaged area:<br>*Fraction* *Isoenzyme* *Tissue*<br>3 MM skeletal muscle<br>2 MB myocardium<br>1 BB brain |
| Creatine<br>24 hr urinary | *24 hr*<br>*creatine* *creatinine*<br>adult male 0-50 mg 25 mg/kg<br>adult female 0-100 mg 21 mg/kg<br><br>found in muscle, brain, blood-increased in catabolic states and muscular dystrophies where rate | High dietary intake of meat<br>Muscle destruction<br>*Muscular dystrophies*<br>1. progressive muscular dystrophy<br>2. myotonia atrophica<br>3. myasthenia gravis<br>*Muscle wasting diseases*<br>1. polio<br>2. amyotrophic lateral sclerosis<br>3. myositis | Hypothyroidism<br>Amyotonia congenita<br>Renal insufficiency | Refrigerate or preserve with toluene or chloroform |

*continued*

**Table 2.** (continued)

| Test | Indicates (or physiologic role) | Normal range | Increased in | Decreased in | Comments |
|---|---|---|---|---|---|
| Creatine 24 hr urinary (continued) | of excretion is increased | | Starvation<br>Hyperthyroidism–normal level almost excludes diagnosis<br>Febrile diseases<br>Active rheumatoid arthritis<br>Testosterone therapy | | |
| Creatinine serum | Derived from creatine, excreted through glomeruli–retention indicates glomerular insufficiency. Creatinine clearance is a measure of glomerular filtration rate | 0.7-1.5 mg/100 ml | Acromegaly and gigantism<br>Diet heavy with roast meat<br>Prerenal azotemia<br>Acute and chronic renal insufficiency<br>Post renal azotemia<br>Urinary tract obstruction<br>Drug induced glomerular inflammation or damage<br>Excess tissue breakdown–fever, burns, cachexia, steroids<br>Congestive heart failure<br>Blood in small bowel<br>Dehydration<br>Shock | Not clinically significant | A more sensitive and specific indicator of renal disease than BUN. Lab results increased by ascorbic acid, barbiturates, sulfobromophthalein methyldopa |
| Glucose serum | | Fasting<br>65-110 mg/100ml | Diabetes mellitus<br>Hemochromatosis<br>Hypothyroidism<br>Adrenocortical hyperactivity (Cushing's syndrome) | Hypothalamic lesions<br>Islet cell tumors<br>Pancreatitis<br>Glucagon deficiency<br>Adrenal carcinoma | Levels vary based on Hematocrit since whole blood [glucose] and plasma [glucose] are different |

| | | | | | |
|---|---|---|---|---|---|
| | | 65-110 mg/100ml | Hyperpituitarism<br>Acromegaly and gigantism<br>Occasionally–liver disease<br>Pheochromocytoma<br>Stress (emotion, burns, shock, anesthesia)<br>Acute and chronic pancreatitis<br>Wernicke's encephalopathy (vit. B deficiency)<br>Some CNS lesions (subarachnoid hemorrhage, convulsive states)<br>*Drugs*<br>corticosteroids<br>chlorthalidone<br>thiazides<br>furosemide<br>ethacrynic acid<br>triamterene<br>indomethacin<br>oral contraceptives<br>isoniazid<br>nicotinic acid<br>phenothiazines<br>paraldehyde<br>ACTH<br>adrenalin | Carcinoma of stomach<br>Fibrosarcoma<br>Hepatic disease-poisoning, hepatitis, cirrhosis, tumor<br>Hypothyroidism<br>Post gastrectomy<br>Hyperinsulinism<br>Malnutrition<br>Adrenal insufficiency (Addison's disease)<br>Early diabetes mellitus<br>Hypopituitarism<br>Hepatic insufficiency (occasionally)<br>Functional hypoglycemia<br>*Drugs*<br>acetaminophen<br>phenacetin<br>pargyline<br>propranolol<br>cyproheptadine | |
| γ-Glutamyl Transpeptidase | Liver disease–a very sensitive indicator. Often | males < 28 mU/ml at 25°C<br>females < 18 mU/ml<br>adolescents < 45 mU/ml | | | An important test in patients with alcoholism and on chronic |

*continued*

**Table 2.** (continued)

| Test | Indicates (or physiologic role) | Normal range | Increased in | Decreased in | Comments |
|---|---|---|---|---|---|
| γ-Glutamyl Transpeptidase (continued) | elevated when alkaline phosphatase and transaminases are normal. Most specific test to indicate liver impairment due to alcoholism since it is induced by alcohol. Present in liver, kidney and pancreas | | Liver disease<br>acute infectious hepatitis<br>toxic hepatitis<br>chronic hepatitis<br>subacute hepatitis<br>cirrhosis<br>intra and extrahepatic obstruction<br>fatty liver<br>primary and metastatic neoplasms<br>alcoholic liver damage<br><br>Barbiturate use<br>Dilantin therapy (chronic)<br>congestive heart failure (occasionally)<br>Post myocardial infarction (50% of patients) begins on 4-5th day, maximum at 8-12th day<br>Pancreatitis–always elevated<br>Pancreatic carcinoma<br>Lipoid nephrosis (some cases)<br>Renal carcinoma (some cases) | | drug therapy. The most sensitive indicator of alcoholism. A very sensitive indicator of liver disease. In acute hepatitis, elevation less marked than other enzymes but last test to return to normal, thus useful as indicator of final recovery. Chronic hepatitis–increased more than in acute hepatitis, higher than SGOT or SGPT in dormant stage. May be only enzyme elevated. Cirrhosis–low levels–if increased by 10-20X suggests superimposed primary carcinoma of liver. Obstructive jaundice –increases are faster and greater than alkaline phosphatase or LAP |

| | | | | | |
|---|---|---|---|---|---|
| Iron serum | Affected by gut absorption and storage in intestine, spleen and marrow<br><br>Breakdown or loss of hemoglobin. Synthesis of new hemoglobin | 60-175 μg/100ml | Hemochromatosis<br>Hemosiderosis<br>Hemolytic disease<br>Pernicious anemia<br>Hypoplastic anemia<br>Viral hepatitis | Iron deficiency<br>Infections<br>Nephrosis<br>Chronic renal insufficiency<br>During periods of active hematopoiesis | |
| Iron binding capacity—serum | Iron transported on globulin-transferrin at rate of 30-40% of capacity to combine with iron. As [iron] goes down, binding capacity goes up | 250-410 μg/100 ml<br><br>Percent saturation 20-55% | Low serum iron<br>Acute or chronic blood loss<br>Pregnancy<br>Acute hepatitis<br>Oral contraceptives | High serum iron<br>Hemochromatosis<br>Hemosiderosis<br>Hemolytic disease<br>Pernicious anemia<br>Acute and chronic s infections<br>Cirrhosis<br>Uremia<br>Malignancy | |
| Lactate dehydrogenase | Distributed throughout body cells and fluids. Elevated by tissue necrosis, particularly acute damage to myocardium, kidneys, lungs, liver, RBC's, skin, skeletal muscle<br><br>Isoenzymes-1,2,3,4,5 | 200-450 Wroblewski °units | Acute myocardial infarction (isoenzymes 1+2↑)<br>Hemolytic anemias<br>Folate deficiency<br>Sickle cell crisis (isoenzyme 1+2↑)<br>Polycythemia vera<br>Pulmonary infarction and embolism<br>Neoplastic disease (50% of patients with carcinoma) | Clofibrate<br>X-ray irradiation | Levels in RBC are 100x those of serum. Hemolysis will produce false elevation. Following myocardial infarction, increases slowly over 3-4 days then declines during next 5-7 days. Levels above 2000 suggest a |

*continued*

**Table 2.** (continued)

| Test | Indicates (or physiologic role) | Normal range | Increased In | Decreased in | Comments |
|---|---|---|---|---|---|
| Lactate dehydrogenase serum (continued) | are found in various concentrations in different organs–help localize site of tissue damage | | Acute phase–infectious hepatitis (isoenzyme 5↑)<br>Renal parenchymal damage (renal cortex–occasional)<br>Dermatomyositis (isoenzyme 5↑)<br>Muscular dystrophies<br>Lymphomas and lymphocytic leukemia (60% of patients–isoenzymes 3+4↑)<br>Disseminated lupus erythematosus (isoenzyme 3+5↑)<br>CA of prostate (isoenzyme 5↑) | | poorer prognosis. Usually not increased in chronic liver disease<br><br>*Alpha enzymes*<br>LDH 1+2 elevated in myocardial infarction, infarction of renal cortex, and hemolytic anemias.<br>See $LDH_1/LDH_2 > 1$ with acute renal infarction. Also elevated in hemolytic anemia, heart valve hemolysis and acute M.I.<br><br>*Gamma enzymes*<br>LDH 4+5 elevated in acute hepatitis, muscular injury, dermatomyositis, muscular |

| | | | | | |
|---|---|---|---|---|---|
| | | | | | dystrophies. With congestive heart failure isoenzymes are normal. LDH 5 increased with chloropromazine hepatitis, carbon tetrachloride poisoning, exacerbation of cirrhosis and biliary obstruction, even when total LDH is normal |
| Lipase serum | Usually low concentration in blood–found in pancreas | 0.2-1.5 units | Acute or exacerbated pancreatitis.<br>Pancreatic obstruction caused by:<br>1. stone<br>2. neoplasm<br>3. inflammation<br>4. drug induced spasm (opiates or codeine)<br>Perforated or penetrating peptic ulcer | | With pancreatitis, lipase remains elevated for up to 14 days after amylase has returned to normal. Usually normal in mumps |
| Magnesium serum | Intracellular electrolyte like potassium, thus serum level remains in normal range till deficiency severe. May have normal serum valve in the face of total body | 1.5-2.5 mEq/l | Renal insufficiency<br>Overtreatment with magnesium salts<br>Diabetic coma<br>Hypothyroidism<br>Addison's disease<br>The controlled diabetes mellitus of older patients<br>Magnesium containing antacids | Idiopathic<br>Lytic tumors of bone<br>Chronic diarrhea<br>Acute loss enteric fluids<br>Excessive lactation<br>Starvation<br>Acute pancreatitis<br>Acute and chronic alcoholism | Low levels associated with mental changes, tetany, weakness, disorientation, somnolence. Magnesium deficiency may cause apparently unexplained hypocalcemia and hypokalemia |

*continued*

**Table 2.** (continued)

| Test | Indicates (or physiologic role) | Normal range | Increased in | Decreased in | Comments |
|---|---|---|---|---|---|
| Magnesium serum (continued) | deficiency, in which case a magnesium loading test is neces- to prove deficit | | | Alcoholic cirrhosis<br>Chronic hepatitis<br>Hepatic insufficiency<br>Diuretic drug treatment with ethacrynic acid or furosemide<br>Excessive renal loss—glomerulonephritis pyelonephritis renal<br>Renal tubular acidosis<br>Hyperthyroidism<br>Hyper and hypoparathy-roidism<br>Aldosteronism<br>When calcium and vit. D being given in high dose<br>G.I. disease with mal-absorption<br>nontropical sprue<br>small bowel resection<br>biliary and intestinal fistulas<br>abdominal irradiation<br>gastric or intestinal aspiration<br>celiac disease | |

| | | | | | |
|---|---|---|---|---|---|
| Phosphatase acid serum | Present in erythrocytes and prostate gland | 0.5-2.0 Bodansky<br>1-5 King-Armstrong units | CA of prostate if cancer has extended beyond capsule or metastasized<br>Infarction of prostate<br>Acute myelocytic leukemia<br>Gaucher's disease<br>Excessive destruction of platelets (I.T.P.)<br>Thromboembolism<br>Hemolytic crises or sickle cell disease<br>Partial translocation trisomy 21<br>Disease of bone<br>advanced Paget's disease<br>metastatic carcinoma of bone<br>multiple myeloma (some patients)<br>hyperparathyroidism<br>Hepatitis<br>Obstructive jaundice<br>Laennec's cirrhosis<br>Acute renal impairment<br>Niemann-Pick disease | | |
| Phosphatase alkaline serum | Present in growing bone, in bile, in placenta.<br>Isoenzymes–liver heat resistant.<br>Bone/placenta-heat sensitive | 2-5 Bodansky units<br>5-13 King-Armstrong units | Children (bone growth)<br>osteoblastic bone disease<br>1. hyperparathyroidism<br>2. rickets<br>3. osteomalacia<br>4. neoplastic bone disease<br>A. osteosarcoma<br>B. metastatic disease | Hypothyroidism<br>Excess vit. D ingestion<br>Milk-alkali syndrome<br>Scurvy<br>Hypophosphatasia<br>Pernicious anemia (1/3 of patients)<br>Celiac disease | One of the most important screening enzymes<br><br>Progressive elevation may be first indication that drug therpy with a particular |

*continued*

**Table 2.** (continued)

| Test | Indicates (or physiologic role) | Normal range | Increased in | Decreased in | Comments |
|---|---|---|---|---|---|
| Phosphatase alkaline | | | 5. myositis ossificans<br>6. Paget's disease<br>7. Boeck's sarcoid<br>8. healing fractures<br>9. osteogenesis imperfecta<br>Hepatic duct or cholangiolar obstruction 2° to stone, stricture, inflammation or neoplasm<br>Children<br>Drug related hepatic disease<br>1. phenothiazines<br>2. methyltestosterone<br>Pregnancy<br>Masked hyperthyroidism<br>Hyperphosphatasia<br>Liver disease–any obstruction of biliary system such as by: T.B., metastatic or primary tumor, cyst, parasite, amyloid, sarcoid, leukemia<br>Primary hypophosphatemia<br>I.V. albumin injection-up to 10x normal levels for days<br>Myocardial or pulmonary infarction (some patients) | Malnutrition | Agent should be stopped |

| | | | | | |
|---|---|---|---|---|---|
| Phosphorus Inorganic–serum | [Phosphorus] controlled by parathyroid gland activity, intestinal absorption, renal function, bone metabolism and nutritional state | Children<br>4-7 mg/100ml<br>adults<br>3-4.5 mg/100ml | Renal insufficiency<br>Hypoparathyroidism<br>Hypervitaminosis D<br>Secondary hyperparathyroidism (renal rickets)<br>Bone disease<br>healing fractures<br>multiple myeloma<br>Paget's disease<br>Osteolytic metastatic tumor in bone<br>Addison's disease<br>Acromegaly<br>Myelogenous leukemia<br>Acute yellow atrophy of liver<br>Upper intestinal obstruction<br>Sarcoidosis<br>Milk-alkali syndrome | Diabetes mellitus*<br>Hyperalimentation*<br>Hyperparathyroidism<br>Nutritional recovery syndrome*<br>Rickets<br>Osteomalacia<br>Prolonged hypothermia<br>Malabsorption syndrome<br>Hypomagnesemia<br>Antacid ingestion (bind phosphate in gut)<br>Starvation<br>Cachexia<br>Chronic alcoholism*<br>I.V. Carbohydrate administration<br>Renal tubular defects<br>Hypokalemia<br>Anabolic steroids<br>Androgens<br>Epinephrine, glucagon,<br>Insulin<br>Thiazide diuretics<br>Acid-base disturbances<br>Diabetic ketoacidosis<br>Genetic hypophosphatemia<br>Pregnancy (occasionally)<br>Hypothyroidism<br>Gout<br>Salicylate poisoning | Asterisks (*) show conditions associated with severe hypophosphatemia. Should be drawn with patient fasting |

*continued*

**Table 2.** (continued)

| Test | Indicates (or physiologic role) | Normal range | Increased in | Decreased in | Comments |
|---|---|---|---|---|---|
| Potassium serum | Intracellular ion regulates neuromuscular and muscular irritability.<br>↑ or ↓ [$K^+$] impair muscle contractility | 3.5-5.0 mEq/l | Renal failure<br>Renal insufficiency<br>Adrenal insufficiency<br>Pseudohypoaldosteronism<br>*Drugs*<br>triamterene<br>phenformin<br>spironolactone<br>Post transfusion hemolytic anemias<br>Iatrogenic–excessive amount in I.V.s<br>excess oral intake of potassium supplements<br>From muscle following trauma<br>status epilepticus<br>periodic paralysis<br>Dehydration<br>Metabolic acidosis | Carcinoma of colon<br>Chronic laxative abuse<br>Starvation<br>Inadequate absorption<br>Vomiting, diarrhea or malabsorption syndromes<br>Gastric suction<br>hyperadrenocorticism<br>2° steroid treatment<br>Metabolic alkalosis<br>Villous adenoma of GI tract<br>Overtreatment with diuretics expecially diazides and mercurials<br>De Toni-Fanconi syndrome<br>Renal tubular acidosis<br>Primary aldosteronism<br>Pseudoaldosteronism<br>Salt loosing nephropathy<br>Cushing's syndrome<br>Acute tubular necrosis (diuretic phase)<br>Chronic pyelonephritis<br>Diuresis following urinary obstruction | An important screening test |

| | | | | | |
|---|---|---|---|---|---|
| | | | | Zollinger-Ellison syndrome<br>*Drugs*<br>tetracycline (degraded)<br>phenothiazines<br>sodium polystyrene sulfonate resin<br>testosterone | |
| Protein serum | Determine plasma colloidal osmotic pressure [ ] determined by livers ability to produce, nutritional state, renal function, certain diseases–i.e., multiple myeloma and metabolic errors | Total protein<br>6-8 g/100 ml<br>albumin<br>3.5-5.5 g/100 ml<br>globulin<br>2-3 g/100 ml<br>fibrinogen<br>0.2-0.6 g/100 ml | *Albumin*<br>dehydration<br>shock<br>hemoconcentration<br>I.V. albumin solution<br>*Globulin*<br>hepatic disease<br>infectious hepatitis<br>cirrhosis<br>biliary cirrhosis<br>hemochromatosis<br>lupus-disseminated<br>acute and chronic infections<br>particularly high with:<br>lymphogranuloma<br>venereum, typhus,<br>leishmaniasis,<br>schistosomiasis and malaria.<br>multiple meyloma<br>Boeck's sarcoid<br>*Fibrinogen*<br>glomerulonephritis<br>nephrosis (occasionally) | *Albumin*<br>malnutrition<br>malabsorption syndrome<br>nephrosis<br>acute and chronic hepatic insufficiency<br>neoplastic disease<br>leukemia<br>*Globulin*<br>malnutrition<br>congenital agammaglobulinemia and acquired hypogammaglobulinemia<br>AID syndrome<br>lymphocytic leukemia<br>*Fibrinogen*<br>disseminated intravascular coagulation<br>1. pregnancy<br>2. meningococcal meningitis | An important screening test |

*continued*

**Table 2.** (continued)

| Test | Indicates (or physiologic role) | Normal range | Increased in | Decreased in | Comments |
|---|---|---|---|---|---|
| Protein serum (continued) | | | infectious disease | 3. metastatic carcinoma or prostate<br>4. metastatic CA<br>5. leukemia<br>acute and chronic hepatic insufficiency<br>congenital fibrinogenopenia | |
| Sodium serum | With its anions $Na^+$ provides the bulk of osmotically active solute in plasma thereby significantly controlling the distribution of body water. Any Na shift to the intracellular compartment or loss of Na from the body decreases the extracellular fluid volume and may thereby affect the circulation, nervous and renal function | 136-145 mEq/l | Essential hypernatremia 2° to hypothalamic lesions<br>Dehydration<br>CNS trauma or disease<br>Hyperaldosteronism<br>Corticosteroid excess<br>Excess water loss–<br>vomiting<br>hyperpnea<br>excessive sweating<br>Excess diuresis<br>diabetes insipidus<br>nephrogenic diabetes insipidus<br>diabetes mellitus<br>diuretics<br>acute tubular necrosis (diuretic phase) | Dilutional-congestive heart failure, nephrosis, cirrhosis with ascites.<br>Addison's disease<br>Renal infufficiency<br>Salt loosing nephropathy<br>Inadequate sodium intake<br>Renal tubular acidosis<br>Physiologic response to trauma or burns<br>GI loss–vomiting, diarrhea, intestinal obstruction or fistula<br>Sweating (profuse) in some patients with cardiac or renal | An important test in psychiatric patients |

| | | | | | |
|---|---|---|---|---|---|
| | | | hypercalcemic nephropathy<br>hypokalemic nephropathy<br>Iatrogenic–I.V.s | disease and edema–serum Na low even though total body Na is increased<br>Excess ADH secretion<br>Hyperglycemia–produces a dilutional hyponatremia | |
| Thyroxine ($T_4$) total serum | Level does not necessarily reflect physiologic effect of thyroxine since level is influenced by carrier protein (thyroxine binding globulin and prealbumin which are effected by pregnancy, drugs, and disease. Carrier protein determined by $T_3$ resin uptake test. The [ ] of free $T_4$ and $T_3$ determines hormonal activity | RIA 5-14 $\mu$g/100 ml<br>CPB 4-11 $\mu$g/100 ml | Hyperthyroidism<br>Thyroiditis (occasionally)<br>Acromegaly<br>Elevation of thyroxine-binding proteins<br>External $T_4$ ingestion | Hypothyroidism (primary or secondary)<br>Decreased thyroxine-binding proteins<br>External $T_3$–inhibits thyrotropin secretion<br>Aminosalicyclic acid, corticosteroids, lithium, thiouracils, methimazole and sulfonamides reduce $T_4$ synthesis<br>Aspirin, chlorpropamide, phenytoin (other anticonvulsants) halofenate and tolbutamide displace $T_4$ from carrier protein binding sites<br>Cholestyramine-interferes with $T_4$s enterohepatic circulation | See Gold (Chapter 2, this text) |

*continued*

**Table 2.** (continued)

| Test | Indicates (or physiological role) | Normal range | Increased in | Decreased in | Comments |
|---|---|---|---|---|---|
| Thyroxine free serum | Determines metabolic activity of $T_4$ which is converted to $T_3$ in peripheral tissue. $T_3$ also directly secreted. Both $T_4$ and $T_3$ are active hormones | 0.8-2.4 ng/100 ml | Hyperthyroidism<br>Active thyroiditis (occasionally)<br>Excess thyroid hormone ingestion | Hypothyroidism<br>External $T_3$<br>Thiouracils<br>Methimazole | See Gold (Chapter 2, this text) |
| Thyroxine binding globulin | Principal carrier for $T_3$ and $T_4$ in plasma. Inherited abnormalities are X linked | RIA 2-4.8 mg/100 ml | Pregnancy<br>Infectious hepatitis<br>Hereditary increases<br>Estrogens<br>Progestins<br>Oral contraceptives<br>Chlormadinone<br>Perphenazine<br>Clofibrate | Major debilitating diseases<br>Hypoproteinemias (globulin)<br>Nephrotic syndrome<br>Cirrhosis<br>Acromegaly (active)<br>Estrogen deficiency states<br>Hereditary deficiency<br>Androgens<br>Anabolic steroids<br>Cortisol<br>Prednisone<br>Corticotropin<br>Oxymetholone | |

| | | | | |
|---|---|---|---|---|
| $T_3$ uptake Resin ($RT_3u$) or Thyroxine-binding globulin assessment (TBG assessment) | Binding saturation of thyroxine binding globulin. Resin takes up non-TBG-bound radioactive $T_3$, thus its activity varies inversely with the number of available TBG sites. The $T_3$ uptake moves in the direction of disease, that is, increased in hyper-thyroidism and decreased in hypo-thyroidism. TBG moves inversely to the direction of disease | 25-36% of uptake of $^{125}I$-$T_3$ by resin<br>0.85-1.15 | *$RT_3U$*<br>hyperthyroidism<br>acromegaly<br>nephrotic syndrome<br>severe hepatic cirrhosis<br>hereditary TBG deficiency<br><br>*TBG (more sites available)*<br>hypothyroidism<br>newborns<br>infectious hepatitis<br>hereditary increase TBG<br><br>*Drug Effects*<br>*$RT_3$ increased-TBG decreased*<br>excess $T_4$<br>androgens<br>anabolic steroids<br>corticosteroids<br>corticotropin<br>heparin<br>warfarin<br>oxymetholone<br>phenytoin<br>phenylbutazone<br>salicylates (high dose) | *TBG*<br>hyperthyroidism<br>acromegaly<br>nephrotic syndrome<br>cirrhosis (severe)<br>hereditary TBG deficiency<br>*$RT_3u$*<br>hypothyroidism<br>newborns<br>infectious hepatitis<br>hereditary increase TBG<br>*Drug Effects*<br>*$RT_3u$ decreased-TBG increased*<br>$T_3$ therapy<br>estrogens<br>progestins<br>oral contraceptives<br>thiouracils<br>perphenazine<br>chlormadinone |

Thyroxine index

estimation of free $T_4 = RT_3u \text{ (in \%)} \times \text{total } T_4 \text{ (in } \mu g/100ml)$

or

$$\frac{\text{Total } T_4\ \mu g/100ml}{\text{TBG assessment}}$$



*continued*

**Table 2.** (continued)

| Test | Indicates (or physiologic role) | normal range | Increased in | Decreased in | Comments |
|---|---|---|---|---|---|
| Transaminases<br>SGOT | Present in high concentrations in muscle, liver and brain. Increases indicate necrosis or disease in these tissues | 5-40 units | Myocardial infarction<br>acute infectious hepatitis<br>Toxic hepatitis<br>Cirrhosis<br>Liver neoplasm–primary and metastatic<br>Transudates associated with neoplastic involvement of serous cavities<br>SGOT also increased in muscular dystrophy<br>dermatomyositis<br>paroxysmal myoglobinuria<br>*Drugs*<br>anabolic steroids<br>androgens<br>clofibrate<br>erythromycin<br>other antibiotics<br>isoniazid<br>methotrexate<br>methyldopa<br>phenothiazines<br>oral contraceptives<br>salicylates<br>acetaminophen<br>phenacetin | Pyridoxine ($B_6$) deficiency<br>Long term isoniazid treatment<br>Pregnancy | Important baselines to obtain before drug treatment is begun |
| SGPT | | 5-35 units | | | |

| | | | | | |
|---|---|---|---|---|---|
| | | | indomethacin<br>acetohexamide<br>allopurinol<br>dicumarol<br>carbamazepine<br>chlordiazepoxide<br>desipramine<br>imipramine<br>codeine<br>morphine<br>meperidine<br>tolazamide<br>propranolol<br>guanethidine<br>pyridoxine | | |
| Triglycerides serum | Fat is hydrolyzed in small intestines, absorbed, resynthesized in mucosal cells → secreted as chylomicrons, transported-stored in adipose tissue→ released, resynthesized in liver | <165 mg/100 ml | *Primary hyperlipoproteinemia*<br>exogenous–type 1<br>hyperbetalipoprotemia–type 2<br>broad beta hyperlipoproteinemia–type 3<br>endogenous hyperlipidemia–Type 4<br>mixed hyperlipidemia–type 5<br>*secondary hyperlipoprotemia*<br>hypothyroidism<br>diabetes mellitus<br>nephrotic syndrome<br>chronic alcoholism with fatty liver | *Primary hypoliproproteinemia*<br>Tangier disease (α-lipoprotein deficiency<br>A-beta-lipoproteinemia<br><br>*secondary hypolipoproteinemia*<br>malnutrition<br>malabsorption<br>paranchymal liver disease (occasionally) | Fast for 12-16 hr before sample drawn |

*continued*

**Table 2.** (continued)

| Test | Indicates (or physiologic role) | Normal range | Increased in | Decreased in | Comments |
|---|---|---|---|---|---|
| Triglycerides serum (continued) | | | oral contraceptives<br>biliary obstruction<br>stress | | |
| Urea nitrogen blood | Urea is the end product of protein metabolism. It is excreted by the kidney with tubular reabsorption varying inversely with the rate of urine flow | 8-25 mg/100ml | Renal insufficiency<br>Nephritis–acute and chronic<br>Acute renal failure (tubular necrosis)<br>Urinary tract obstruction<br>Increased nitrogen metabolism with decreased renal blood flow ex–dehydration, gastrointestinal bleeding<br>Decreased renal blood flow–<br>acute myocardial infarction<br>shock<br>congestive heart failure<br>Addison's disease<br>renal artery stenosis<br>Antibiotics that impair kidney<br>Guanethidine<br>Methyldopa<br>Indomethacin<br>Isoniazid<br>Propranolol<br>Potent diuretics | Hepatic failure 2° drugs, poisoning, hepatitis<br>Nephrosis without renal insufficiency<br>Cachexia<br>Late pregnancy<br>Acromegaly<br>Low protein–high carbohydrate diet<br>Celiac disease<br>Nephrotic syndrome (some patients) | In chronic renal disease, BUN correlates better with uremic symptoms that does serum creatinine |

| | | | | | |
|---|---|---|---|---|---|
| Uric acid serum | End product of nucleoprotein metabolism-excreted by kidney | males 3-8 mg/100 ml<br>females 1.5-6 mg/100ml | Gout<br>25% of relatives of patients with gout<br>Toxemia of pregnancy<br>Lymphoma–especially post radiation<br>Leukemia<br>Multiple myeloma<br>Polycythemia vera<br>Treatment with anti-leukemic drugs<br>Drug treatment–many cancers<br>Resolving pneumonia<br>Renal insufficiency and failure<br>Psoriasis (1/3 of patients)<br>Glycogen storage disease (type I)<br>Hemolytic anemia, sickle cell anemia<br>Lesch-Nyhan syndrome<br>Toxemia of pregnancy<br>Down's syndrome<br>Disseminated neoplasma<br>*Drugs*<br>salicylates (low dose)<br>thiazides<br>ethacrynic acid<br>spironolactone<br>furosemide | Acute hepatitis (occasionally)<br>Treatment with<br>allopurinol<br>probenecid<br>*Drugs*<br>salicylates (high doses)<br>methyldopa<br>clofibrate<br>phenylbutazone<br>cinchophen<br>sulfinpyrazone<br>phenothiazines<br>ACTH<br>cortisone<br>coumarin<br>glyceryl guaiacolate<br>Wilson's disease<br>Fanconi's syndrome<br>Acromegaly (some patients)<br>Celiac disease<br>Pernicious anemia in relapse (some patients)<br>Xanthinuria<br>Neoplasma–<br>carcinomas<br>Hodkin's disease | An important screening test.<br>hyperuricemia–incidence higher in Filipinos and Blackfoot Indians than whites<br><br>Levels very labile. Increased by emotional stress and total fasting<br><br>Serum uric acid is increased in 80% of patients with elevated serum triglycerides |

*continued*

**Table 2.** (continued)

| Test | Indicates (or physiologic role) | Normal range | Increased in | Decreased in | Comments |
|---|---|---|---|---|---|
| Uric acid serum (continued) | | | triamterene<br>ascorbic acid<br>cancer chemotherapeutics<br>Patients with arteriosclerosis and hypertension<br>Diet-high protein or diet high in nucleoprotein (ie.., sweetbreads, liver)<br>Lead poisoning<br>Von Gierke's disease<br>Maple sugar urine disease<br>Polycystic kidneys<br>Calcinosis universalis and circumscripta<br>Hypoparathyroidism<br>Primary hyperparathyroidism<br>Alcoholism (some patients)<br>Hypothyroidism<br>Sarcoidosis<br>Chronic berylliosis | | |

[a]This table is modified, adapted and reproduced with permission from the following sources.

1. Krupp MA, Chatton MK: Current Medical Diagnosis & Treatment. Lange Medical Publications, Los Altos, California, copyright 1980.
2. Wallach J: Interpretation Of Diagnostic Tests. A Handbook Synopsis Of Laboratory Medicine. Third edition, Little, Brown and Company, Boston copyright 1978.

We thank both publishers for their kind permission permitting us to reproduce this material.

employed in admission evaluations and batteries. The reader should bear in mind that this is an abbreviated summary and is not intended to exhaust all diagnostic possibilities; rather, it is provided as a guide of the major physiologic states and conditions which have a high probability of altering a specific test or pattern of tests. It is hoped that it will be of use as a ready reference for the practicing clinician.

## CONCLUSION

The routine laboratory evaluation of acutely demented psychotic patients on admission to hospital is a necessary and indicated part of their treatment. Careful evaluation provides the physician with the information necessary to appropriately diagnose and treat his patient. It ensures the patient's safety, provides baselines necessary to evaluate the effects of pharmacological treatment, and provides data to diagnose unrecognized physical illness. A negative workup is a source of reassurance to both the patient and the physician, while positive findings direct subsequent diagnostic evaluation and consultation. This workup also indirectly ensures that the patient's civil rights will be appropriately protected and in a positive way protects the physician from charges of negligence or malfeasance.

Arguments that the routine screening of hospitalized patients is ineffective or inefficient, in our opinion, do not apply to the acutely psychotic patient as we hope we have demonstrated. Studies as to the specific yield of routine admission tests in various subpopulations of acutely ill psychiatric patients are desparately needed and have recently begun to appear in the literature. (see Gold's excellent chapter in this volume.) It is hoped that the use of admission laboratory evaluation for acutely psychotic and demented patients will become routine in our psychiatric hospitals and that through these procedures we will be able to eliminate a variety of unrecognized physical disorders while providing better care for patients suffering from functional disease. The data provided by these tests will also help us evaluate the long term effects of our medications and prevent or minimize the effect of subsequent or concurrent illnesses which may develop and afflict our patients.

## REFERENCES

1. Bernstein RA, Andrews EM: The hospitalized psychiatric patient and the primary care physician. Psychosomatics 22:11:959–970, 1981
2. Blustein JE: Further observations on brain tumors presenting as functional psychiatric disturbances. Psychiatric Journal of the University of Ottawa I:21–26, 1976
3. Boston Collaberative Drug Surveillance Program. Boston University Medical Center. Psychiatric side effects of non-psychiatric drugs. Seminars in Psychiatry 3:406–420, 1971

4. Browning CH, Miller SI, Tyson RL: The psychiatric emergency: A high risk medical patient. Compr Psychiatry 15:153–156, 1974
5. Comroe BI: Follow-up study of 100 patients diagnosed as neurotic. J Nerv Ment Dis 83:679–684, 1936
6. Davidson R: Paranoid symptoms in organic disease. Geront Clin 6:93–100, 1964
7. Davies DW: Physical illness in psychiatric outpatients. Br J Psychiatry 111: 27–33, 1965
8. DeVaul RA, Hall RCW: Hallucinations. In Hall RCW (ed): Psychiatric Presentations of Medical Illness: Somatopsychic Disorders. New York, Spectrum Publications, 1980
9. DiSclafani A, Hall RCW, Gardner ER: Drug induced psychosis: Emergency diagnosis and management. Psychosomatics 22:10:845–855, 1981
10. Dulfano NJ, Ishikawa S: Hypercapnia: Mental changes and extra pulmonary complications: An expanded concept of the CO2 intoxication syndrome. Ann Intern Med 63:829–841, 1965
11. Eastwood MR, Trevelyan MH: Relationship between physical and psychiatric disorder. Psychol Med 2:363–372, 1972
12. Freyhan FA, Giannelli S, Jr., O'Connell RA, et al: Psychiatric complications following open heart surgery. Compr Psychiatry 12:3:181–195, 1971
13. Ganz VH, Gurland BJ, Deming WE, et al: The study of the psychiatric symptoms of systemic lupus erythematosus: A biometric study. Psychosom Med 34:207–220, 1972
14. Gardner ER, Hall RCW: Psychiatric symptoms produced by over-the-counter drugs. Psychosomatics 23:2:186–190, 1982
15. Gifford S, Gunderson JG: Cushing's disease as a psychosomatic disorder: A selective review of the clinical and experimental literature and a report of ten cases. In Perspectives in Biology and Medicine, Winter:169–221, 1970
16. Gold MS, Pottash ALC, Extein I: "Symptomless" autoimmune thyroiditis in depression. Psychiatry Res 6:261-269, 1982
17. Gold MS, Pearsall HR: Covert hypothyroidism presenting as depression. Presented at the American Psychiatric Association, Annual Scientific Meeting, Toronto, Canada 1982
18. Gould J: Virus disease and psychiatric ill-health. Br J Clin Pract 11:12:918–922, 1957
19. Gurland BJ, Ganz VH, Fleiss JL, et al: The study of the psychiatric symptoms of systemic lupus erythematosus. Psychosom Med 34:3:199–206, 1972
20. Hall RCW (ed) Psychiatric Presentations of Medical Illness. New York, Spectrum Publications, 1980
21. Hall RCW, Popkin MK, DeVaul RA, et al: Physical illness presenting as psychiatric disease. Arch Gen Psychiatry 35:1315–1320, 1978
22. Hall RCW, Beresford TP, Popkin MK, et al: Medical basis of psychiatry: A reexamination of values and principles. Psychiatric Medicine 1(1):3–20, 1983
23. Hall RCW, Beresford TP, Gardner ER: Psychiatric symptoms of medical illness. Physician & Patient I:I:32–38, 1982
24. Hall RCW, Beresford TP, Gardner ER, et al: The medical care of psychiatric patients. Hosp Community Psychiatry 33:1:25–34, 1982
25. Hall RCW, Popkin MK, DeVaul R, et al: Psychiatric manifestations of Hashimoto's thyroiditis. Psychosomatics 23:4:337–342, 1982

26. Hall RCW: Psychiatric effects of thyroid hormone disturbance. Psychosomatics 24:1:7–18, 1983
27. Hall RCW, Gardner ER, Popkin MK, et al: Unrecognized physical illness prompting psychiatric admission: A prospective study. Am J Psychiatry 138: 5:629–635, 1981
28. Hall RCW, Stickney SK, Gardner ER, et al: Psychiatric reactions to long-term intravenous hyperalimentation. Psychosomatics 22:5:428–443, 1981
29. Hall RCW, Feinsilver DL, Holt RE: Anticholinergic psycosis: Differential diagnosis and management. Psychosomatics 22:7:581–587, 1981
30. Hall RCW, Zisook S: Paradoxical reactions to benzodiazepines. Br J Clin Pharm 11:99s–104s, 1981
31. Hall RCW, Zisook S: Psychological effects of therapeutic abortion. The Female Patient 9:168–178, 1984
32. Hall RCW, Levenson AJ: Depression in the elderly female. The Female Patient, 7:8:14–24, 1982
33. Hall RCW: Impact of medical illness on sexual-marital relationships. Med Aspects Hum Sex 14:2:25–30, 1980
34. Hall RCW, Stickney SK, Gardner ER: Psychiatric symptoms in patients with systemic lupus erythematosus. Psychosomatics 22:1:15–24, 1981
35. Hall RCW, Gruzenski WP, Popkin MK: Differential diagnosis of somatopsychic disorders. Psychosomatics 20:6:381–389, 1979
36. Hall RCW, Levenson AJ, LeCann AF. Evaluation and assessment of non-functional psychiatric illness in the elderly. In Levenson AJ, Hall RCW (eds): Neuropsychiatric Manifestations of Physical Disease in the Elderly. New York, Raven Press, 1981
37. Hall RCW, Popkin MK: Hallucinogens: A chemical trip to wonderland. In Mule SJ (ed): Behavior In Excess, New York, MacMillan Publishing Company, 1981
38. Hall RCW, Gardner ER, Stickney SK, et al: Physical illness manifesting as psychiatric disease–II: Analysis of a state hospital inpatient population. Arch Gen Psychiatry 37:989–995, 1980
39. Hall RCW, Popkin MK, Stickney SK, et al: Presentation of steroid psychosis. J Nerv Ment Dis 167:229–236, 1979
40. Hall RCW: Medically induced psychiatric disease–an overview. In Hall RCW (ed): Psychiatric Presentations of Medical Illness: Somatopsychic Disorders. New York, Spectrum Publications, 1980
41. Hall RCW: Anxiety. In Hall RCW (ed) Psychiatric Presentations of Medical Illness: Somatopsychic Disorders. New York, Spectrum Publications, 1980
42. Hall RCW: Depression. In Hall RCW (ed): Psychiatric Presentations of Medical Illness: Somatopsychic Disorders. New York, Spectrum Publications, 1980
43. Hall RCW, Stickney SK, Gardner ER: Behavioral toxicity of non-psychiatric drugs. In Hall RCW (ed): Psychiatric Presentations of Medical Illness: Somatopsychic Disorders. New York, Spectrum Publications, 1980
44. Hall RCW, Popkin MK, DeVaul R, et al: Physical illness presenting as psychiatric disease. Arch Gen Psychiatry 35:11:1315–1320, 1978
45. Hall RCW, Popkin MK: Psychological symptoms of physical origin. The Female Patient 2:10:43–47, 1977
46. Hall RCW, Stickney SK: Postpartum psychiatric disorders. The Female Patient 3:3:86–89, 1978

47. Hall RCW: Psychological factors affecting routine medical care. Md State Med J 21:62–63, 1972
48. Herridge CF: Physical disorders in psychiatric illness. Lancet 2:949–951, 1960
49. Hill JB: Salicylate intoxication. New Eng J Med 228:1110–1113, 1973
50. Hinkle LE, Wolff HG: Health in the social environment: Experimental investigation. In Leighton A, Klausen J, Wilson R (eds): Explorations in Social Psychiatry. New York, Basic Books, 1957
51. Hoffman RS: Diagnostic errors in the evaluation of behavioral disorders. JAMA 2:48:8:964–967, 1982
52. Holt RE, Rawat S, Beresford TP, et al: Computed tomography of the brain and the psychiatric consultation. Psychosomatics 23:10:1007–1019, 1982
53. Jefferson JW, Marshall JR (eds): Neuropsychiatric Features Of Medical Disorders. New York, Plenum Publishing Corp. 1981
54. Johnson DAW: The evaluation of routine physical examination in psychiatric cases. Practitioner 200:686–691, 1968
55. Kellner R: Psychiatric ill health following physical illness. Br J Psychiatry 112:71–73, 1966
56. Kirkpatrick B, Hall RCW: Seizure disorders. In Hall RCW (ed): Psychiatric Presentations of Medical Illness: Somatopsychic Disorders. New York, Spectrum Publications, 1980
57. Koranyi EK: Morbidity and rate of undiagnosed physical illnesses in a psychiatric clinic population. Arch Gen Psychiatry 36:414–419, 1979
58. Koranyi EK: Somatic illness in psychiatric patients. Psychosomatics 21:887–891, 1980
59. Kornfeld DS, Zimberg S, Malm JR: Psychiatric complications of open heart surgery. N Engl J Med 273:287–292, 1965
60. Leff MJ, Roatch JF, Bunney WE, Jr: Environmental factors preceeding the onset of severe depressions. Psychiatry 33:293–311, 1970
61. Levenson AJ, Hall RCW (eds): Neuropsychiatric Manifestations Of Physical Disease In The Elderly, New York, Raven Press, 1981
62. Lipowski ZJ: Psychiatry of somatic diseases: Epidemiology, pathogenesis, classification. Compr Psychiatry 16:2:105–124, 1975
63. Lucente FE, Fleck S: A study of hospitalization anxiety in 408 medical and surgical patients. Psychosom Med 34:4:304–312, 1972
64. Maguire GP, Granville-Grossman KL: Physical illness in psychiatric patients. Br J Psychiatry 115:1365–1369, 1968
65. Marshall H: Incidence of physical disorders among psychiatric inpatients. Br Med J 2:468–470, 1949
66. Meyer E, III, Derogatis LR, Miller MJ, et al: Medical clinic patients with emotional disorders. Psychosomatics 19:10:611–622, 1978
67. Perl M, Hall RCW, Dudrick SJ, et al: Psychological aspects of long-term home hyperalimentation. J Parenter Enter Nutr 4:6:554–560, 1980
68. Perl M, Hall RCW, Gardner ER: Behavioral toxicity of psychiatric drugs. In Hall RCW (ed): Psychiatric Presentations of Medical Illness: Somatopsychic Disorders. New York, Spectrum Publications, 1980
69. Peroutka SJ, Sohmer BH, Kumar AJ, et al: Hallucinations and delusions following a right temporoparietooccipital infarction. Johns Hopkins Med J 151:4:181–185, 1982
70. Peterson LG, Popkin MK, Hall RCW: Psychiatric aspects of cancer. Psychosomatics 22:9:774–793, 1981

71. Pless IB, Roghmann KJ: Chronic illness and its consequences: Observations based on three epidemiologic surveys. J Pediatr 79:351-359, 1971
72. Popkin MK, Moldow CF, Hall RCW, et al: Psychaitric aspects of allogeneic bone marrow transplantation for aplastic anemia. Dis Nerv Syst 38:11:925-927, 1977
73. Rabins PV: The prevalence of reversible dementia in a psychiatric hospital. Hosp Community Psychiatry 32:7:490–492, 1981
74. Raskin NH, Fishman RA: Neurological disorders in renal failure. N Engl J Med 294:143–148, 1976
75. Roessler R, Greenfield N: Incidence of somatic disease in psychiatric patients. Psychosom Med 23:413–419, 1961
76. Rogers MP, Dubbey D, Reich P: The influence of the psyche and the brain on immunity and disease susceptibility: A critical review. Psychosom Med 41:147–164, 1979
77. Schwab JJ, et al: Social Order In Mental Health. New York, Brunner/Mazel, 1979
78. Schwab JJ: Psychiatric illness in medical patients. Presented at the 28th annual meeting of the Academy of Psychosomatic Medicine, Dallas, Texas, November 2, 1981
79. Smith CK, Barish J, Correa J, et al: Psychiatric disturbance in endocrinologic disease. Psychosom Med 34:69–86, 1972
80. Struve FA: Utilization of clinical electroencephalographic assessment in the psychiatric hospital: Considerations concerning the issue of routine screening versus selective physician referrel. J Psychiatr Treat Eval 2:55–62, 1980
81. Tonks CM: Mental illness in hypothyroid patients. Br J Psychiatry 110:706–710, 1964
82. Vaillant G: Natural history of male psychological health, IV what kinds of men do not get psychosomatic illness. Psychosom Med 40:5:420–431, 1978
83. Vaillant FH: Adaptation To Life. Boston, Massachusetts, Little, Brown, 1978
84. Watson CG, Buranen C: The frequency and identification of false positive conversion reactions. J Nerv Ment Dis 167:243–247, 1979
85. Koranyi EK (ed): Physical Illness In The Psychiatric Patient. Springfield, Illinois, Charles C. Thomas, 1982
86. Koranyi EK: Physical health and illness in a psychiatric outpatient department population. Can Psychiatr Assoc J 17:109–116, 1972
87. Phillips RJ: Physical disorder in 164 consecutive admissions to a mental hospital. Br Med J 2:363–366, 1937
88. Slater ET, Glitherow E: Follow-up of patients diagnosed as suffering from hysteria. J Psychosom Res 9:9–13, 1965
89. Burke AW: Physical illness in psychiatric patients in Jamaica. Br J Psychiatry 121:321–322, 1972
90. Burke AW: Physical disorder among day hospital patients. Br J Psychiatry 133:22–27, 1978
91. Summers WK, Munoz RA, Read MR: The physical examination–Part II: Findings in 75 unselected psychiatric patients. J Clin Psychiatry 42:99–102, 1981
92. Malzberg B: Mortality Among Patients With Mental Disease. Utica, New York, New York State Hospital Press, 1934
93. Odegard O: The excess mortality of the insane. Acta Psychiatr Neurol Scand 27:353–367, 1952

94. LaBruzza AL: Physical illness presenting as psychiatric disorder: Guidelines for differential diagnosis. J Operational Psychiatry 12:24–31, 1981
95. Anderson WH: Differential diagnosis of acute psychosis. In Manschreck TC (ed): Psychiatric Medicine Update: MGH Review For Physician. Amsterdam, Elsevier North Holland, 1979
96. Karasu TB, Waltzman SA, Lindermayer J, et al: The medical care of patients with psychiatric illness. Hosp Community Psychiatry 31:464–471, 1980
97. Kampmeier RH: Diagnosis and treatment of physical disease in the mentally ill. Ann Intern Med 86:637–645, 1977
98. Bibring GL: Psychiatry and medical practice in a general hospital. N Engl J Med 254:366–372, 1956
99. Goodwin JM, Goodwin JS, Kellner R: Psychiatric symptoms in disliked medical patients. JAMA 241:1117–1120, 1979
100. Talbott JA, Linn L: Reactions of schizophrenics to life-threatening disease. Psychiatr Q 50:218–227, 1978
101. Marchand WE: Occurrence of painless myocardial infarction in psychotic patients. N Engl J Med 253:51–55, 1955
102. Schwab JJ, Bialow MR, Clemmons RS, et al: Hamilton rating scale for depression with medical in-patients. Br J Psychiatry 113:83–88, 1967
103. Stewart MA, Drake F, Winokur G: Depression among medically ill patients. Dis Nerv Syst 26:8:479–485, 1965
104. Helsborg HC: Psychiatric investigations of patients in a medical department. Acta Psychiatr Neurol Scand 33:303–335, 1958
105. Maguire GP, Julier DL, Hawton KE, et al: Psychiatric morbidity and referral on two general medical wards. Brit Med J 1:268–270, 1974
106. Payson HE, Davis JM: The psychosocial adjustment of medical inpatients after discharge: A follow-up study. Am J Psychiatry 123:1220–1225, 1967
107. Culpan R, Davis B: Psychiatric illness at a medical and surgical outpatient clinic. Compr Psychiatry 1:228–235, 1960
108. Hilkevitch A: Psychiatric disturbance in outpatients of a general medical outpatient clinic. Int J Neuropsych 1:371–375, 1965
109. Rosen BM, Locke BZ, Goldberg ID, et al: Identification of emotional disturbance in patients seen in general medical clinics. Hosp Community Psychiatry 23:364–370, 1972
110. Schwab JJ, Bialow M, Brown JM, et al: Diagnosing depression in medical inpatients. Ann Intern Med 67:695–707, 1967
111. Cay EL, Vetter N, Philip AE, et al: Psychological status during recovery from an acute heart attack. J Psychosom Res 16:425–435, 1972
112. Dovenmuehle RH, Verwoerdt A: Physical illness and depressive symptomatology. I. Incidence of depressive symptoms in hospitalized cardiac patients. J Am Geriatr Soc 10:932–947, 1962
113. Kurland HD, Hammer M: Emotional evaluation of medical patients. Arch Gen Psychiatry 19:72–78, 1968
114. Johns MW: Symptoms of neurotic illness in general hospital patients. Med J Aust 2:41–44, 1972
115. Shulman R: The present status of vitamin $B_{12}$ and folic acid deficiency in psychiatric illness. Can Psychiatr Assoc J 17:205–216, 1972
116. Fras I, Litin EM, Pearson JS: Comparison of psychiatric symptoms in carcinoma of the pancreas with those in some other intraabdominal neoplasms Am J Psychiatry 123:1553–1562, 1967

117. Gifford S, Gunderson JG: Cushing's disease as a psychosomatic disorder: A selective review of the clinical and experimental literature and a report of ten cases. Perspect Biol Med 13:169–221, 1970
118. Williams RH: Metabolism and mentation. J Clin Endocr 31:461–479, 1970
119. Goodwin FK, Bunney WE: Depressions following reserpine: A reevaluation. Semin Psychiatry 3:435–448, 1971
120. Peterson P: Psychiatric disorders in primary hyperparathyroidism. J Clin Endocrinol Metab 28:1491–1495, 1968
121. Brown GL, Wilson WP: Parkinsonism and depression. South Med J 65:540–545, 1972
122. Zaphiropoulos G, Burry HC: Depression in rheumatoid disease. Ann Rheum Dis 33:132–135, 1974
123. Richards DH: Depression after hysterectomy. Lancet 2:430–433, 1973
124. Guze SB: The occurrence of psychiatric illness in systemic lupus erythematosus. Amer J Psychiatry 123:1562–1570, 1967
125. Carpenter WT, Strauss JS, Bunney WE: The psychobiology of cortisol metabolism: Clinical and theoretical implications. In Shader RI (ed): Psychiatric Complications Of Medical Drugs, New York, Raven Press, 1972
126. Malamud N: Psychiatric disorder with intracranial tumors of limbic system. Arch Neurol 17:113–123, 1967
127. Flor-Henry P: Psychosis of temporal lobe epilepsy. Epilepsia 10:363–395, 1969
128. Greiber MF: Psychoses associated with the administration of atabrine. Am J Psychiatry 104:306–314, 1947
129. McFarland HR: Addison's disease and related psychoses. Compr Psychiatry 4:90–95, 1963
130. Roth N: The psychiatric syndromes of porphyria. Int J Neuropsychiat 4:32–44, 1968
131. Marks V, Ross CF: Hypoglycemia. Philadelphia, Davis, 1965
132. Whybrow PC, Prange AJ, Treadway CR: Mental changes accompanying thyroid gland dysfunction. Arch Gen Psychiatry 20:48–63, 1969
133. Victor M: The amnesic syndrome and its anatomical basis. Can Med Assoc J 100:1115–1125, 1969
134. Lipowski ZJ: Delirium, clouding of consciousness and confusion. J Nerv Ment Dis 145:227–255, 1967
135. Eilenberg MD: Psychiatric illness and pernicious anemia: A clinical re-evaluation. J Ment Sci 106:1539–1548, 1960
136. Nauta WJH: The problem of the frontal lobe: A reinterpretation. J Psychiatr Res 8:167–187, 1971
137. Davison K, Bagley CR: Schizophrenia-like psychosis associated with organic disorders of the central nervous system: A review of the literature. In Herrington RN (ed): Current Problems In Neuropsychiatry. Ashford, Kent; Headley, 1969
138. Achte KA, Hillbom E, Aalberg V: Post-traumatic psychoses following war brain injuries. Helsinki, Kirjapaino Yrjo Levikoski, 1967
139. Stone MH: Drug-related schizophrenic syndrome. Int J Psychiatr Med 11: 391–437, 1973
140. Verwoerdt A: Psychopathological responses to the stress of physical illness. In Lipowski ZJ (ed): Psychosocial Aspects Of Physical Illness. Basel, Karger, 1972

141. Lipowski ZJ, Kiriakos RZ: Borderlands between neurology and psychiatry: Observations in a neurological hospital. Psychiatr Med 3:131–147, 1972
142. Zubek JP, MacNeil M: Studies on immobilization: Behavioral and EEG effects. Can J Psychol 20:316–336, 1966
143. Levy R: The immobilized patient and his psychologic well-being. Postgrad Med 40:73–77, 1966
144. Karacan I, Salis PJ, Williams RL: Clinical disorders of sleep. Psychosomatics 14:77–88, 1973
145. Feinsilver DL, Hall RCW, Gardner ER: Emergency room psychiatry: Role conflicts, future directions. In Masserman JH (ed): Current Psychiatric Therapies, Vol. 21. New York, Grune & Stratton, 1982
146. Feinsilver DL, Hall RCW: The new crisis psychiatry: An overview. Psychiatr Ann 12:757–761, 1982
147. Groves JE: Taking care of the hateful patient. N Engl Med 298:883–887, 1978
148. Hossenlopp CM, Holland J: Ambulatory patients with medical and psychiatric illness: Care in a special medical clinic. Int J Psychiatr Med 8:1–11, 1977–1978
149. Hackett TP, Cassem NH, Wishnie HA: The coronary care unit: An appraisal of its psychological hazards. N Engl J Med 279:1365–1370, 1968
150. Stern MJ: Psychosocial adaptation following an acute myocardial infarction. Paper presented at the Annual Meeting of the American Psychosomatic Society, Philadelphia, March 29, 1974
151. McKegney FP: Intensive care syndrome: Definition, treatment and prevention of new "disease of medical progress." Conn Med 30:633–636, 1966
152. Cassem NH, Hackett TP' Psychiatric consultation in a coronary care unit. Ann Intern Med 75:9–14, 1971
153. Hackett TP: The Lazarus complex revisited. Ann Intern Med 76:135–136, 1972
154. Klein RF, Kliner WA, Zipes DP: Transfer from a coronary care unit: Some adverse responses. Arch Intern Med 122:104–108, 1968
155. Koumans AJR: Psychiatric consultation in an intensive care unit. JAMA 194: 633–637, 1965
156. Gombos EA, Lee TH, Harton R, et al: One year's experience with an intermittent dialysis program. Ann Intern Med 61:462–469, 1964
157. Shea EJ, Bogdan DF, Freeman RB, et al: Hemodialysis for chronic renal failure. IV. Psychologic considerations. Ann Intern Med 62:558–563, 1965
158. Abram HS: Survival by machine: Psychological aspects of chronic dialysis. Psychiatr Med 1:37–50, 1970
159. Cooper AJ: Hypomanic psychosis precipitated by hemodialysis. Compr Psychiatr 8:168–174, 1967
160. Abram HS, Moore GL, Westervelt FB, Jr.: Suicidal behavior in chronic dialysis patients. Am J Psychiatry 127:1199–1204, 1971
161. Abram HS: Psychotherapy in renal failure. Curr Psychiatr Ther 10:86–92, 1969
162. Alfrey AC, Mishell JM, Bruks J, et al: Syndrome of dyspraxia and multifocal seizures associated with chronic hemodialysis. Trans Am Soc Artif Intern Organs 18:257–261, 1972
163. Abram HS, Wadlington WW: On the selection of patients for artificial and transplanted organs. Ann Intern Med 69:619–620, 1968

164. Cobb S, Lindemann E: Neuropsychiatric observations. Ann Surg 117:814–824, 1943
165. Lewis SR, Goolishian HA, Wolf CW, et al: Psychological studies in burn patients. Plast Reconstr Surg 31:323–332, 1963
166. Jorgensen JA, Brophy JJ: Psychiatric treatment of severely burned adults. Psychosomatics 14:331–335, 1973
167. Andreason NJC, Noyes R, Jr., Hartford CE, et al: Management of emotional reactions in seriously burned adults. N Eng J Med 286:65–69, 1972
168. Hamburg DA, Hamburg B, DeGonza S: Adaptive problems and mechanisms in severely burned patients. Psychiatry 16:1–20, 1953
169. McDaniel J: Physical Disability And Human Behavior. New York, Pergamon Press, 1969
170. Munro D: Rehabilitation of patients totally paralyzed below the waist with special reference to making them ambulatory and capable of earning their own living: An end result study of 445 cases. N Engl J Med 250:4–14, 1954
171. Conomy JP: Disorders of body image after spinal cord injury. Neurology 23: 842–850, 1973
172. Wachs H, Zaks M: Studies of body image in men with spinal cord injury. J Nerv Ment Dis 131:121–127, 1960
173. Reich P, Kelly M: Suicide attempts by hospitalized medical and surgical patients. N Engl J Med 294:298–301, 1976
174. Weiss AJ: Reluctant patient-special problems in psychologic treatment of patients with myelopathy. NY State J Med 68:2049–2053, 1968
175. Schwab JJ, Brown JM, Holzer CE: Depression in medical inpatients with gastrointestinal diseases. Am J Gastroenterol 49:146–152, 1968
176. Schwab JJ, Marder L, Clemmons RS, et al: Anxiety, severity of illness and other medical variables. J Psychosom Res 10:297–303, 1966
177. Weisman AD, Hackett TP: Organization and function of a psychiatric consultation service. Int Rec Med 173:306–311, 1960
178. Lipowski ZJ: Review of consultation-liaison psychiatry and psychosomatic medicine: II. Clinical aspects. Psychosom Med 29:201–224, 1967
179. Lipowski ZJ: Consultation-liaison psychiatry in a general hospital. Compr Psychiatr 12:461–465, 1971
180. Lipowski ZJ: Psychosomatic medicine in a changing society: Some current trends in theory and research. Compr Psychiatr 14:203–215, 1973
181. Lipowski ZJ: Psychiatric consultations in medical and surgical outpatient clinics. Can Psychiatr Assoc J 14:239–245, 1969
182. Petersen HW, Martin MJ: Organic disease presenting as a psychiatric syndrome. Postgrad Med 54:78–83, 1973
183. Lipowski ZJ: Consultation-liaison psychiatry: An overview. Am J Psychiatry 131:623–630, 1974
184. Stoeckle JD, Davidson GE: Bodily complaints and other symptoms of a depressive reaction, its diagnosis and significance in a medical clinic. JAMA 180:134–139, 1962
185. Stoeckle JD, Zola IK, Davidson GE: The quantity and significance of psychological distress in medical patients. J Chronic Dis 17:959–970, 1964
186. Bunce DFM, II, Jones LR, Badger LW, et al: Medical illness in psychiatric patients: Barriers to diagnosis and treatment. South Med J 75:941–944, 1982
187. Statistical Note 68. Department of Health Education and Welfare. Washington, D.C., February 1973

188. Durbridge TC, Edwards F, Edwards RJ, et al: The evaluation of benefits of screening tests done immediately on admission to hospital. Clin Chem 22: 968–971, 1976
189. Physicians Group Evaluates Lab Tests. Lab World, p14, April, 1981
190. McKegney PF: The incidence and characteristics of patients with conversion reactions: I. A general hospital consultation service sample. Am J Psychiatry 124:542–545, 1967
191. Plumb MM, Holland J, Park SK, et al: Depressive symptoms in patients with advanced cancer: A controlled assessment. Paper presented at the Annual Meeting of the American Psychosomatic Society, Philadelphia, March 29-31, 1974
192. Lishman WA: Organic Psychiatry: The Psychological Consequences of Cerebral Disorder. London, Blackwell Scientific Publications, 1980
193. Sher PP: Diagnostic effectiveness of biochemical liver-function test, as evaluated by discriminant function analysis. Clin Chem 23:627–630, 1977
194. Truett J, Cornfield J, Kannel W: A multivariate analysis of the risk of coronary heart disease in Framingham. J Chronic Dis 20:511–524, 1967
195. Amenta JS, Harkins ML: The use of discriminant functions in laboratory medicine. Evaluation of phosphate clearance studies in the diagnosis of hyperparathyroidism. Am J Clin Pathol 55:330–341, 1971
196. Glick JH: Serum lactate dehydrogenase isoenzyme and total lactate dehydrogenase values in health and disease and clinical evaluation of these tests by means of discriminant analysis. Am J Clin Pathol 52:320–328, 1969
197. Werner M, Brooks SH, Cohnen G: Diagnostic effectiveness of electrophroesis and specific protein assays evaluated by discriminate analysis. Clin Chem 18: 116–123, 1972
198. Baron DN: A critical look at the value of biochemical liver function tests with special reference to discriminant function analysis. Ann Clin Biochem 7:100–103, 1970
199. Conn RB: Optimal utilization of the laboratory in making clinical decisions. Hum Pathol 11:407–412, p411, 1980
200. Fraser CG, Smith BC, Peake MJ: Effectiveness of an outpatient urine screening program. Clin Chem 23:2216–2218, 1977
201. Report For Analytical Chemists. Anal Chem 43:29A–31A, July 1971
202. Spratt DI, Pont A, Miller MB, et al: Hyperthyroxinemia in patients with acute psychiatric disorders. Am J Med 73:41–48, 1982
203. Wallach JB: Interpretation of Diagnostic Tests: A Handbook Synopses of Laboratory Medicine, Third Edition. Boston, Little Brown, p537–557, 1978
204. Henry JB: Clinical Diagnosis And Management By Laboratory Methods, 16th Edition. Philadelphia, W.B. Saunders Co. 1979
205. Cole GW: Biochemical test profiles and laboratory system design. Hum Pathol 11:424–434, 1980 (p. 431)
206. Steele C, Lucas MJ, Tune LE: An approach to the management of dementia syndromes. Johns Hopkins Med J 151:362–268, 1982
207. Popkin MK, McKenzie TB: The provisional diagnosis of dementia: Three phases of evaluation. In Hall RCW, Beresford TP: Handbook of Psychiatric Diagnoses, vol. 2. New York, Spectrum Publications, 1984

CHAPTER 11

# Psychiatric Diagnostic Procedures in the Emergency Department

DONALD L. FEINSILVER

Many emergency room visits are not planned in advance. Previous records may be unavailable or the patient may be completely unknown at the facility. Collateral informants may or may not be available. Many psychiatric patients arrive at the emergency department in a state that hardly allows for providing an informative history. Other patients, such as the drug seeker, may intentionally falsify the history. Yet, no matter how sparse the information, a presumptive diagnosis must be made. Psychiatric interviewing expertise is essential for eliciting a comprehensive history and various psychiatric diagnostic procedures, used in conjunction with the history, can maximize diagnostic accuracy in the emergency department setting.

Usually an exhortation to physicians to order diagnostic tests is unnecessary. Emergency department physicians, along with physicians of other specialties, utilize laboratory investigations and consultation in an almost defensive manner. One might assume that many diagnostic procedures would be ordered for psychiatric patients in the emergency department. This has generally not been the case. Often psychiatric emergencies have been managed at non-medical "crisis intervention services."

*Handbook of Psychiatric Diagnostic Procedures*, vol. 1, edited by R. C. W. Hall and T. P. Beresford. 

Now psychiatry is moving towards the general hospital setting, with greater laboratory capabilities [1]. Changing reimbursement patterns will encourage avoiding hospitalization [2]. A push to maximize emergency room diagnostic capabilities will result. This should lead to greater preliminary diagnostic accuracy, spare some patients hospitalization, and enable a more rapid initiation of appropriate treatment.

The emergency psychiatrist is not simply a triage officer, but rather a medical specialist who must constantly exercise clinical judgement in ordering diagnostic procedures for emergency department patients. Often the patient is removed to a psychiatric hospital where some laboratory modalities will not be as readily available. For the purpose of discussion, we will group diagnostic procedures into three categories: first, the physical examination; second, laboratory investigations; and third, special diagnostic procedures.

## THE PHYSICAL EXAMINATION

Perhaps it seems puzzling that the physical examination warrants mention as a diagnostic procedure. But it does, since only a minority of psychiatrists perform one [3]. Often an emergency department physician "medically clears" a patient who then is turned over to the psychiatrist. This is unsatisfactory for several reasons. First, it demeans the image of the psychiatrist. If the psychiatrist acquiesces to this sort of system, he or she is not acting as a physician and recommendations the psychiatrist may offer, such as recommending laboratory examinations, will be taken less seriously. Second, and of even greater concern, many of these "medically clear" patients are, in fact, medically ill. This warrants elaboration.

As early as 1936, Comroe investigated this phenomenon. He followed 100 patients who were diagnosed as "psychoneurotic" and found that 24 of these patients developed significant organic disease within eight months. This seminal work indicated that patients' psychiatric symptoms often serve as early indicators of impending physical disorders [4].

Marshall, in 1949, surveyed 175 psychiatric inpatients and found that 44% of these patients had a physical illness that required treatment [5]. Presumably these patients had passed through some initial screening, analagous to an emergency department "clearance."

Davies examined 36 outpatients who were referred to a psychiatrist and found that 21 of these (58%) had a physical illness. Fifteen (41%) of these patients had a medical disorder related to their psychiatric condition [6].

Johnson, in 1968, reported that among 250 consecutive admissions to a psychiatric inpatient facility, twelve percent were there because of a physical illness that was producing their psychiatric symptoms [7]. Maguire and Granville-Grossman, in the same year, found 34% physical morbidity among 200 consecutive psy-

chiatric inpatient admissions. Furthermore, they demonstrated that 60% of the medically ill patients had abnormal physical findings at the time of admission. This graphically demonstrated the necessity for physical examination as part of the admission process [8]. Psychiatric patients presenting to emergency departments are at high risk for having concommitant or causative physical illness. This has now been demonstrated several times. One cannot argue that performing emergency department physical examinations is not productive [4–9,11].

Hall, in 1978, studied 658 consecutive outpatients at a community mental health center and demonstrated that 9.1% had medically induced psychiatric symptoms. Forty-six percent of these patients were suffering from a medical illness of which they were unaware and that their family physician had not diagnosed [9]. The presence of a screening physician, either at a clinic or in the emergency department, does not guarantee the psychiatric patient's physical health. Some argue that it falls within the jurisdiction of the emergency department psychiatrist to be the guarantor of the psychiatric patient's physical status, by performing a physical examination and requesting consultation as appropriate [10].

In the largest study to date, Koranyi evaluated 2090 psychiatric clinic patients and demonstrated one "major medical illness" (defined as causing active symptoms, causing concern on medical grounds, or requiring medical treatment) in 43% [11].

The components of a physical examination fall outside the purview of this chapter. The examination, though, should especially focus on the neurological, endocrinological, and cardiovascular systems. One should be especially reluctant to ascribe a functional label to patients who complain of visual hallucinations, distortions, or who evidence unusual physical symptoms [9,12].

## LABORATORY INVESTIGATIONS

Standard laboratory examinations such as the CBC, blood chemistries, thyroid functions, urinalysis, and chest x-ray can provide a useful data base for this group of patients who present with higher rates of physical illness. These laboratory studies should be available. Thus, linkage of services rendering treatment for "psychiatric emergencies" with general hospitals is necessary. The appendix of this text lists the normal values for these laboratory tests. Access to a radiologist, or a physician knowledgeable in reading x-rays, should be available at a site where psychiatric emergencies are managed.

### CAT Scan

The CAT scan procedure is expensive and should not be ordered indiscriminantly. However, it can provide worthwhile information. Many emergency departments now have immediate access to a CAT scan machine or even a machine of

**Table 1. Emergency Department Indications for CAT Scanning[a]**

1. Clinical suspicion of intracranial focal lesions based on focal signs and symptoms.
2. Severe head trauma with mental status changes
3. Patient with history of prior neurological insult presenting with altered mental status
4. Suspected cerebrovascular accident

[a]Note: A physical examination and mental status examination should always precede ordering a CAT scan.

their own. Table 1 summarizes emergency guidelines. Abnormal CAT scans have been described in conditions as diverse as schizophrenia and phencyclidine intoxication [14,15]. The most practical emergency department use is in searching for an anatomically defined neurological abnormality. Currently I know of no emergency department which has ready access to a PET scan or NMR equipment. Who knows what the future will hold?

### Examination of the Cerebrospinal Fluid

Any patient presenting with a sudden alteration in mental status accompanied by fever or signs of meningeal irritation such as Kernig or Brudzinski's sign should receive a lumbar puncture with subsequent examination of the cerebrospinal fluid [16]. Unfortunately, all too often no one takes the psychiatric patient's temperature in the emergency department. Vital signs should be taken for every patient unless the patient specifically refuses or is so agitated that it is impossible. (In that case, the vital signs should be taken as soon as the agitation subsides sufficiently that it becomes possible.) Even the patient who comes to the emergency department "just to talk to the psychiatrist" should have vital signs taken. If nothing else, the vital signs will serve as a screening for hypertension. Recent advances in neurology's high technology have not rendered examination of the cerebrospinal fluid obsolete. Normal cerebrospinal fluid values are presented in Table 2 as well as clinical conditions associated with various abnormalities.

## TESTING FOR PORPHYRIA

Porphyria is a relatively rare condition, although one that has interesting historical links. Acute intermittent porphyria is the most frequent form. The usual acute presentation is psychosis accompanied by abdominal pain. Acutely, the urine has a marked increase in porphobilinogen. The urine may be of normal color when fresh, but becomes brown, red, or black after standing for several hours due to an

**Table 2. Cerebrospinal Fluid (CSF)**

| | Range of normal values | Conditions potentially productive of psychiatric symptoms to be considered if outside of normal range |
|---|---|---|
| Appearance | Clear | (If not traumatic tap)<br>Subarachnoid hemorrhage<br>Intracranial bleeding<br>Metastatic melanoma<br>Subdural hematoma |
| Cells | None | Subarachnoid hemorrhage infection<br>Thrombosis<br>Tumor<br>Meningitis<br>Parasitic infestation (Eosinophils) |
| Glucose | 45–80 mg/100 ml | If decreased:<br>Bacterial meningitis<br>Tuberculous meningitis<br>Fungal meningitis<br>Sarcoidosis |
| Total protein | 15–45 mg/100 ml | If increased:<br>Diabetes<br>Brain tumor<br>Spinal cord tumor<br>Multiple sclerosis<br>Syphylis |
| Gamma globulin | 19% (IgB 2.0–5.9 mg/dl) | If increased:<br>Multiple sclerosis<br>Subacute sclerosing panencephalitis<br>General paresis<br>Herpes encephalitis<br>Myxedema |

Table 3. Substances Potentially Detectable in a Toxicology Screening (Emergency Department Specimen)

1. Alcohols
2. Aromatic solvents
3. Carbon monoxide
4. Chlorinated solvents
5. Drugs[a]: acetominophen, allyisobaltabarbital, amitryptiline, amobarbital, amphetamine, barbital, butabarbital, carbamazepine, chlordiazepoxide, chlorpromazine, codeine, cocaine, desipramine, diazepam, diphenhydarmine, diphenylhydantoin, doxepin, ephidrine, ethosuximide, flurazepam, glutethimide, imipramine, lidocaine, meperidine, mephenytoin, meprobamate, methadone, methamphetamine, methapyrilene, methagualone, methyprylon, morphine, nortryptiline, oxazepam, oxycodone, pentazocaine, pentobarbital, perphenazine, phenacentin, phencyclidine, phenobarbital, phenylbuatzone, primidone procaine, prochlorperazine, propoxyphene, salicyclic acid, scopolamine, secobarbotal, thioridazine, trifluoperazine

Courtesy Clinical Toxicology Laboratory–The Medical College of Wisconsin [39].
[a]For drug screens, an initial screening by an appropriate procedure (e.g. thin layer chromatography) is followed by a confirmatory procedure (usually GC mass spectrometry).

increase in porphobilinogen, coporoporphyrin, or uroporphyrin. In a 24 hour collection, normal values are: porphyrins–less than 300 mcg, and urobilinogen–0 to 4 mcg. The serum sodium and chloride are often decreased during an acute attack. Laboratory findings and clinical symptoms may be precipitated by drugs such as barbiturates or alcohol [17].

Since the treatment for acute porphyria is not unlike that of an acute functional psychosis–phenothiazine administration–a possible strategy is to collect the urine, treat the patient, and then observe the urine for color changes. Using barbiturates is to be avoided.

### Toxicology Screens

Distinguishing a functional from a toxic psychosis is often problematic. Fortunately, most emergency departments have the capability of toxicology screening whether this be for "sedative-hypnotics" in a most general way (which usually can yield results with a minimal delay) or for qualitative and even quantitative analyses for specific compounds. A list of compounds potentially detectable by toxicology screening is given in Table 3.

Toxicology screens are often underutilized [18]. Serum, urine, or even gastric lavage specimens can be subjected to these analyses. The cost of the analysis may not be inconsiderable, but the whole course of treatment may hinge on the results. Assuming that the patient is suffering from a functional psychosis and immediately introducing treatment with an antipsychotic agent may be diagnostically incorrect, may result in drug interaction and, if the correct diagnosis is never made and this treatment continues for some time, may needlessly expose the patient to adverse side effects. Late adolescence and early adulthood show a high incidence of acute schizophrenia, but so too are they prime ages for a toxic psychosis. The widespread prevalence of drug-induced psychoses may be unappreciated. One report, for example, indicates that phencyclidine (PCP) abuse is reaching epidemic proportions in some populations, and is usually misdiagnosed [19].

The number and diversity of agents found present in accident and poisoning victims of this age group is great. Horwitz et al in 1976 found more than 85 different drugs and other agents in the body fluids of approximately 1000 victims of accidental or deliberate poisonings. Nineteen percent of these patients had two or more drugs present [20].

When using only history, mental status findings, and physical examination, clinicians have had only moderate success determining which drugs patients had taken. In one study, 74 biological fluids were submitted for laboratory toxicology analysis. Drugs implicated in the clinical history were compared to those actually found by the laboratory in order to evaluate the diagnostic utility of toxicology screening. The laboratory found either some or all of the drugs suspected from the history in 68% of the laboratory-analyzed cases. In an additional 16%, the laboratory found none of the implicated drugs but did find other drugs not suggested by the history. In 25% of the cases at least one drug not implicated by history was found [21].

Street drug abusers are often more up to date on new patterns of drug abuse than are emergency room clinicians. We recently have seen a series of Limbitrol® abusers [22].

Studying patients presenting to a university hospital emergency room with suspected drug abuse, Bailey found an average of 1.7 different drugs per patient on the admission toxicology screen (usually ethanol, barbiturates, opiates, or phenothiazines). When the same patient would return a subsequent time, one-third of the previously detected drugs were again present [23].

### Alcohol Levels

No drug is so commonly abused as alcohol. Most visits to emergency departments by intoxicated patients are unplanned, but result from prior plans going awry—perhaps because of trauma. The clinician should suspect possible alcohol abuse, if not addiction, in the case of some traumatized patients. Silent alcoholism often goes undiagnosed in general hospital settings. The emergency department might serve as an initial screening area for some patients. Beresford et al developed a laboratory screening battery, for general hospital use, that identifies with 80% accuracy individuals at risk for alcohol addiction [24].

**Table 4. Clinical Correlates at Varying Serum Alcohol Concentrations**

| | |
|---|---|
| .040–.050% | disinhibition begins, impairment of judgement begins. |
| .100% | legal intoxication in most localities; ataxia usually noticeable. |
| .150–.250% | motor area of the brain markedly depressed; possible marked emotional dysfunction. |
| .300% | signs of acute brain syndrome evident: confusion, possible disorientation, possible lowered level of consciousness. |
| .400% | coma and risk of death. |

Intoxicated patients are often undiagnosed or misdiagnosed in emergency departments. This situation could be remedied somewhat. The serum alcohol level is an often available, often underutilized emergency room diagnostic procedure [25]. One need only think of the large number of undiagnosed intoxicants to confirm this. Generally, serum alcohol levels of .100 mg% constitute legal intoxication. The finding of .300 mg.% is considered marked intoxication and suggests chronic alcoholism. Typical clinical findings found at various serum alcohol concentrations are listed in Table 4. The individual who chronically abuses alcohol will be tolerant, however, and show decreased clinical signs at a given serum concentration. In fact, the paucity of clinical findings in the presence of a high serum concentration indicates tolerance and chronic abuse.

In a 1981 British study, Holt et al found that 40% of the emergency department accident cases had a positive blood alcohol level and that 82% of these had a level of .080 mg.% or greater on breath alcohol analysis [26]. They suggested that alcoholism treatment facilities need to be integrated with accident and emergency services. Champion et al, studied the relation between serum osmolality and blood alcohol level in 565 acute trauma patients and found a close correlation [27]. Breath tests with a fuel cell alcometer give immediate results. A high correlation is present between breath test results and serum concentration [28].

## SPECIAL DIAGNOSTIC PROCEDURES

Special diagnostic procedures are procedures in which the results are obtained by a clinical observation rather than by a laboratory measurement. It is probable that these procedures are underutilized in emergency department settings. Used judiciously and with the necessary precautions, they provide much useful diagnostic information.

## Naloxone (Narcan®) Challenge

The naloxone challenge is a simple and safe diagnostic procedure that tests for opiate use or addiction. The use of opiates can be determined by the IV administration of one ampule (0.4 mg) of naloxone (Narcan®), an opiate antagonist. Occasionally more than one ampule will be necessary. Other than idiosyncratic allergy to naloxone, there are basically no contraindications to this test. No response is seen in the nonopiate using patient. (If the patient has overdosed on something else, no harm is done.) However, in the case of the opiate user, the unconscious patient awakens. In the case of the addicted patient, naloxone induces a narcotic abstinence syndrome, marked by diaphoresis, "gooseflesh," general discomfort and the initiation of a "flu-like" syndrome. The patient can then be referred to an appropriate drug treatment program and, in some cases, methadone detoxification might be started. Naloxone is essentially without narcotic properties of its own [29].

## Administration of 50% Dextrose

There is essentially no contraindication to the IV administration of 50% dextrose. This procedure can prevent cerebral damage and loss of life in a patient suffering from hypoglycemia. Most protocols for "coma of unknown etiology" require this administration [30]. Patients with milder forms of hypoglycemia may show normalization of the mental status on receiving the dextrose solution. It is not necessary that the patient be a proven diabetic prior to receiving the ampule. The presence of signs of hypoglycemia—such as altered mental status, agitation, anxiety, diaphoresis, low blood pressure, tachycardia or tremor may serve as indications. Prior to the IV administration, a blood specimen should usually be drawn for a serum glucose determination and sent off, marked STAT, to the laboratory. Acutely intoxicated alcoholics and alcoholics in withdrawal will sometimes become hypoglycemic as well.

The diabetic patient with a high blood sugar will not be further injured by the 50% dextrose administration since the hyperosmolar state will be treated anyway. While this procedure will not be curative for the majority of emergency department patients, it can be diagnostic and life-saving for an occasional patient. Milder forms of hypoglycemia can be treated orally, such as by having the patient drink orange juice with sugar added. Prior to this, a blood sample should be drawn to confirm the diagnosis (since one would not want to overlook some other cause of altered mental or physical status). The administration of IV dextrose or having the patient take a sugar solution orally is well known to emergency department physicians as a curative procedure. It can also diagnose a cause of altered mental status.

**Table 5. Side Effects of Physostigmine**

Pulmonary (contraindications: bronchitis, asthma)
- Parasympathetic:
  - Bronchial gland secretion
  - Bronchial smooth muscle contraction

Cardiovascular (containdications: heart block, arrhythmia, coronary artery disease)
- Sympathetic:
  - Elevation of blood pressure
  - Increased automaticity of pacemaker
  - Vasoconstriction
- Parasympathetic:
  - Decrease in conduction velocity

Gastrointestinal (contraindications: peptic ulcer or colitis)
- Parasympathetic:
  - Increased gastric acid secretion
  - Increased smooth muscle contraction

Genitourinary (contraindications: urinary or renal obstruction)
- Parasympathetic:
  - Increased smooth muscle contraction

Occular (contraindication: glaucoma)
- Dilatation of fine blood vessles and increased permeability of the blood-aqueous humor barrier

Other contraindications: thyroid disease; pregnancy

## The Physostigmine Challenge

Physostigmine is an anticholinesterase drug that readily reverses signs and symptoms of central anticholinergic delirium. Since over 600 drugs are potentially productive of central anticholinergic delirium, the physostigmine challenge may be used as a diagnostic as well as a therapeutic procedure. The patient who responds to physostigmine with the normalization of mental and physical states is suffering from an anticholinergic delirium, whereas the patient who does not have a response is suffering from some other condition.

Physostigmine 1 to 2 mg IV or IM is given and a response is sought within 30 to 40 minutes. If the patient's sensorium clears and normalization of vital signs occurs, the presumptive diagnosis is anticholinergic delirium. Often a single dose of physostigmine will not be sufficient to permanently clear the sensorium, since physostigmine is a relatively short acting drug, and many anticholinergic drugs are fairly long acting. Among anticholinergic drugs are tricyclic antidepressants, especially amitriptyline, and various over-the-counter cold preparations. Low potency neuroleptics, such as thioridazine, also possess anticholinergic properties. Unlike naloxone or 50% dextrose, physostigmine is not an innocuous drug. In fact, there are many conditions that preclude its use. Among these are gangrene, asthma, uncontrolled diabetes, and cardiac ischemia [31]. Side effects of physostigmine are listed in Table 5.

## Barbiturate Tolerance Tests

Many barbiturate abusing patients will deny or minimize the quantity of barbiturates they are taking. Protocols have been devised for barbiturate tolerance tests [32,33]. The basic theory is that patients who are at risk for withdrawal can be identified by identifying their pre-existing tolerance for barbiturates. The goal of the barbiturate tolerance test is to determine the milligram equivalent of a short acting barbiturate that approximates the patient's daily consumption. After this determination, the patient may begin a regimen of detoxification in which the daily dose decreases by either 10% or 100 mg per day.

Either of two methods may be employed to determine tolerance. In the first method, the one we employ, a fixed barbiturate dose is given and the patient is observed 90 minutes later for signs of barbiturate intoxication. According to the severity of the apparent intoxication, an estimate of the patient's daily barbiturate consumption is made. The estimation process begins by giving the patient 200 mg orally of a short acting barbiturate such as pentobarbital. Approximately 90 minutes later the patient is again observed. A sleeping but arousable patient is assumed to have no tolerance for barbiturates and thus not be addicted. If the patient is alert but demonstrating dysarthria, the estimate is that the patient has been taking the equivalent of approximately 500 to 600 mg per day of a short acting barbiturate. If the patient demonstrates no signs of intoxication other than slight nystagmus, the patient is assumed to have been taking 700 to 800 mg per day of a short acting barbiturate. If the patient demonstrates no signs of intoxication whatsoever, the assumption is that about 900 mg per day of barbiturates are being consumed. If the patient is actually showing signs of barbiturate withdrawal, the estimated daily consumption is at least the equivalent of 1200 mg of a short acting barbiturate. The usual daily decrease is 100 mg. Commonly 32 mg of phenobarbtal, a long acting barbiturate, is substituted for each 100 mg of the short acting barbiturate and the dose decreased by 32 mg per day. Contraindications to a barbiturate tolerance test are known barbiturate allergy, porphyria, respiratory depression, or known intoxication with another substance such as alcohol.

The second method for a barbiturate tolerance test employes holding the end point of intoxication constant and seeing how many hourly doses of a short acting barbiturate are necessary to achieve this level. In one protocol, the patient receives 200 mg of pentobarbital upon arrival but, barring severe withdrawal symptoms, receives no further drugs while observed for 6 hours. If the patient is agitated or tremulous six hours later, another 200 mg of pentobarbital is given. This is repeated every six hours for 24 hours. The medication is withheld if the patient becomes intoxicated or if any unusual complaints or signs develop. If intoxication occurs as manifested by nystagmus, ataxia, or dysarthria, no further drug is given. The formula applied is adding the total amount of pentobarbital consumed in the 24 hours preceding intoxication, and then subtracting 100 mg from the total. The sum is divided by four and this amount is given every six hours for 48 hours. The daily intake is then decreased by 100 mg every 24 hours until the patient is drug-free. However, if the patient is not intoxicated after 24 hours on the previously stated regimen, the dose is increased to 300 mg every 6 hours or until intoxication occurs. If intoxication does not occur on 300 mg every six hours for 24 hours, the dosage is increased to 400 mg every six hours. The formula of subtracting 100, dividing by four and giving this dose every six hours until the patient is drugfree is again applied [34]. These procedures are important since the incidence of covert barbiturate abuse is high [34–36].

### The Amytal Interview

The amytal interview refers to the intravenous administration of sodium amytal followed by a psychiatric interview. This interview can be used for either diagnostic or therapeutic purposes in the emergency department.

Administering sodium amytal necessitates some precautions. One should be cautious in administering this drug to a patient with a history of drug dependence or abuse. Barbiturates induce liver microsomal enzyme activity which accelerates the biotransformation of various drugs and is probably part of the mechanism for the tolerance encountered with barbiturates. Thus all barbiturates should be used with caution in patients with decreased liver functions. Elderly or debilitated patients may become markedly excited or depressed as a response to barbiturates. Also this drug may diminish the effects of exogenous cortisol and thus caution should be exercised with the hypoadrenal patient.

In an emergency department setting, probably the most important considerations are that the patient has not already taken other sedative-hypnotics, that the patient is not pregnant, and that the possibility of respiratory arrest be considered and thus the capability for intubation be present. Regarding the ability to rapidly intubate if necessary, an emergency department setting is often ideal.

The theoretical basis for the amytal interview is that the disinhibiting effect of the intravenous barbiturate will enable the patient to speak more freely or will relieve an hysterical symptom. The amytal interview can aid in the differential diagnosis of such conditions as catatonia, hysteria, and elective mutism.

We employ the following procedure. First, the patient must be free of medical contraindications to the use of sodium amytal. These would include: history of porphyria, barbiturate addiction; instability of vital signs, most especially hypotension or fever; hepatic impairment; and respiratory compromise. As mentioned, a physician should be available who is capable of intubating the patient if this rare necessity arises.

The patient must consent to the procedure. The patient reclines and an IV is started with an indwelling line. Although various modifications exist, we slowly infuse 5% dextrose and water through this IV line. A solution of 5% sodium amytal (500 mg of sodium amytal dissolved in 10 cc of sterile water) can then be pushed into this IV line at a rate not exceeding 50 mg per minute. The patient is asked to slowly count backwards from 50. The IV administration of sodium amytal is stopped when the patient forgets the task, becomes dysarthric, or loses track of the numbers. In any event, we rarely exceed 500 mg and often use far less.

A psychiatric interview is then begun using a neutral topic as the starting point. If mute, the patient is given the suggestion that he or she will probably feel like talking soon. The mute patient receives sodium amytal until some sign of barbiturate intoxication, such as nystagmus, appears, or until 500 mg has been administered. The interview then proceeds in the normal manner and ends when sufficient diagnostic material has been elicited. In the case of the patient with organic impairment, no improvement occurs and only sedation is observed. In hysterical conversion, alleviation of the symptom occurs which may prove diagnostic. Various studies indicate that up to 50% of previously mute patients begin to talk during an amytal interview [37]. Summarizing, the amytal interview is a useful, but not totally risk-free procedure. Since medical back-up is accessible, the emergency department is often the ideal locale.

## MEDICO-LEGAL CONSIDERATIONS

Emergency department psychiatrists see patients in the most acute stages of illness. At these times, the patient may be unwilling to follow the psychiatrist's recommendations. Issues regarding the right to refuse treatment are presently hot medicolegal issues [38]. The usual issue, though, is involuntary treatment. What of refusing diagnostic procedures?

The medico-legal situation is simple. Any patient, competent or incompetent, can refuse a purely diagnostic (as opposed to therapeutic) procedure. Thus, often the psychiatrist will be thwarted in his or her plans to optimize the emergency department diagnostic work-up. All the psychiatrist can do is try to develop sufficient rapport that the patient becomes willing to participate in (or submit to) the diagnostic procedure. It may not be within the patient's best medical interests to refuse a lumbar puncture, but it is within his legal rights. Thus, emergency department psychiatric diagnostic procedures are virtually always voluntary.

Some procedures may require written informed consent. Informed consent is often requested, for example, for an amytal interview (assuming the patient is not catatonic). Here, the risks and benefits of the procedure and alternative methods of diagnosing are explained to the patient. (The silent patient is often assumed to be consenting.)

Other procedures, such as a chest x-ray, or the drawing of a CBC or electrolytes may require only implied consent. Nothing is specifically signed, nor are the risks and benefits of these procedures specifically explained. The assumption is that unless the patient protests he or she is consenting. Usually, these procedures are presumed covered under the general consent for treatment that the patient signed upon arrival at the emergency department. When a patient cannot—as opposed to will not—sign this general consent, as in the case of a child or an incapacitated adult, proxy consent from the patient's closest available relative is usually sought.

The physician must obey the law, but practicing good medicine dictates that appropriate diagnostic procedures at least be recommended. In short, psychiatric diagnostic procedures may not be administered involuntarily and the correct level of consent must be previously obtained.

## SUMMARY

Increasingly, psychiatric emergencies are being managed in the emergency departments of general hospitals. Greater diagnostic capabilities will be available to psychiatrists working in these settings. The traditional triage and gatekeeper functions will be complemented, if not replaced, by enhanced diagnostic capabilities. Accordingly, psychiatrists will have to be familiar with the various psychiatric diagnostic procedures available and to judiciously perform or order the appropriate investigations. Some patients' agitation will render certain procedures impractical. Some procedures are not innocuous and all require some cost and time expenditure. The psychiatrist has to use considerable judgement—weighing the possible advantages of the diagnostic procedure against the possible disadvantages of prolonging the patient's stay in the emergency department, and the risks and cost of the procedure.

## REFERENCES

1. Brook Lodge Conference on Consultation Liaison Psychiatry, Kalamazoo, Michigan, December 1, 1981
2. Hospital Statistics, 1979, Chicago, American Hospital Association. 1979
3. McIntyre J, Romano J: Is there a stethoscope (and is it used?) Arch Gen Psychiatry 34:1147–1151, 1977
4. Comroe B: Follow-up of 100 diagnosed as neurotic. J Nerv Ment Dis 83: 679–684, 1936
5. Marshall H: Incidence of physical disorders among psychiatric inpatients. Br Med J 2:468–470, 1949
6. Davies DH: Physical illness in psychiatric outpatients. Br J Psychiatry 111: 27–33, 1965

7. Johnson DAW: The evaluation of routine physical examination in psychiatric cases. Practitioner 200:686–691, 1968
8. Maguire C, Granville-Grossman KL: Physical illness in psychiatric patients. Br J Psychiatry 115:1365–1369, 1968
9. Hall RCW, Popkin MK, DeVaul R, et al: Physical illness presenting as psychiatric disease. Arch Gen Psychiatry 35:1315–1320, 1978
10. Feinsilver DL, Hall RCW: The new crisis psychiatry: An overview. Psychiatr Ann 12:757–761, 1982
11. Koranyi EK: Morbidity and role of undiagnosed physical illness in a psychiatric clinic population. Arch Gen Psychiatry 36:414–419, 1979
12. Jefferson JW, Marshall R: Neuropsychiatric Features of Medical Disorders. New York: Plenum Medical Book Co., 1981
13. Holt RE, Rawat S, Beresford TP, et al: Computed tomography of the brain and the psychiatric consultation. Psychosomatics 23:1007–1019, 1982
14. Pearlson GD, Veroff RE: Computerized tomographic scan changes in manic-depressive illness. Lancet II:470, 1981
15. Beeson HA: Intracranial hemorrhage associated with phencyclidine abuse. JAMA 248:585–586, 1982
16. Berkow R: The Merck Manual of Diagnosis and Therapy. Rahway, NJ: Merck Sharpe and Dohme Research Laboratories, 1982
17. Marver HS, Schmid R: The porphyrias in Stanbury JB, Wyngaarden JB, Fredrickson DS (eds.) The Metabolic Basis of Inherited Disease. New York: McGraw-Hill,1972
18. Lundberg GD, Malberg CB, Pantlik VA: Frequency of clinical toxicology test-ordering and results in a large urban general hospital. Clin Chem 20:121–125, 1974
19. Pitts FN, Allen RE, Aniline O, et al: The dilemma of the toxic psychosis: Differential diagnosis and the PCP psychosis. Psychiatr Ann 12:762–768, 1982
20. Horwitz JP, Hills EB, Andrezejewski D, et al: Adjunct hospital emergency toxicology service. JAMA 235:1708–1712, 1976
21. Bailey DN, Manoguerra AS: Survey of drug-abuse patterns and toxicology analysis in an emergency-room population. J A Toxicol 4:199–203, 1980
22. Feinsilver DL, Beresford TP, Hall RCW, et al: Limbitrol as a new street drug. (Ltr. to ed.) Am J Psychiatry 139:1377–1378, 1982
23. Bailey DN: Survey of admission toxicology panels in patients with multiple hospitalizations. J A Toxicol 4:204–206, 1980
24. Beresford TP, Low D, Hall RCW, et al: A computerized diagnostic biochemical profile for the detection of alcoholism. Psychosomatics 23:713–720, 1982
25. Keeley K: Emergency room treatment of alcohol abuse and alcoholism in Pattison EM, Kaufman E (eds.) Encyclopedic Handbook of Alcoholism, New York: Gardner Press, 1982
26. Holt S, Stewart IO, Dixon JM, et al: Alcohol and the emergency service patient. Br Med J 6:638–640, 1981
27. Champion AR, Baker SP, Benner C et al: Alcohol intoxication and serum osmolality. Lancet 1:1482–1484, 1975
28. Evans RP, McDermott FT: Use of an alcometer in a casualty department. Med J Aust 1:185–186, 1981
29. Physician's Desk Reference. Oradell, NJ: Medical Economics Company, 1983.
30. Smith BH: Differential Diagnosis Neurology. New York: Arco, 1979
31. Feinsilver DL: Antipsychotic medications: Guidelines for use in emergencies. Hosp Prac 17:92A–H, 1982

32. Gorelick DA: Pharmacotherapy of alcohol and drug abuse. Psychiatr Ann 13: 71–79, 1983
33. Khantzian EJ, McKenna GJ: Acute toxic and withdrawal reactions associated with drug use and abuse. Ann Intern Med 90:361–372, 1979
34. Blumberg AG, Cohen M, Heaton AM, et al: Covert drug abuse among voluntary hospitalized psychiatric patients. JAMA 217:1659–1661, 1971
35. Bakewell WE, Wikler A: Nonnarcotic addiction: Incidence in a university hospital psychiatric ward. JAMA 196:710–713, 1966
36. Butzer SC, Cline DW: Covert drug abuse among young hospitalized psychiatric patients. Minn Med 961–962, 1974
37. Perry JC, Jacobs D: Overview: Clinical applications of the amytal interview in psychiatric emergency settings. Am J Psychiatry 139:552–559, 1982
38. Stone AA: Mental Health and Law: A System in Transition. New York: Jason Aronson, 1976
39. Wu A: Personal communication

# Index